STEROIDS - FROM PHYSIOLOGY TO CLINICAL MEDICINE

Edited by **Sergej M. Ostojic**

Steroids - From Physiology to Clinical Medicine
http://dx.doi.org/10.5772/46119
Edited by Sergej M. Ostojic

Contributors

Dai Mitsushima, Hajime Ueshiba, Rosário Monteiro, Cidália Pereira, Maria João Martins, Paul Dawson, Zulma Tatiana Ruiz-Cortés, Anna Kokavec, Seung-Yup Ku, Sanghoon Lee, Marko D Stojanovic, Sergej Ostojic, Emad Al-Dujaili

Published by InTech

Janeza Trdine 9, 51000 Rijeka, Croatia

Publishing Process Manager Ana Pantar
Technical Editor InTech DTP team
Cover InTech Design team

Additional hard copies can be obtained from orders@intechopen.com

Steroids - From Physiology to Clinical Medicine, Edited by Sergej M. Ostojic
p. cm.
ISBN 978-953-51-0857-3

For EU product safety concerns:
IN TECH d.o.o., Prolaz Marije Krucifikse Kozulić 3, 51000 Rijeka, Croatia,
info@intechopen.com or visit our website at intechopen.com.

Meet the editor

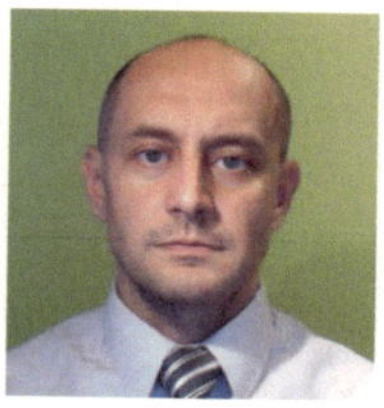

Professor Sergej M. Ostojic received his medical degree from the Faculty of Medicine, University of Belgrade, Serbia in September 1996. He then pursued his post-graduate training in exercise science & medicine and obtained PhD at the University of Belgrade in 2003. In 2002, he joined the faculty of the Institute of Sports Medicine at Sports Academy Belgrade. Currently he is the Director of Human Performance Laboratory at the Center of Health, Exercise and Sport Sciences, Belgrade and Professor at Faculty of Sport and Physical Education at the University of Novi Sad. His research is focused on physiological responses to maximal and submaximal exercise, and evaluation of the ergogenic properties of dietary agents. He is a member of American College of Sports Medicine, European Physical Conditioning Association and International Federation of Sports Medicine. He has a number of publications in different journals in medicine, physiology & sport science.

Contents

Preface

Understanding complex mechanisms of action and key roles in different biological processes in the body has moved steroid science and medicine to expand rapidly in the past decades. Dozens of distinct steroids are identified as both control and target molecules, with regulation of physiological and pathophysiological steroidogenesis recognized as one of the essential research topics in the field. On the other hand, steroids have been practiced as both medical agents and clinical markers for many purposes, from bone marrow stimulation to growth monitoring. This book covers contemporary basic science on steroid research, along with steroid practical application in endocrinology and clinical medicine.

The book is divided in two parts. The first part deals with physiological and pathophysiological roles of steroids, with reference to production and action of gonadal steroids, role of steroid sulfonation in mammalian growth and development, sex specific and steroids-dependent mechanism of hippocampal function, and the importance of hydroxysteroid dehydrogenases for the modulation of tissue glucocorticoid availability. The second part will cover different aspects of steroids application in clinical environment. Topics covered in the second part include the endocrine function after ovarian transplantation in terms of sex steroid production from the cryopreserved and reimplanted ovaries, the diagnostic significance of collection, storage and measurement of androgens in saliva of females, main drawbacks of steroids use in sport and exercise, analysis of serum steroid hormone profiles in patients with adrenocortical tumors, and correlation between salivary and serum cortisol responses after alcohol intake.

In response to the need to address novel and valuable information on steroids science and medicine, we sincerely hope that this book will enable readers to comprehend this fast-growing and exciting scientific field.

Sergej M. Ostojic, MD, PhD
Professor of Biomedical Sciences in Sport & Exercise
Center for Health, Exercise and Sport Sciences, Belgrade
Faculty of Sport and Physical Education, University of Novi Sad
Serbia

Section 1

Physiology and Pathophysiology of Steroids

Chapter 1

Gonadal Sex Steroids: Production, Action and Interactions in Mammals

Zulma Tatiana Ruiz-Cortés

Additional information is available at the end of the chapter

http://dx.doi.org/10.5772/52994

1. Introduction

There are five major classes of steroid hormones: testosterone (androgen), estradiol (estrogen), progesterone (progestin), cortisol/corticosterone (glucocorticoid), and aldosterone (mineralocorticoids). Testosterone and its more potent metabolite dihydrotestosterone (DHT), progesterone and estradiol are classified as sex-steroids, whereas cortisol/corticosterone and aldosterone are collectively referred to as corticosteroids.

Sex steroids are crucial hormones for the proper development and function of the body; they regulate sexual differentiation, the secondary sex characteristics, and sexual behavior patterns. Sex hormones production is sexually dimorphic, and involves differences not only in hormonal action but also in regulation and temporal patterns of production. Gonadal sex steroids effects are mediated by slow genomic mechanisms through nuclear receptors as well as by fast nongenomic mechanisms through membrane-associated receptors and signaling cascades. The term *sex steroids* is nearly always synonymous with *sex hormones* (Wikipedia).

Steroid hormones in mammals regulate diverse physiological functions such as reproduction, mainly by the hypothalamic-pituitary-gonadal axis, blood salt balance, maintenance of secondary sexual characteristics, response to stress, neuronal function and various metabolic processes(fat, muscle, bone mass). The panoply of effects, regulations and interactions of gonadal sex steroids in mammals is in part discussed in this chapter.

2. Production of gonadal steroids

Cholesterol is found only in animals; it is not found in plants although they can produce phytoestrogens from cholesterol-like compounds called phytosterols.

Because cholesterol cannot be dissolved in the blood, it must be carried through the body on a "carrier" known as a lipoprotein. A lipoprotein is cholesterol covered by protein. There are two types of liproproteins-LDL (low density lipoprotein) and HDL (high density lipoprotein). All steroid hormones are synthesized from cholesterol through a common precursor steroid, pregnenolone, which is formed by the enzymatic cleavage of a 6-carbon side-chain of the 27- carbon cholesterol molecule, a reaction catalyzed by the cytochrome P450 side-chain cleavage enzyme (P450scc, CYP11A1) at the mitochondria level (Figure 1a). The ovarian granulosa cells mainly secrete progesterone (P4) and estradiol (E2); ovarian theca cells predominantly synthesize androgens,and ovarian luteal cells secrete P4 (and its metabolite 20α-hydroxyprogesterone (Hu et al., 2010). Progesterone is also synthesized by the corpus luteum and by the placenta in many species as it will be mentioned later. Testicular Leydig cells are the site of testosterone (T) production. The brain also synthesizes steroids *de novo* from cholesterol through mechanisms that are at least partly independent of peripheral steroidogenic cells. Such *de novo* synthesized brain steroids are commonly referred to as neurosteroids. In mammals, the adrenal or suprarrenal glands are endocrine glands that produce at the outer adrenal cortex androgens such as androstenedione.

All these steroidogenic tissues and cells have the potential to obtain cholesterol for steroid synthesis from at least four potential sources: a) cholesterol synthesized *de novo* from acetate;b) cholesterol obtained from plasma low-density lipoprotein (LDL) and high-density lipoprotein (HDL); c) cholesterol-derived from the hydrolysis of stored cholesterol esters in the form of lipid droplets; and d) cholesterol interiorized from the plasma membrane, all this mechanisms implicating cell organels such as smooth endoplasmic reticuli, endosomes and of course mitochondria (Figure 1b). Although all three major steroidogenic organs (adrenal, testis and ovary) can synthesize cholesterol de novo under the influence of the tropic hormone, the adrenal and ovary preferentially utilize cholesterol supplied from plasma LDL and HDL via the LDL-receptor mediated endocytic pathway.

The use of LDL or HDL as the source of cholesterol for steroidogenesis appears to be species dependent; rodents preferentially utilize the SR-BI/selective pathway; this is a process in which cholesterol is selectively absorbed while the lipoprotein (mainly HDL) remains at the cell surface. The discovery of a specific receptor for this process (scavenger receptor class B, type I, known as SR-BI) has revolutionized the knowledge about the selective uptake pathway as a means of achieving cholesterol balance (Azhar et al., 2003).

Humans, pigs and cattle primarily employ the LDL/LDL-receptor endocytic pathway to meet their cholesterol need for steroid synthesis. In contrast, testicular Leydig cells under normal physiological conditions rely heavily on the use of endogenously synthesized cholesterol for androgen (testosterone) biosynthesis (Hu et al., 2010).

2.1. Ontogeny and sexual dimorphism

Steroidogenesis of gonadal sex hormones is by definition sexually dimorphic in hormonal action and also in regulation and temporal patterns of production.

http://dx.doi.org/10.5772/52994

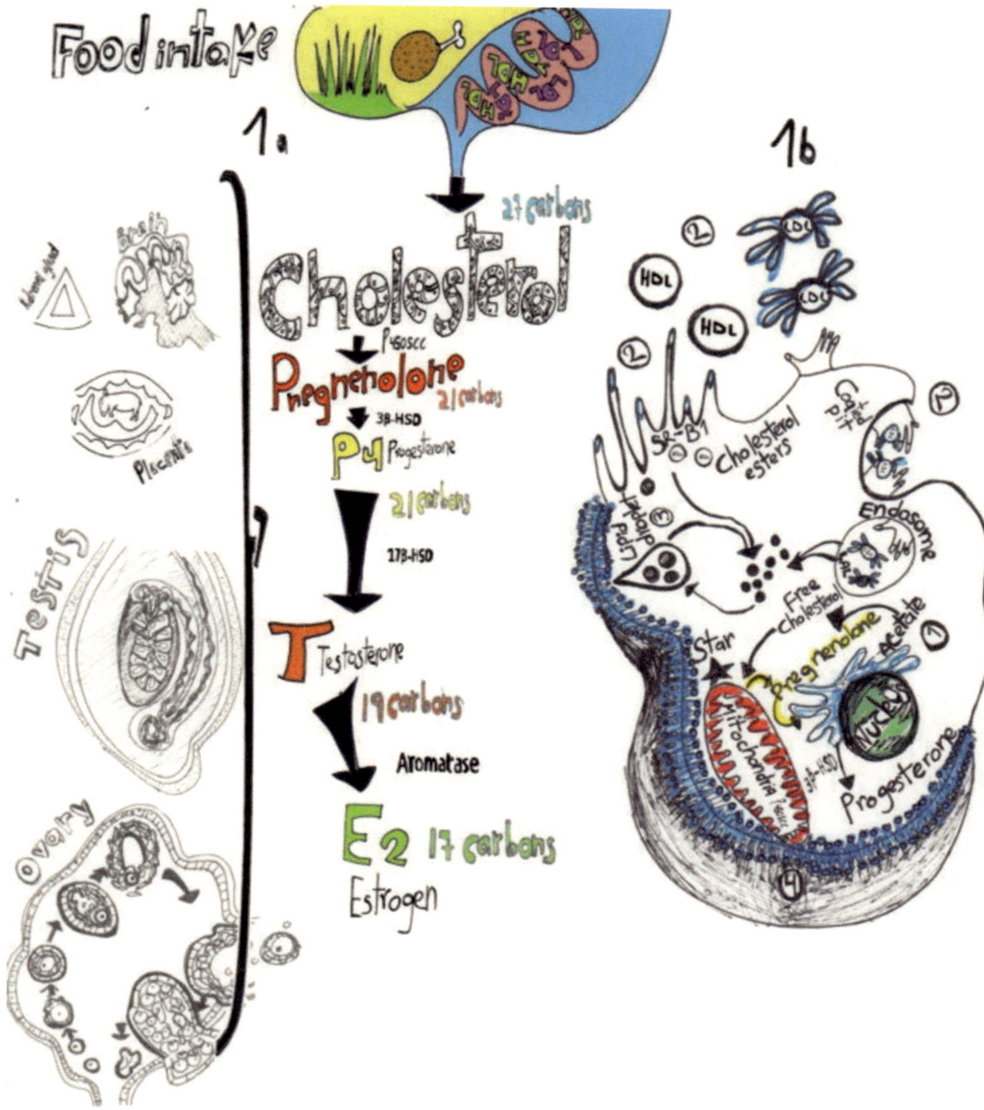

Ser: Smooth endoplasmic reticulum

Figure 1. Gonadal Steroids Synthesis Pathway. Modified from (Stocco, 2006; Senger, 2006). a) Steroidogenic tissues: adrenal gland, placenta, ovary, testis. Cholesterol from food intake is used (as LDL and HDL in plasma) by different cells in those tissues to synthesize the commune precursor: pregnenolone. The cascade continue with the androgens and estrogens production. b) Production of pregnenolone from four potential cholesterol sources: 1. synthesized *de novo* from acetate; 2. from plasma low-density lipoprotein (LDL) and high-density lipoprotein (HDL); 3. from the hydrolysis of stored cholesterol esters in the form of lipid droplets; and 4. Interiorized from the plasma membrane; cell organels implicated: smooth endoplasmic reticuli, endosomes and mitochondria

2.1.1. Males

The mesoderm-derived epithelial cells of the sex cords in developing testes become the Sertoli cells which will function to support sperm cell formation. A minor population of non-epithelial cells appears between the tubules by week 8 of human fetal development. These are Leydig cells. Soon after they differentiate, Leydig cells begin to produce androgens as mentioned before. In humans, Leydig cell populations can be divided into fetal Leydig cells that operate prenatally, and the adult-type Leydig cells that are active postnatally. Fetal Leydig cells are the primary source of testosterone and other androgens which regulate not only the masculinization of external and internal genitalia but also neuroendocrine function affecting behavioral and metabolic patterns.

Interestingly, adrenocortical and gonadal steroidogenic cells seem to share an embryonic origin in the coelomic epithelium, and they may exist as one lineage before divergence into the gonadal and adrenocortical paths. A common origin is also supported by the testicular adrenal rest tumours that are often found in male patients with congenital adrenal hyperplasia. Although much rarer, adrenal rests tumours have also been found in the ovary, also supporting the concept of a common origin of the steroidogenic cells. Those prenatal steroidogenic Leydig cells undergo degeneration and it is not well know which paracrine or endocrine factor(s) in the human fetal testis control this involution. Experiments on rodents have indicated that the regression of fetal Leydig cells occurs when plasma levels of LH remain high, suggesting that this gonadotropin cannot protect the cells from involution. It has been suggested that several factors – e.g. tumour growth factor b (TGFb), anti-Müllerian hormone (AMH), gonadotropin-releasing hormone (GnRH) –might play a role in fetal Leydig cell degeneration in rodents. TGFb is an attractive candidate for this purpose, since this factor is expressed by fetal Leydig cells during late fetal life and potently inhibits fetal Leydig-cell steroidogenesis in vitro.

It has been suggested that the development of human Leydig cells is triphasic and comprises fetal Leydig cells that function during the fetal period, neonatal Leydig cells that operate during the first year of life, and adult-type Leydig cells that appear from puberty onwards. This hypothesis is based on the triphasic developmental profile of plasma testosterone levels during human development.

All morphological modifications are accompanied by cellular growth and increasing expression of steroidogenic enzymes and LH receptors. These cellular events significantly enhance the capacity of mature Leydig cells to produce testosterone. Interestingly, reports in humans and experimental animals demonstrate that fully mature Leydig cells can dedifferentiate to previous stages of their development. These cellular events involve several morphological changes such as a reduction of the smooth endoplasmic reticulum and numbers of mitochondria, and impairment of T secretion. Paracrine control of Leydig cells steroidogenesis have been reported. Ghrelin appear to be appropriate markers for estimating the phase of Leydig-cell differentiation and the functional state of the cells. Leptin is another endocrine/ paracrine factor that can modulate Leydig-cell steroidogenesis signalling transduction pathway(s) as a negative control in human Leydig cells. In a recent work we suggested a possible direct effect of leptin on calves gonads until the onset of puberty. The correlation

http://dx.doi.org/10.5772/52994

between the expression of leptin receptors (OBR) isoforms and their association with leptin and testosterone concentrations also indicated the complementary action of receptors and those hormones in peripubertal calves testis (Ruiz-Cortes and Olivera, 2010). Platelet-derived growth factor (PDGF), vascular endothelial growth factor (VEGF) and endothelin and their receptors have been reported to be expressed in normal human Leydig cells, and have been suggested to play a role in the autocrine/paracrine regulation of human Leydig cell physiology (Svechnikov and Söder, 2008).

2.1.2. Females

In the ovary, the cellular contribution to steroidogenesis is very different from that in the testis, and both granulosa cells and theca cells contribute to steroidogenesis. In the testis supporting cell lineage gives rise to Sertoli cells which are nurse cells for spermatogenesis. For ovarian histogenesis, the supporting cell lineage gives rise to granulosa cells. Theca cells develop from stromal steroidogenic precursor cells outside the follicles and are ovarian counterparts of Leydig cells. The theca cells synthesize androgen in response to human chorionic gonadotropin, hCG and pituitary LH, but are not capable of producing estrogen since they lack expression of CYP19 aromatase, the enzyme converting androgen to estrogen. This enzyme is expressed by granulosa cells and these cells can produce estrogen and progesterone in response to LH and FSH stimulation. Thus, both theca cells and granulosa cells are required for estrogen synthesis by the ovary, and both gonadotropins (LH, FSH) are needed. These joint actions form the basis of the two cell, two-gonadotropin hypothesis for biosynthesis of estrogen. This is much more complex than the straight forward situation in the testis where Leydig cells produce androgen in response to LH (or hCG)(Svechnikov and Söder, 2008).

In the female, as in male, leptin excerts important action on steroidogenesis. We proved that Leptin, acting through STAT-3, modulates steroidogenesis in a biphasic and dose-dependent manner, and SREBP1 induction of StAR expression may be in the cascade of regulatory events in porcine granulosa cells (Ruiz-Cortes et al., 2003).

2.2. Androgens and anabolic steroids

2.2.1. Androgens

Scientists have studied androgens since the 18th century. Androgens are dubbed the male hormones mainly because males make and use more testosterone and other androgens than females. These steroid hormones confer masculinity by triggering and controlling body programs that govern male sexual development and physique. In females, androgens play more subtle roles (Tulane University).

The androgens, as paracrine hormones, are required by the Sertoli cells in order to support sperm production. They are also required for masculinization of the developing male fetus (including penis and scrotum formation)(Table 1). Under the influence of androgens, remnants of the mesonephron, the Wolffian ducts, develop into the epididymis, vas deferens and seminal vesicles. This action of androgens is supported by a hormone from Sertoli cells,

MIH (Müllerian inhibitory hormone), which prevents the embryonic Müllerian ducts from developing into fallopian tubes and other female reproductive tract tissues in male embryos. MIH and androgens cooperate to allow for the normal movement of testes into the scrotum. Two weak androgens, dehydroepiandrosterone and androstenedione are mostly synthesized in adrenal glands (in small amounts also in the brain). Androstenedione is converted into T mainly in testis Leydig cells and peripheral tissue, or aromatized into estradiol. Testosterone is metabolized by 5a-reductase in the potent androgen 5a-dihydrotestosterone and like androstenedione in estradiol by P450-aromatase (also called estrogen synthase) (Figure 1) (Michels and Hoppe, 2008).

In humans, the role of androgens with respect to breast growth and neoplasia was evaluated. Measurement of circulating sex steroids and their metabolites demonstrates that androgen activity is normally quite abundant in healthy women throughout the entire life cycle. Epidemiological studies investigating T levels and breast cancer risk have major theoretical and methodological limitations and do not provide any consensus. The molecular epidemiology of defects in pathways involved in androgen synthesis and activity in breast cancer holds great promise but is still in early stages. Clinical observations and experimental data indicate that androgens inhibit mammary growth and have been used with success similar to that of tamoxifen to treat breast cancer. Given these considerations, it is of concern that current forms of estrogen (E) treatment in oral contraceptives and for ovarian failure result in suppression of endogenous androgen activity. Thus, there is need for studies on the efficacy of supplementing both oral contraception and E replacement therapy with physiological replacement androgen, perhaps in a non aromatizable form, to maintain the natural E–androgen ratios typical of normal women (Dimitrakakis et al., 2002).

2.2.2. *Anabolic steroids*

Anabolic steroids are synthetic derivatives of testosterone and are characterized by their ability to cause nitrogen retention and positive protein metabolism, thereby leading to increased protein synthesis and muscle mass. Primary therapeutic use of testosterone is for replacement of androgen deficiencies in hypogonadism. These compounds are used for gynecologic disorders, anemia, osteoporosis, aging and treatment of delayed puberty in boys. Anabolic steroids have also been taken to improve athletic performance to enhance muscle development and to reduce body fat (Sevin et al., 2005).

According to surveys and media reports, the legal and illegal use of these drugs is gaining popularity. Testosterone restores sex drive and boosts muscle mass, making it central to 2 of society's rising preoccupations: perfecting the male body and sustaining the male libido. Testosterone has potent anabolic effects on the musculoskeletal system, including an increase in lean body mass, a dose-related hypertrophy of muscle fibers, and an increase in muscle strength. For athletes requiring speed and strength and men desiring a cosmetic muscle makeover, illegal steroids are a powerful lure, despite the risk of side effects. Recent clinical studies have discovered novel therapeutic uses for physiologic doses of anabolic-androgens steroids (AAS), without any significant adverse effects in the short term. In the wake of important scientific advances during the past decade, the positive and negative effects of AAS warrant reevaluation (Evans, 2004). In 1991 testosterone and related AAS were declared controlled substances. However, the relative abuse and dependence liability of AAS have not been fully characterized. In humans, it is difficult to separate the direct psychoactive effects of AAS from reinforcement due to their systemic anabolic effects. However, using conditioned place preference and self-administration, studies in animals have demonstrated that AAS are reinforcing in a context where athletic performance is irrelevant. Furthermore, AAS share brain sites of action and neurotransmitter systems in common with other drugs of abuse. In particular, recent evidence links AAS with opioids. In humans, AAS abuse is associated with prescription opioid use. In animals, AAS overdose produces symptoms resembling opioid overdose, and AAS modify the activity of the endogenous opioid system (Wood, 2008).

Antiandrogens prevent or inhibit the biological effects of androgens. They are often indicated to treat severe male sexual disorders such as paraphilias, as well as use as an antineoplastic agent in prostate cancer. They can also be used for treatment prostate enlargement, acne, androgenetic alopecia and hirsutism. The administration of antiandrogens in males can result in slowed or arrested development or reversal of male secondary sex characteristics, and hyposexuality (Sevin et al., 2005).

2.3. Estrogens and progestogens

Estrogens, or oestrogens, are a group of compounds named for their importance in the estrous cycle of humans and other animals. They are the primary female sex hormones. Natural estrogens are steroid hormones, while some synthetic ones are non-steroidal. Estrogen can be broken down into three distinct compounds: estrone, estradiol and estriol. During a mammal reproductive life, which starts with the onset of puberty and continues until andropause and /or menopause (in human), the main type of estrogen produced is estradiol. Enzymatic actions produce estradiol from androgens. Testosterone contributes to the production of estradiol, while the estrogen estrone is made from androstenedione. Phytoestrogens have analogous effects to those of human estrogens in serving to reduce menopausal symptoms, as well as the risk of osteoporosis and heart disease. In Animal husbandry (sheep and cattle) they may also have important physiological and sometimes deleterious reproductive effects as they are present in some pastures plants such as soybean, Alfalfa, red clover, white clover, subterranean clover, Berseem clover, birdsfoot trefoil and in native American legumes such as Vicia americana and Astragalus serotinus (Adams, 1995). Other estrogen containing foods Include: Anise seed, Apples, Baker's yeast, Barley, Beets, Carrots, Celery, Cherries, Chickpeas, Clover, Cucumbers, Dates, Eggs, Eggplant, Fennel, Flaxseed, Garlic, Lentils, Licorice, Millet, Oats, Olives, Papaya, Parsley, Peas, Peppers, Plums, Pomegranates, Potatoes, Pumpkin, Red beans, Rhubarb, Rice, Sesame seeds, Soybean sprouts, Soybeans, Split peas, Sunflower seeds, Tomatoes, Wheat, Yams.

Progestogens are characterized by their basic 21-carbon skeleton, called a pregnane skeleton (C21). In similar manner, the estrogens possess an estrane skeleton (C18) and androgens, an andrane skeleton (C19) (Figure 1). Progestogens are named for their function in maintaining pregnancy (pro-gestational), although they are also present at other phases of the estrous and menstrual cycles. The progestogen class of hormones includes all steroids with a pregnane skeleton, that is, both naturally occurring and synthetic ones. Exogenous or synthetic hormones are usually referred to as progestins.

Progesterone is the major naturally occurring human progestogen. Progesterone (P4) is produced by the corpus luteum in all mammalian species. Luteal cells possess the necessary enzymes to convert cholesterol to pregnenolone (P5), which is subsequently converted into P4. Progesterone is highest in the diestrus phase of the estrous cycle as is going to be explained.

2.3.1. Estradiol

Estradiol (E2 or 17β-estradiol, also oestradiol) is a sex hormone. Estradiol has 17 carbons (C17) and 2 hydroxyl groups in its molecular structure, estrone has 1 (E1) and estriol has 3 (E3). Estradiol is about 10 times as potent as estrone and about 80 times as potent as estriol in its estrogenic effect. Except during the early follicular phase of the menstrual cycle, its serum levels are somewhat higher than that of estrone during the reproductive years of the human female. Thus it is the predominant estrogen during reproductive years both in terms of absolute serum levels as well as in terms of estrogenic activity. During menopause, estrone is the predominant circulating estrogen and during pregnancy estriol is the predominant circulating estrogen in terms of serum levels. Estradiol is also present in males, being produced as an active metabolic product of testosterone. The serum levels of estradiol in males (14 - 55 pg/mL) are roughly comparable to those of postmenopausal women (< 35 pg/mL). Estradiol *in vivo* is interconvertible with estrone; estradiol to estrone conversion being favored. Estradiol has not only a critical impact on reproductive and sexual functioning, but also affects other organs, including the bones (Table 1).

There is scientific literature that may be relevant about the use of estradiol from the point of view of food safety. In cattle for example Estradiol benzoate (10-28 mg) or estradiol-17ß (estradiol; 8-24 mg) is administered (orally) to cattle to increase the rate of weight gain (i.e. growth promotion) and to improve feed efficiency. Estradiol valerate is also administered by subcutaneous or intramuscular injection to synchronize estrus in cattle. Estradiol is generally considered to be inactive when administered orally due to gastrointestinal and/or hepatic inactivation.

Circulating estradiol, like T, is bound to sex hormone-binding globulin (SHBG, in Figure 4) and, to a lesser extent, serum albumin. Only 1-2% of circulating estradiol is unbound; 40% is bound to SHBG and the remainder to albumin. Plasma SHBG is secreted from the liver; a similar, non-secretory form is present in many tissues, including reproductive tissues and the brain.

Urinary and faecal metabolites of estrogens in animals and humans have been studied for use as possible indicators of risk for hormone-dependent cancers or for infertility. There is at present no consensus about the importance of specific metabolites or metabolite ratios as prognostic factors, with the possible exception of estriol as a marker of the well-being of the feto-placental unit (World Health Organization International Programme on Chemical Safety, 2000).

Estrogens have been isolated from testes of stallion, bulls, boars, dogs and men. Estrogens may play a role in the pathogenesis of prostatic hyperplasia common in aged dogs, and estrogens receptors are present in prostatic urethra and prostatic glands of dogs. Estrogens like androgens, are transferred from testicular vein to the testicular artery. In several species, levels of estrogens in the blood of testicular artery are consistently higher than the levels in systemic blood. The mechanisms involved in the transfer of estrogens from vein to artery in the pampiniform plexus and its physiology role are not clear. Estrogens may be playing important role in regulating the pituitary-gonadal axis. In several species, estrogens inhibit Leydig cell secretion of testosterone (Pineda, 2003) as it will be mentioned.

Name of Steroid (abbrev.)	Steroidogenic Tissues	Target Tissue (male and female)	Physiological functions (male and female)
Estradiol (E2)	Granulosa cells of follicle Placenta Sertoli cells of testis	Brain, hypothalamus Bones Entire female reproductive tract and mammary gland	Sexual behavior (male and female) Secondary female sex characteristics GnRH regulation, Ovulation Elevated secretory activity of the entire female tract Enhanced uterine motility Regulation of cardiovascular physiology Bone integrity and neuronal growth
Progesterone (P4)	Luteinized/luteal cells Placenta Adrenal	Hypothalamus Uterine endometrium, myometrium Mammary gland Leydig cells	Follicular growth and ovulation Endometrial secretion Inhibits GnRH release Inhibits reproductive behavior Promotes maintenance of pregnancy
Testosterone (T)	Leydig cells of testis Theca interna cells of ovary	Accesory sex glands (male) Tunica dartos of scrotum Seminiferous epithelium Skeletal muscle Brain (female) Granulosa cells	Anabolic growth (male), Increase muscle mass Promotes spermatogenesis Promotes secretion of accessory sex glands Substrate for E2 synthesis (female) Secondary sex characteristics Decrease risk of osteoporosis

Table 1. Sex steroids: Source, Target tissues and Physiological Functions. Modified from (Hu et al., 2010; Senger, 2006)

2.3.2. *Progesterone*

Progesterone, also known as P4 (pregn-4-ene-3,20-dione), is a C-21 steroid hormone involved in the female menstrual/estral cycle, pregnancy and embryogenesis of humans and other species. Progesterone is produced in the ovaries, the adrenal glands (suprarenal), and, during pregnancy, in the placenta. Progesterone is also stored in adipose (fat) tissue. Progesterone is synthesized by the ovarian corpus luteum, but during pregnancy the main source of P4 is the placenta as in woman,mare and ewe; in cow, the time of placenta takeover is 6-8months of pregnancy. In other species (goat, sow, queen, bitch,rabbit, alpaca,camel, llama) there is no placenta P4 production at all, the ovarian CL is in charge of the entire P4 for gestation. In mammals, P4, like all other steroid hormones, is synthesized from pregnenolone, which in turn is derived from cholesterol. Androstenedione can be converted to testosterone, estrone and estradiol (Figure 1)(Wikipedia). Important functions of P4 are (1) inhibition of sexual behavior; (2) maintenance of pregnancy by inhibiting uterine contractions and promoting glandular development in the endometrium; and (3) promotion of alveolar development of the mammary gland. The synergistic actions of estrogens and progestins are notable in preparing the uterus for pregnancy and the mammary gland for lactation (Table 1).

In at least one plant, *Juglans regia*, progesterone has been detected. In addition, progesterone-like steroids are found in *Dioscorea mexicana*. It contains a steroid called diosgenin that is taken from the plant and is converted into progesterone. Diosgenin and progesterone are found in other *Dioscorea* species as well.

The switch from the principal steroid product of the maturing follicle (estrogens) to that of the developing and mature corpus luteum (P4) is one of the amazing hallmarks of the ovary sex steroids production occurring during luteinization as described later.

Of interest, we have reported that during the differentiation of granulosa cells into luteal cells *in vitro*, it exists an inverse modulation between the expression of LH receptors (LHR) and the concentration of LH, and this expression of LHR could be regulated by P4 produced by luteinized granulosa cells (Montaño et al., 2009).

3. Functional organization of the hypothalamic-pituitary-gonadal axis: sex steroids control of reproduction

Gonadal secretory activites involve two special cell types responsive to FSH and LH. Ovarian granulosa cells and testicular Leydig cells are responsive primarily to LH and synthesize androgens. Ovarian thecal cells and testicular Sertoli cells as well as Leydig cells respond to FSH with conversion of androgens into estrogens (P450aromatase activity). FSH also stimulates Sertoli cells to synthesize inhibin, activin, and other local bioregulatory factors (Norris, 2007).

3.1. Gonadal steroids and female reproductive cyclicity

Anatomically in the female hypothalamus, there are two GnRH neurons centers. The first, the surge center, consists of three nuclei called the preoptic nucleus, the anterior hypothalamic area and the suprachiasmatic nucleus. This center releases basal levels of GnRH until it receives the appropriate positive stimulus. This stimulus is known to be a threshold level of estrogen in the absence of P4. When the estrogen concentration in the blood reaches a certain level, a large quantity of GnRH is released from the terminals of neurons, the cells bodies of which are located in the surge center. In natural condition, the preovulatory surge of GnRH occurs only once during the estrous or menstrual cycle. The second, the tonic center, releases small episodes of GnRH in a pulsatile fashion similar to a driping faucet. This episodic release is continuous and throughout reproductive life and during the entire estrous cycle (Senger, 2006).

The female in various species have two important periods that mark the reproductive cycle: follicular and luteal phases. The follicular phase begins after luteolysis that causes the decline in P4. Gonadotropins (FSH and LH) are therefore produced and cause follicles to produce E2. The follicular phase is dominated by E2 produced by ovarian follicles and ends at ovulation. The luteal phase begins after ovulation and includes the development of corpus luteum that produces P4, and luteolysis that brought about by prostaglandin F2α. In women, the follicular phase is divided into menses and proliferative period (5 and 9 days respectively); luteal phase is the secretory phase (14 days). In domestic animals, the follicular phase is divided in pro-estrus (2 days) and estrus (1 day), and the luteal phase in metestrus (4 days) and diestrus (14 days). At the pro-estrus, as P4 drops, FSH and LH increase together in response to GnRH. FSH and LH cause the production of E2 by ovarian follicles (Figure 2). When recruited follicles develop dominance, they produce E2 and inhibin that suppresses FSH secretion from the anterior lobe of the pituitary. Thus, FSH does not surge with the same magnitude as LH. The pre-ovulatory surge of GnRH is controlled by high E2 and low P4. In mammals, including humans, E2 in the presence of low P4 exerts a differential effect on GnRH. Thus, E2 in low concentrations causes a negative feedback (suppression) on the preovulatory center. That is, low estrogen reduces the level of firing GnRH neurons in the preovulatory-surge center. However, when E2 levels are high (estrus), as they would be during the mid-to late follicular phase (figure 2), the preovulatory center responds dramatically by releasing large quantities of GnRH. This stimulation in response to rising concentrations of E2 is referred to as positive feedback. During the middle part of the cycle, when E2 levels are low and P4 is high (metestrus, diestrus), there is negative feedback on the preovulatory center, thus preventing high amplitude pulses of GnRH. Interesting, when comparing human vs. other mammals, the P4 does not influence sexual receptivity but in domestic animals, those high levels of P4 inhibit it (Senger, 2006) (Figure 2).

As reviewed by Murphy, luteinization is a remarkable event involving cell proliferation, cell differentiation, and tissue remodeling that is unparalleled in the adult mammal. It comprises two major processes: (a) the terminated proliferation plus rapid hypertrophy and differentiation of the steroidogenic cells of follicle into the luteal cells of the CL. Luteinization is both a qualitative and quantitative change because the mammalian CL produces up to 100-fold greater amounts of steroid (P4) than the follicle. Luteolysis results in cessation of P4 production, in structural regression to forma corpus albicans and into a follicular development and entrance into a new follicular phase.

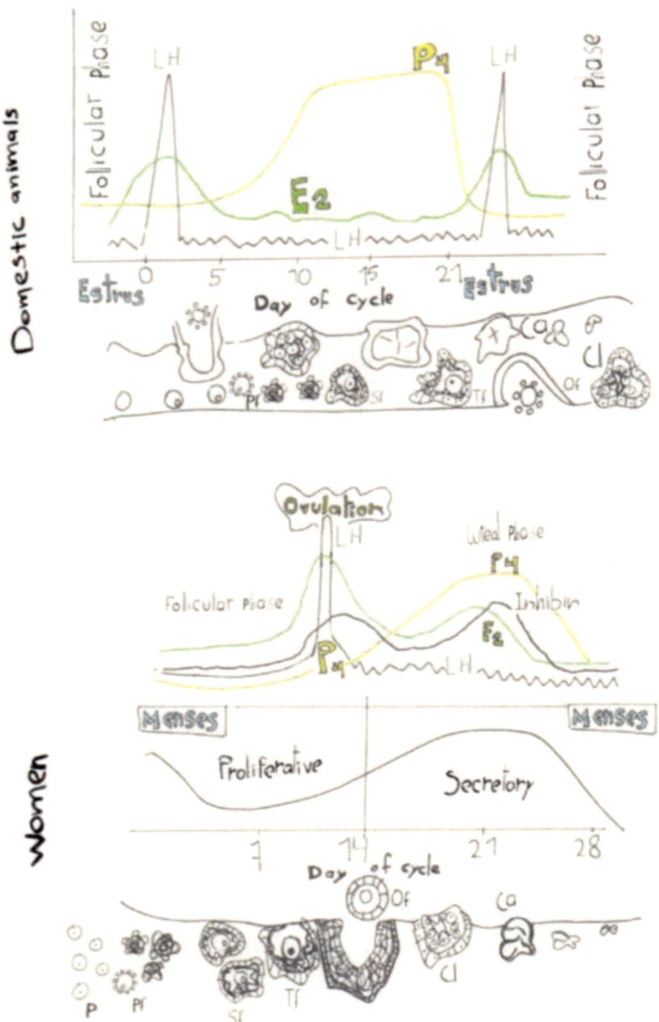

P: Primordial follicle, PF: Primary follicle, SF: Secondary follicle, TF: Tertiary follicle, OF: Ovulatory follicle, Cl: Corpus luteum, Ca: Corpus albicans

Figure 2. Female cyclicity and gonadal steroids. Modified from (López et al., 2008; Senger, 2006) The two types of reproductive cycles are the estrus and the menstrual cycles. Each cycle consists of a follicular and a luteal phase. The follicular phase is dominated by the hormone E2 from ovarian follicles. E2 causes marked changes in the female tract for pregnancy. Anestrus stands for periods of time when estrous cycles cease. Pregnancy, season of the year, lactation, forms of stress and pathology cause anestrus. Amenorrhea refers to the lack of menstrual periods and is caused by many of the same factors that cause anestrus. A menstrual cycle consists of the physiological events that occur between successive menstrual periods (about 28 days). No endometrial sloughing (menstruations) occurs in animal with estrous cycles.Lutealphase is dominated by P4 from corpus luteum.

As the main steroid produced during luteal phase is the P4 it is important to mention about the manipulation of the estrous and menstrual cycles by exogenous administration of P4. It serves indeed as an "artificial corpus luteum" (ear subcutaneous implants or intravaginal devices). Exogenous P4 suppresses estrus and ovulation. When this exogenous P4 is removed or withdrawn, the animal will enter pro-estrus and estrus within 2 to 3 days after removal. This application is intended to increase the convenience of artificial insemination programs and to facilitate fertility in domestic husbandry animal (improving pregnancy rates). In contrast, the use of exogenous P4 in humans (oral, transdermal,injectable, implants) is intended to block ovulation and minimize pregnancy probability (contraception)(Senger, 2006).

3.2. Gonadal steroids and spermatogenesis

Upon stimulation by LH, the Leydig cells of the testes produce androgens. Dihydrotestosterone is found in high enough concentration in peripheral tissue to be of functional importance. Functions of T, as states before, include (1) development of secondary sex characteristics; (2) maintenance of the male duct system; (3) expression of male sexual behavior (libido); (4) function of the accessory glands; (5) function of the tunica dartos muscle in the scrotum; and (6) spermatocytogenesis. The role of T in regulating the release of hypothalamic and gonadotropic hormones is similar to that described for P4 in the female. High concentrations of T inhibit the release of GnRH, FSH, and LH, a negative feedback control. Conversely, when T concentrations are low, higher levels of GnRH, FSH, and LH are released. Thus, reciprocal action of T with the hypothalamic and gonadotropic hormones is necessary for regulation of normal reproduction in the male (Figure 3)(Gyeongsang National University). Luteinizing hormone acts on the Leydig cells within the testes. These cells are analogous to the cells of the theca interna of antral follicles in the ovary. They contain membrane bound receptors for LH. When LH binds to their receptors, Leydig cells produce P4, most of which is converted to T. The production of T takes place by the same intracellular mechanism as in the female. The Leydig cells synthesize and secrete T less than 30 minutes after the onset of an LH episode (Figure 3). This T secretion is short and pulsatile, lasting for a period of 20 to 60 minutes. It is believed that pulsatile discharge of LH is important for two reasons. First, high concentration of T within the seminiferous tubule is essential for spermatogenesis (Senger, 2006). Second, Leydig cells become unresponsive to sustained high levels of LH believed to be caused by reduction in the number of LH receptor. In fact, continual high concentrations of LH result in reduced secretion of T. Intratesticular levels of T are 100-500 times higher than that of systemic blood. However, testicular T is diluted over 500 times when it reaches the peripheral blood (Senger, 2006). This dilution added to a short half-life of the T (here, there is considerable variation in the half-life of testosterone as reported in the literature, ranging from 10 to 100 minutes; it is metabolized in the liver) keep systemic concentrations well below that which would cause down-regulation of the GnRH/LH feedback. The role of the pulsatile nature of T is not fully understood. It is believed that chronically high systemic concentrations of T suppress FSH secretion. Sertoli cells function is FSH dependent. Thus, their function is compromised when FSH is reduced. The periodic reduction in T allows the negative feedback on FSH to be removed. But the exact role of this FSH diminution it is not clear as well as the physiological role of paracrine/

autocrine inhibin effects within the testis has not been clarified. While the α subunit knock-out mouse model suggests that this protein protects against the development of testicular tumours, there is no evidence for a physiological role of paracrine/autocrine inhibin signalling on spermatogenesis or steroidogenesis (de Kretser et al., 2001). Sertoli cells also produce inhibin that, as in the female, suppresses FSH secretion from the anterior lobe of the pituitary. The physiologically important hormone that exerts tonic negative feedback upon FSH secretion in men is inhibin B (Illingworth et al., 1996). Inhibin and androgen binding protein are produced by Sertoli cells under the influence of FSH. As in the female, inhibin selectively inhibits the release of FSH while not affecting the release of LH. Androgen binding protein binds T, making it available for its functions in spermatozoa production.

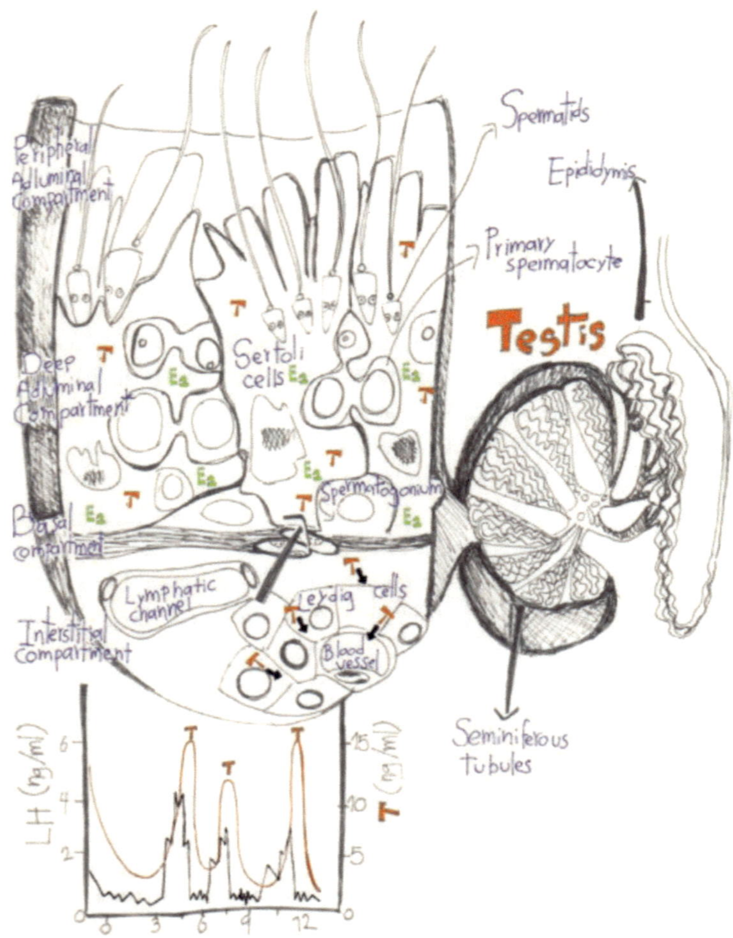

Figure 3. Spermatogenesis and steroids. Modified from (Senger, 2006). There is a pulsatile discharge of LH. Leydig cells produce important concentrations of testosterone (T).High concentration of T within the seminiferous tubule, essential for spermatogenesis. Sertoli cells aromatize T from Leydig cell into E2.

Under the influence of FSH the Sertoli cells convert T to E2 and other estrogens (Figure 3). The stallion and the boar secrete large amount of E2 but since they are secreted as molecules with low physiologic activity they seem to be of little consecuence. Sertoli cells convert T to E2 utilizing a mechanism identical to the granulosal cell of the antral follicle in the female (Senger, 2006). The exact role of E2 in male reproduction it is not clear. The finding of both aromatase and E2 receptors (ERs) in the developing fetal testis implies a possible involvement of estrogens in the process of differentiation and maturation of developing rodent testis from an early stage of morphogenesis, probably ERβ having a major role than ERα (Luconi et al., 2002; Rochira et al., 2005). Also, T and E2 in the blood act on the hypothalamus and exert a negative feedback on GnRH and, in turn, LH and FSH are reduced.

3.3. Sex steroids molecular pathways in target tissues

Steroid hormones regulate cellular processes by binding to membrane, intracellular and/or nuclear receptors that, in turn, interact with discrete nucleotide sequences to alter gene expression. Because most steroid receptors in target cells are located in the cytoplasm, they need to get into the nucleus to alter gene expression. This process typically takes at least 30 to 60 minutes. In contrast, other regulatory actions of steroid hormones are manifested within seconds to a few minutes. These time periods are far too rapid to be due to changes at the genomic level and are therefore termed nongenomic or rapid actions, to distinguish them from the classical steroid hormone action of regulation of gene expression. The rapid effects of steroid hormones are manifold, ranging from activation of mitogen-activated protein kinases (MAPKs), adenylyl cyclase (AC), protein kinase C and A (PKC,PKA), and heterotrimeric guanosine triphosphate-binding proteins (G proteins) (in Figure 4 and 5). In some cases, these rapid actions of steroids are mediated through the classical steroid receptor that can also function as a ligand-activated transcription factor, whereas in other instances the evidence suggests that these rapid actions do not involve the classical steroid receptors. One candidate target for the nonclassical receptor-mediated effects are G protein-coupled receptors (GPCRs), which activate several signal transduction pathways. One characteristic of responses that are not mediated by the classical steroid receptors is insensitivity to steroid antagonists, which has contributed to the notion that a new class of steroid receptors may be responsible for part of the rapid action of steroids. Evidence suggests that the classical steroid receptors can be localized at the plasma membrane, where they may trigger a chain of reactions previously attributed only to growth factors. Identification of interaction domains on the classical steroid receptors involved in the rapid effects, and separation of this function from the genomic action of these receptors, should pave the way to a better understanding of the rapid action of steroid hormones (Cato et al., 2002; Simoncini et al., 2004) (Figure 4 and 5).

3.3.1. Androgens

The biological activity of androgens is thought to occur predominantly through binding to intracellular androgen-receptors, a member of the nuclear receptor family, that interact with specific nucleotide sequences to alter gene expression. This genomic-androgen effect typically takes at least half an hour. In contrast, the rapid or non-genomic actions of androgens are manifested within in seconds to few minutes. This rapid effect of androgens are manifold, ranging from activation of G-protein coupled membrane androgen receptors or sex hormone-binding globulin receptors, stimulation of different protein kinases, to direct modulation of voltage- and ligand gated ion-channels and transporters. The physiological relevance of these non-genomic androgen actions has not yet been determined in detail. However, it may contribute to modulate several second messenger systems or transcription factors, which suggests a cross-talk between the fast non-genomic and the slow genomic pathway of androgens (Michels and Hoppe, 2008) (Figure 4).

The rapid actions of androgens are mediated by direct binding to the target protein (e.g., ion-channel) or by a specific association to different receptors. The non-genomic androgen action based on receptor level can be mediated by at least three androgen-binding proteins, the classical intracellular androgen receptor, the transmembrane androgen receptor and the transmembrane sex hormone-binding globulin receptor. For both transmembrane receptors, the non-genomic effect is converted via a G-protein coupled process, whereas binding to intracellular androgen receptors may lead to an activation of several cytosolic pathways. All rapid androgen actions are predominantly mediated by second messenger signaling (especially Ca2+) and phosphorylation events, including different intracellular signal routes, e.g., PKA, MAPK, phospholipase:PLC, phosphatidylinositol-3 kinase:PI-3K, steroid receptor co-activator:Src pathways. Although some studies implicated benefits of the non-genomic androgen actions on the cardiovascular and neuropsychiatric systems, more detailed research and clinical studies are still required (Michels and Hoppe, 2008).

Increasing evidence suggests that nongenomic effects of testosterone and anabolic androgenic steroids (AAS) operate concertedly with genomic effects. Classically, these responses have been viewed as separate and independent processes, primarily because nongenomic responses are faster and appear to be mediated by membrane androgen receptors, whereas long-term genomic effects are mediated through cytosolic androgen receptors regulating transcriptional activity. Numerous studies have demonstrated increases in intracellular Ca2+ in response to AAS. These Ca2+ mediated responses have been seen in a diversity of cell types, including osteoblasts, platelets, skeletal muscle cells, cardiac myocytes and neurons. The versatility of Ca2+ as a second messenger provides these responses with a vast number of pathophysiological implications. In cardiac cells, testosterone elicits voltage-dependent Ca2+ oscillations and inositol-1,4,5-triphosphate receptors:IP3R mediated Ca2+ release from internal stores, leading to activation of MAPK and the serine/threonine protein kinase regulating cell growth, cell proliferation, cell motility, cell survival, protein synthesis, and transcription: mTOR. In neurons, depending upon concentration, testosterone can provoke either physiological Ca2+ oscillations, essential for synaptic plasticity, or sustained, pathological Ca2+ transients that lead to neuronal apoptosis. It was proposed that Ca2+ acts as an important point of crosstalk between nongenomic and genomic AAS signaling, representing a central regulator that bridges these previously thought to be divergent responses (Vicencio et al., 2011).

http://dx.doi.org/10.5772/52994

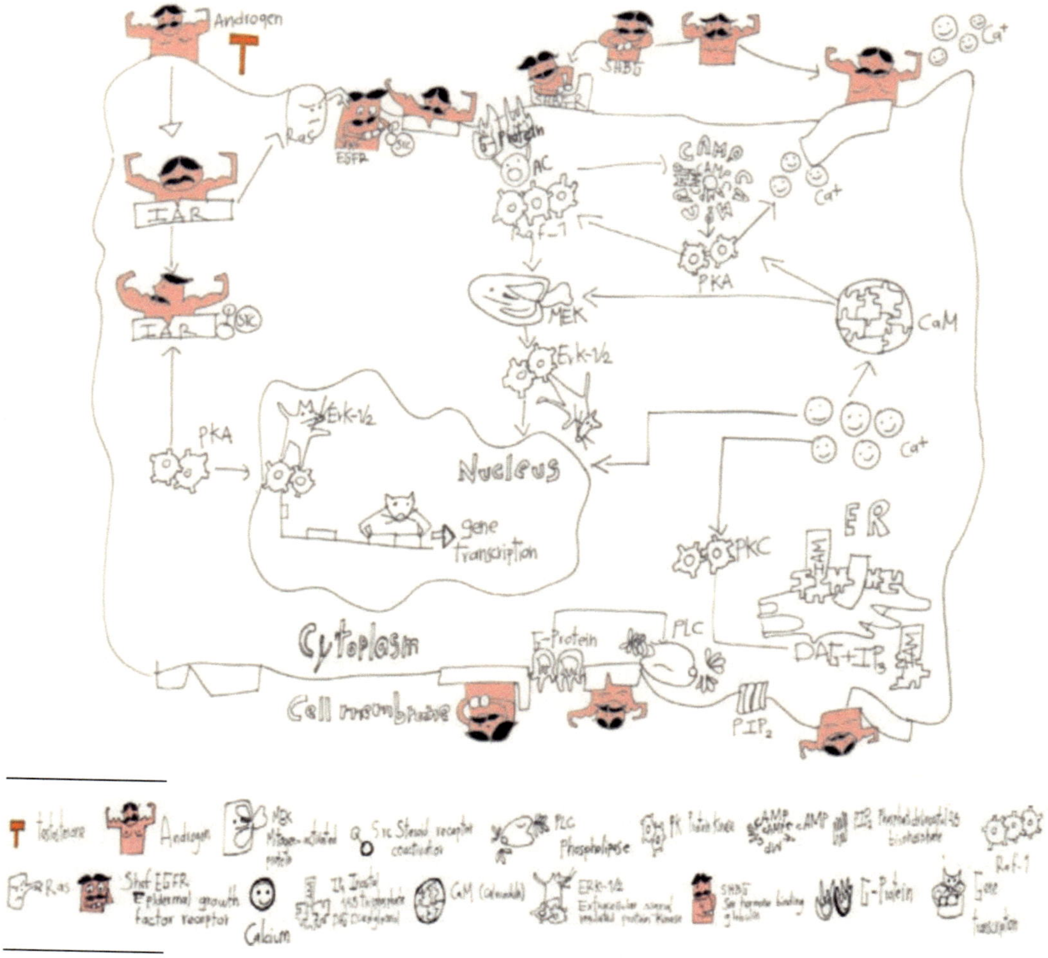

Figure 4. Actions and pathways of androgens. Modified from (Michels and Hoppe, 2008). The rapid effects of steroid hormones are mediated by he activation of mitogen-activated protein kinases (MAPKs), adenylyl cyclase (AC), protein kinase C and A (PKC,PKA), and heterotrimeric guanosine triphosphate-binding proteins (G proteins). The cross-talk between the fast non-genomic and the slow genomic pathway by androgens binding to their internal androgens receptors (IAR) is mediated in part by intracellular Ca2+.

3.3.2. Estrogens

In 2009 Charidıti et al. described four main pathways of estrogen receptors (ERs) alpha (a) and beta (b) signaling as a matter of "sophisticated" control systems necessary to obtain a tight equilibrium in estrogen action and regulation of ER expression in tissues and cells (Charitidi et al., 2009).

The first well known molecular mechanism is the classic ligand dependent pathways. Estrogen receptors are kept inactive in the nucleus and cytoplasm of the cell forming a complex with various heat shock proteins (hsp) that act as chaperones when the cell is not exposed to estrogens. Such proteins are hsp90, hsp70 and hsp56 and by forming a complex with the ERs they are believed to prevent them from binding to their response elements EREs, but also keep them capable of binding to their ligands (estrogens) with high affinity. When the estrogens diffuse across the cell and nuclear membrane they interact with the inactive form of the ERs and separate them from the hsp-complex. ERs are now activated and can form homodimers and to a lesser extent heterodimers to bind to their estrogens EREs. The EREs are commonly located in the promoter regions of estrogen target genes and make it possible for the ERs to specifically bind to the DNA and regulate transcription either as enhancers or repressors.

Once the complex of the activated ERs together with co-activator proteins (such as ligand-dependent activation function-1 and 2: AF-1 and AF-2) is bound to the ERE it can either up- or down-regulate the expression of the target gene. This is decided by whether the ERE is "positive" or "negative" in the particular cell type for the ERs as well as by the cellular milieu (Figure 5).

The second molecular mechanism is the ligand independent. It is possible that the ERs get activated even in the absence of their ligands with the aid of intracellular second messengers. Growth factors are able to activate MAPKs and they subsequently become phosphorylated and thus activate the ERs. This ligand-independent ER activation is still dependent on AF-1. Another intracellular path that can lead to ER activation in the absence of ligands is via cAMP, a second messenger for G-protein coupled receptors and activates the PKA pathway. AF-2 is needed for cAMP activation of ERs. In this type of ligand-independent activation of ERs, growth factors and second messengers take over estrogens part to induce/elicit the same response from ERs (Figure 5).

The third signaling pathway is the ERE independent one. Estrogens exert their actions through the two ERs but also through other transcription factors. In this case the ligand-activated ERs do not bind to their EREs but anchor instead to other transcription factors directly bound to DNA in their specific response elements. In this mechanism ERs act more as co-regulators than actual transcription factors (activating protein-1 (AP-1), (Fos/Jun) or the stimulating protein-1 (Sp1)). Thus this, pathway is also referred to as transcription factor cross-talk (Figure 5)). Furthermore, the two ERs differ in their capacity to interact with different transcription factors. For example in the presence of 17beta-estradiol, ERa induces AP-1 driven gene transcription, while ERb has an inhibitory effect. This contrasting transcriptional activity is another example of the opposing actions of each ER.

The last mechanism is the non-genomic plasma-membrane pathway. The above mentioned mechanisms include the relatively long processes of gene transcription and mRNA translation and are thus insufficient to explain the short-term effects of estrogens that are found. Intracellular pathways that increase intracellular calcium, cAMP, or the phosphorylation of the cAMP response element binding protein (CREB), can result in an instantaneous response of the cell. This pathway does not require transcription of genes via the ERs and is referred to as non-genomic mechanisms of estrogen action, similar to the non-genomic pathways of androgens (Charitidi et al., 2009) (Figure 5).

In adults, the interaction of estrogen genomic and nongenomic mechanisms may act to maintain physiology or signal transduction pathways as hormone levels fluctuate across the estrus cycle. As such, a disruption of the hormone/receptor system through a loss of hormone, decreased receptor expression, or uncoupling of receptor-transcriptional activity due to chronically elevated estrogen levels, would contribute to age-related changes that underlie the progressive senescence of physiological processes. Treatments designed to increase ER activity around the time of menopause, such as cyclic estrogen replacement, may be more beneficial than chronic hormone replacement (Foster, 2005).

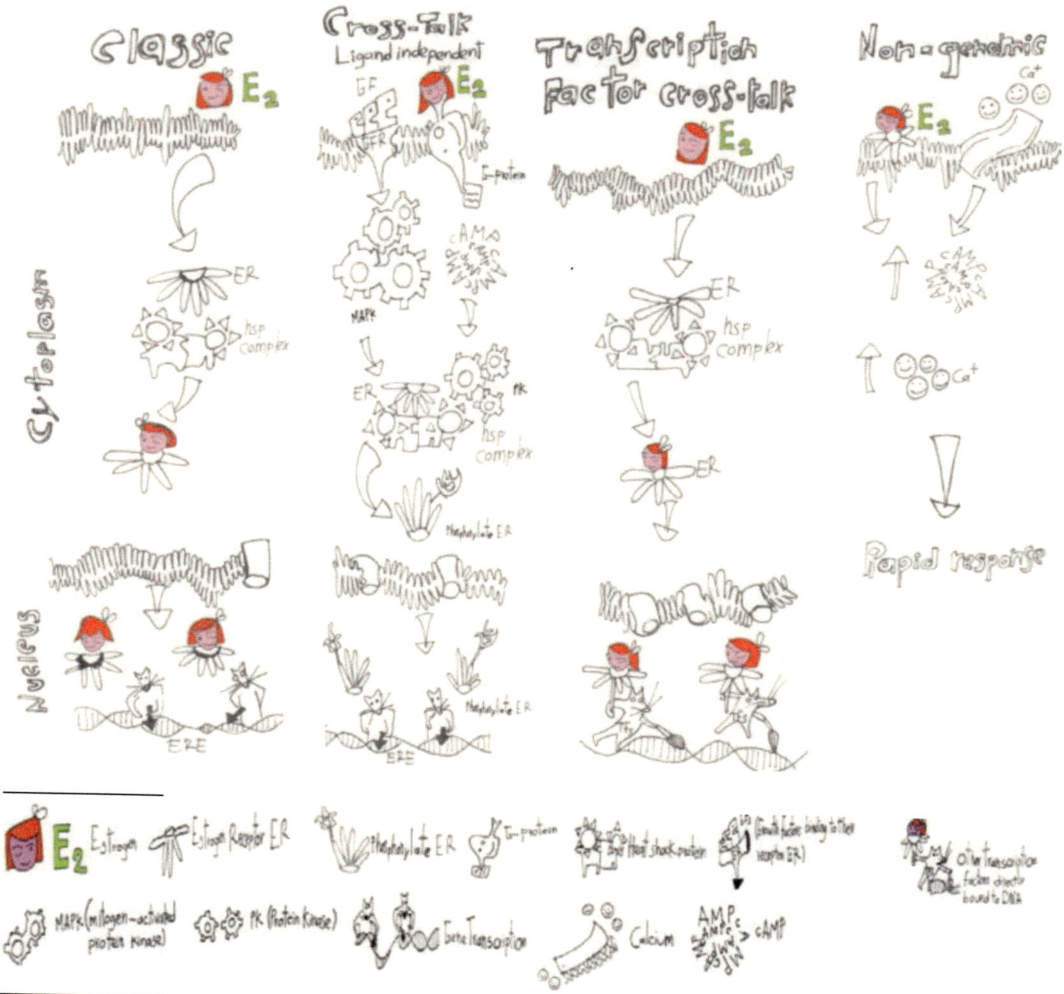

Figure 5. Actions and pathways of estrogens. Modified from (Charitidi et al., 2009). Four molecular mechanisms of E2 signaling in target cells. The first is the classic ligand dependent pathways. Estrogen receptors (ER) are liberated from heat shock proteins complex (hsp) and can continue their nuclear-DNA effect. The second is the ligand independent. It is possible that the ERs get activated even in the absence of their ligands with the aid of intracellular second messengers. The third is the ERE independent. In this case the ligand-activated ERs do not bind to their EREs but anchor instead to other transcription factors. The fourth is the non-genomic plasma-membrane pathway and does not require transcription of genes via the ERs. Besides those well documented genomic and non- genomic molecular pathways, it is important to mention the epigenetic regulation.

Recently, it was published a review about the overlapping nongenomic and genomic actions of thyroid hormone and estrogens and androgens. Authors concentrate on the tumor cell model, where, for example, estrogens and thyroid hormone have similar MAPK-dependent proliferative actions and where dihydrotestosterone also can stimulate proliferation. Steroids and thyroid hormone have similar anti-apoptotic effects in certain tumors; they also have overlapping or interacting nongenomic and genomic actions in heart and brain cells.

Their possible clinical consequences seem of crutial importance for the potential endocrine therapy targeting steroids receptors directly or indirectly (hormone or protein with overlapping effects) as reported for breast cancer and the nuclear and citoplasmic estrogen receptor and aromatase (Davis et al., 2011; Levin and Pietras, 2008).

Estradiol epigenetic effects have been reported with results providing evidence for mitotic regulation in follicle development by estrogen and demonstrate a previously undiscovered mechanism for induction of cell proliferation in ovarian and mammary gland cells. This epigenetic mark is induced by both FSH and 17beta-estradiol (E2), acting independently. E2-induced H3 phosphorylation fails to occur in mice with inactivated alpha-isoform of the nuclear estrogen receptor. E2 induction of histone phosphorylation is attenuated by cell cycle inhibition. Further, E2 induces the activity of the mitotic kinase, Aurora B, in a mammary tumor cell model where mitosis is estrogen receptor-alpha dependent (Ruiz-Cortes et al., 2005).

3.4. Reproductive moments and steroids

3.4.1. Puberty

Sex steroids regulation of the initiation of puberty was reported since 1979 in murine studies. Immature female rats presented evidence of oestrogen secretion by day 32 of life and an increased sensitivity of the pituitary to LHRH by day 34. These data suggested that in addition to the increased release of GnRH during puberty, a sex steroid induced alteration in the pituitary's responsiveness to GnRH may also be a significant contributory factor in the increase in secretion of gonadotropins at puberty. The stimulatory effect appeared to be related both to the quantity of sex steroid and the challenging dose of GnRH. These studies show that in addition to changes in sensitivity at the level of the hypothalamus, the CNS and gonads steroid and GnRH modulation of the response of the pituitary gland, are important events in the onset of puberty (Mahesh and Nazian, 1979).

Puberty is associated with an increasing production of androgenic steroids. Adrenal androgen formation (adrenarche), may precede gonadal testosterone synthesis. Both adrenal and gonadal androgens exert their biological effects via the androgen receptor, a nuclear transcription factor modulating a specific transcription regulation of largely unknown genes. During puberty, virilizing actions such as genital enlargement and sexual hair growth can be distinguished from anabolic action such as the gain in muscle strength and general changes in body composition. Furthermore, androgens play a major role in the initiation and maintenance of spermatogenesis. Thus, different androgenic steroids play an important role in the process of puberty (Hiort, 2002)(Table 2).

Male infants have a surge in T levels during the first few months of life. These levels fall to quite low (but greater than in female infants and children) until the pubertal rise. Nighttime elevations in serum T concentration are detectable even before the onset of the external signs of pubertal development following the sleep-entrained rises in serum LH. The daytime levels rise later as the testis volume increases.Testosterone is a substrate for 5-a reductase (conversion to dihydrotestosterone) and for aromatase (conversion to estradiol). The effects on muscle are likely in part due directly to T and indirectly to E2 because of the marked increase in growth hormone-GH and IGF-I levels due to an action of E2 on the hypothalamus and pituitary (Rogol, 2002).

In domestic animals, Senger and his team very appropriately mentioned in his book how the "story on the onset of puberty is not complete". It is about many factors that may be controlling this important physiological process of acquiring reproductive and productive competence. This capability is influenced by achieving the appropriated energy metabolism/body size and appropriated exposure to external modulators such as photoperiod (goat, sheep, horse), size of social groups (pig, cow) and the presence of the male (cow, goat). Genetics of the animal likely play a role in how these cues are generated within the animal (metabolic signals) and /or perceived (external cues, metabolic signals). The exact mechanisms that enable E2 to control GnRH secretion by the hypothalamus during the peripubertal period are still unknown even if since 1979 this effect was porposed as mentioned at the beginning of this apart. Other factor that need better understanding is the effect of ferhormones (as social clue), including steroids hormones, on the control of puberty onset; olfactory and vomeronasal organs are implicated but the exact pathways is not well defined. Finally, from a genetic improvement/reproductive management standpoint, is of interest the goal of shortening the time of onset of puberty, mainly in the male, in order to fasten the availability of spermatozoa production (particulary for artificial insemination in bulls, swine and poultry), the generation interval could be reduced and genetic improvement accelerated. Since female must maintain a successful pregnancy, deliver live offspring and lactate, there a clearly physiological limit to hastened puberty in females (Senger, 2006). The use of exogenous sex steroids for those purposes (male and female) is possible but also very questioned because of the secondary effects and the potential food residues (meat and milk) for human. Interestingly, Nelson proposed three potential predictors (i.e., biomarkers) of longevity in mammals (1) age of pubertal onset, (2) concentrations of gonadal steroids and (3) timing of age-related infertility. Ages of pubertal onset and of declining fertility are hypothesized to be positively correlated with longevity. Concentrations of androgens and estrogens are proposed to be inversely and positively correlated, respectively, with life span (Nelson, 1988).

3.4.2. Fertilization

Thirty years ago research results about the effect of follicular steroids on the maturation and fertilization of mammalian oocytes was reported. Pronuclear development was used to measure the effects on ovine oocytes of altering follicular steroidogenesis during maturation *in vitro*. Follicular steroid secretion was altered using enzyme inhibitors and exogenous steroid supplementation. Abnormalities induced during maturation were measured 24 h after transfer of oocytes to the oviducts of inseminated hosts. The authors concluded that oocytes require a specific intra-follicular steroid environment for the completion of the full maturation process. Alterations to the steroid profile during maturation induce changes in the oocyte which are expressed as gross abnormalities at fertilization (Moor et al., 1980).

Similarly, in other study, oocytes were collected by aspiration of preovulatory follicles from 55 women. After collection and culture, the oocytes were inseminated with the spermatozoa of the husband. The levels of progesterone, oestradiol-17β and androstenedione in the clear follicular fluid were measured by radioimmunoassay. A multivariate analysis containing these three hormone levels together with two ratios of progesterone with each of the other hormones indicated reasonable discrimination between the oocytes which fertilized and those which remained unfertilized after insemination. The discriminant analysis suggested that the fertilization of the oocytes could have been predicted on the basis of these hormonal profiles with a success rate which exceeded 90% (Fishel et al., 1983).

More recently, an academic article presents the result of a study on the correlation among sex steroids in follicular fluid (FF) and cultured granulosa cells and fertilization. The study examined the levels of E2, P4, and T in follicular fluid from stimulated cycles and their granulosa cell cultures after oocyte retrieval and the correlation between these levels. It revealed that there is no link among fertilization and sex steroid levels in FF and granulosa cells (FertilityWeekly, 2011). This is an important recent report taking in account that now a day in some in vitro fertilization –IVF- protocols, sexual steroids are commonly used as factor of fertilization improvement. Also, high follicular fluid E2 may be a marker for oocytes that will fertilize normally with intracytoplasmic sperm injection (ICSI) (Lamb et al., 2010).

At the spermatozoa level, in human it was demonstrated the expression of a functional surface estrogen receptor (of 29 KDa). Luconi et al., suggested that this receptor and of course its ligand, may play a role in the modulation of non-genomic action (via calcium modulation) of P4 in spermatozoa during the process of fertilization: E2 stimulates tyrosine phosphorylation of several sperm proteins, including the 29-KDa protein band, and determines a reduction of calcium response to P4, finally resulting in modulation of P4-stimulated sperm acrosome reaction in a dose-response manner (Luconi et al., 1999) (Table 2).

3.4.3. *Gestation and placentation*

The ontogeny and functional role of steroidogenesis during mammalian gestation is poorly understood. A 2002 review provides a summary of findings on the spatio-temporal expression of key steroidogenic genes controlling progesterone synthesis in the uterus during mouse pregnancy. Authors have shown that onset of P450scc and an identified isoform of murine 3beta-hydroxysteroid dehydrogenase/isomerase type VI (3betaHSD VI) expression occurs upon decidualization of the uterine wall induced by implantation. This unexpected early expression of the enzymes in the maternal decidua is terminated at mid-pregnancy when the steroidogenic ability reappears in the extraembryonic giant cells at the time of placentation. The giant cells express the StAR protein. Unlike the human placenta, the steroidogenic genes are not expressed in the cells of the mature mouse placenta during the second half of gestation. The results suggested that, during early phases of pregnancy, local P4 synthesis in the maternal decidua and the trophoblast layers surrounding the embryonal cavity is important for successful implantation and/or maintenance of pregnancy. It was proposed that the local production of progesterone acts as an immunosuppressant at the materno fetal interface preventing the rejection of the fetal allograft (Ben-Zimra et al., 2002).

Strauss III et al. published in 1996 a review on the placental steroidogenesis capacity including the evidence for a dialogue between the ovary and the pituitary and placenta. In some mammals, the placenta eclipses the pituitary in the maintenance of ovarian function (e.g., mouse and rat). In human and in sheep, horse, cat, and guinea pig, the placenta acquires the ability to substitute for the ovaries in the maintenance of gestation at various times during pregnancy. They noted that even though the placentae of other species cannot substitute for ovarian function, all placentae critically studied expressed steroidogenic enzymes. Therefore, the ability to elaborate or metabolize steroid hormones is one common feature of trophoblast cells despite the marked differences in placental morphologies. In human, rhesus monkey, baboon, and horse, the placenta does not express 17a-hydroxylase. Placental estrogen synthesis in these species depends upon a source of androgen precursor from the fetus; the fetal adrenal glands in the case of primates, the gonadal interstitial cells in the case of the horse. In contrast, the trophoblast cells of rat, pig, sheep and cow express 17a-hydroxylase and are able to synthesize androgens and in some species estrogens.

In the rat, estrogen, synthesized by the ovaries, suppresses placental expression of 17a-hydroxylase. Since the rat placenta elaborates androgens that are potential precursors for ovarian aromatization, a dialogue between the placenta and ovary may take place in this species. Estrogens not only regulate 17a-hydroxylase expression, they control placental mass. The rat placenta hypertrophies in response to ovariectomy, and this hypertrophy is blocked by exogenous estrogen. These findings support the notion of an ovarian-placental interaction (Strauss et al., 1996) (Table2).

3.4.4. Parturition

Since 1983, Meinecke-Tillnann et al. described the changes in the plasma levels of estrone and E2 during the estrous cycle, gestation and puerperium in the goat. Estrone sulphate and E2 concentrations rose until the 12th week of gestation and then declined to about 50% of the former ranges of concentrations before rising again to high values at weeks 17–20 of gestation. Increasing plasma levels of estrone sulphate and E2 were determined during the last ten days preceding parturition. The concentrations of estrone sulphate returned to basal levels by the 2nd-4th day post partum whereas oestradiol-17β values reached base values 24 hours after parturition. Both estrogen concentrations remained constant during the puerperium until day 51 post partum (Meinecke-Tillrnann et al., 1983). This complete described estrogene pattern is now a day well understood. In 2006, Senger clearly described the removal of "progesterone block" that occurs during mammals gestation and necessary to start parturition. Fetal cortisol promotes the synthesis of three enzymes that convert P4 to E2. Progesterone, that is high at the placenta interface (from gonadal or placental origin depending on the species, as explained before), is converted to 17 alpha-hydroxy-P4 by the enzyme 17alpha-hydroxylase. Fetal cortisol also induce the production of 17-20 desmolase to produce androstenedione from the 17 alpha-hydroxy-P4 and then the induced enzyme aromatase converts androstenedione to estrogens; that is at the end a dramatic drop in P4 and a dramatic elevation in E2. The consecuences are that myometrium becomes increasingly more active and displays noticeable contractions. At the same time, fetal cortisol induces placental production of PGf2a which initiates the luteolytic process, contributing to the decrease of gonadal P4 production. Sex steroids and oxytocin (OT) produced within intrauterine tissues have been implicated in the regulation of parturition. Fang et al. performed very complete studies to determine the relationships among E2, P4, OT, and their receptors in uterine tissues during late gestation and parturition in the rat; to observe the effects of the estrogen antagonist tamoxifen (TAM) on these factors; and to evaluate the rat as a potential model for events at human parturition. Serum E2 increased throughout late gestation accompanied by an increase in uterine OT mRNA and ER. Serum P4 declined after day 19, and uterine PR did not change significantly. Uterine PGE2 increased progressively, reaching peak levels the evening before delivery. Uterine OTR did not increase until the morning of delivery, and uterine OT peptide concentrations increased only during parturition. Parturition was significantly delayed by 24 h in the TAM-treated group. TAM inhibited the increase in serum E2, uterine ER, and OT mRNA and peptide, but had no effect on serum P4 or uterine PR levels. With TAM, the responses of uterine OTR and prostaglandin E2 (PGE2) were significantly delayed, but still underwent a significant increase before the delayed parturition. These results supported that indeed E2 stimulates the synthesis of ER, OT, and OTR within the rat uterus and is essential for normal parturition. P4 withdrawal may be more important to the increases in OTR and PGE2, but these are delayed in the absence of estrogen (Fang et al., 1996). The precise temporal control of uterine contractility is essential for the success of pregnancy. For most of pregnancy, progesterone acting through genomic and non-genomic mechanisms promotes myometrial relaxation. At parturition the relaxatory actions of progesterone are nullified and the combined stimulatory actions of estrogens and other factors such as myometrial distention and immune/inflammatory cytokines, transform the myometrium to a highly contractile and excitable state leading to labor and delivery. Steroid hormone control myometrial contractility and parturition as part of the parturition cascade. (Mesiano and Welsh, 2007). The compulsory progesterone withdrawal necessary for delivery take place is mediated by changes in myometrial expression of progesterone receptors (PRs)-a and –b. This withdrawal in human parturition may be mediated by an increase in the myometrial PR-a to PR-b ratio due to increased PR-a expression affecting myometrial cell progesterone responsiveness (Merlino et al., 2007) (Table2).

3.4.5. Puerperium or postpartum

In domestic animals, puerperium begins immediately after parturition and lasts until reproductive function in restored so that another ovulation occurs and other potential pregnancy can take place. The time required for complete uterine repair and ovarian activity to resume in the postpartum female varies significantly among species (beef cows: 30d and 50-60d; dairy cows: 45-50d and 25d; ewe: 30d and 180d; mare: 28d and 12 d; sow: 30d and 7d; queen: 30d and 30d; bitch: 90d and 150d, a long natural postpartum anestrus). In beef cow, sows and women, the lactation inhibits ovarian activity (Senger, 2006). Also, manipulation of abnormal anestrus in ruminants with sex steroids implants (P4,E2), intra muscular or intravaginal devices during postpartum are intended in order to shortening or at least to be near the normal period required to re-produce.

In beef cows (zebu-Bos indicus cattle), in some environmental conditions, the interval parturition-ovarian reactivation (anestrous period) and the abnormal sex steroids production represent a big economical problem (180-240 d, vs. 60d theorical proposed (Senger, 2006)) because animals are not producing during this large interval and the "physiological" goal of one calf a cow a year is not reached at all. This was investigated many years ago in the follicular morfological and steroids dynamics aspects concluding about very individual patterns and about the potential early capacity of initiating ovarian activity depending on many factors (Ruiz-Cortes and Olivera-Angel, 1999). The return to the ovarian activity postpartum, is determined by the recovery of the hipotalamic-hipofisis-ovary axis and mainly by three factors: (a) nutrition, by the secretion of leptin from adipocites, (b) suckling, by prolactin production and (c) the cow-calf link, mediated by the senses of the vision and smell. In addition, after ovarian recovery postpartum, the cows present low fertility associated with corpus luteum of short duration and low production of P4. The induction of estrus with progestins has generated corpus luteum of normal duration, in response to the weaning or to the injection of gonadotrophins. Zebu cows postpartum, were treated with progestins and with temporal suckling interruption (TSI):calves-cows separation, for 72 hours. We could conclude that the treatment with TSI solely or in combination with progestins, can induce estrus, ovulation and corpus luteum of good quality, in postpartum Zebu cows. This useful tool for shortennig calving intervals is now a day used with success by local farmers (Giraldo Echeverri et al., 2005).

Those features indicate mainly the multifactorial effects of the peripartum on the sex steroids production, but also the gonadal steroids important role in the pospartum cyclicity reactivation.

High levels of E2 near the delivery and some days after are also regulating the OTR expression and the OT and effects myometrium. Thus contractions needed for the placenta membranes and lochia (blood-tinged fluid containing remnants of the fetal placenta and endometrial tissue) discharge in the early postpartum occurs (Table 2).

Studies in primates have suggested that pre- and peripartum sex steroid hormones may be important determinants of maternal behavior and motivation, since higher levels of prepartum estrogen are associated with maternal competency and infant survivorship. The researchers found that high concentrations of prepartum E_2 in callitrichid primates are not necessarily associated with competent maternal behavior and may instead be associated with poor infant survivorship and inadequate maternal care. That appears to be convergent with research focusing on human mothers and may represent a common underlying mechanism linking prepartum estrogen and postpartum affect and behavior in some primates. Similary, in males of this specie, T, and possibly E2, play an important role in balancing the expression of paternal care with that of other reproductive behavior (Fite and French, 2000; Nunes et al., 2000).

3.4.6. Lactation

The importance of the sex steroid hormones E2 and P4 for normal development of the mammary gland was recognized several decades ago and has been unequivocally confirmed since. This influence is not restricted to mammogenesis, but these hormones also control involution. Growth factors also have been shown to modulate survival (epidermal growth factor, amphiregulin, transforming growth factor α, insulin like growth factor, and tumor necrosis factor α) or apoptosis (tumor necrosis factor α, transforming growth factor β) of mammary cells. Lamote et al. published in a review about the interaction between both groups of modulators as an important functional role for sex steroid hormones in the lactation cycle in co-operation with growth factors. At that time the molecular mechanism underlying the influence of sex steroid hormones and/or growth factors on the development and function of the mammary gland remained largely unknown (Lamote et al., 2004).

Nevertheless, in a model of *in vitro* mammary gland involution (mammary epithelial cells – MEC) where authors were interested in the autophagy and the apoptosis occurring during involution, they concluded about important molecular pathways explaining the sex steroids-growth factors cross-talk during lactation and involution. They investigated the effects of insulin-like growth factor-1 (IGF-I) and epidermal growth factor (EGF) signaling, as well as sex steroids on autophagy focusing about the role regulatory role of mTOR. The kinase mTOR links IGF-I and EGF signaling in inhibiting the autophagy pathways. Contrary to IGF-I and EGF, E2 and P4 exerted stimulatory effects on autophagy in bovine MEC. At the same time, it was a suppressive effect of both steroids on mTOR activation/phosphorylation. In conclusion, autophagy in bovine MEC undergoes complex regulation, where its activity is controlled by survival pathways dependent on IGF-I and EGF, which are involved in suppression of autophagy, and by pregnancy steroids, which act as inducers of the process (Sobolewska et al., 2009). Probably mammogenesis is also regulated by similar kinase pathway, and this is a clue finding to better understand sex regulation of mammalian lactation (Table 2).

Ovarian steroids (E2 and P4) diffuse directly from the blood into milk by passive diffusion because they are lipid soluble. All steroids hormones can be found in milk. The concentration of E2 and P4 in milk reflects cyclic hormone production by the ovaries and is highly correlated with blood concentrations. Such a phenomenon enables steroids (particulary P4) to be easely assayed in milk to determine the reproductive status of the female. In cows, the ELISA technology enables P4 levels in milk to be determined. The measurement of P4 in each milking through the use of "in-line" assay technology in the milking parlor is a revolutionary goal to achieve for research and for farmers producers management. The development of such technology would enable the producer to determine whether a cow is cycling, the stage of estrous cycle, pregnancy status and some form of ovarian pathology (v.g. cystic ovarian desease), for each cow, on a daily basis (Senger, 2006).

3.4.7. Menopause and andropause

Menopause is defined as the permanent cessation of menstruation resulting from the loss of ovarian follicular activity and marks the end of natural female reproductive life. Menopause is preceded by a period of menstrual cycle irregularity, known as the menopause transition or peri-menopause, which usually begins in the mid-40s. The menopause transition is characterized by many hormonal changes predominantly caused by a marked decline in the ovarian follicle numbers. A significant decrease in inhibin B appears to be the first endocrine marker of the menopause transition with FSH levels being slightly raised. Marked decreases in estrogen and inhibin A with significant increases in FSH are only observed in the late stage of menopause transition. At the time of menopause, FSH levels have been shown to increase to 50% of final post-menopausal concentrations while estrogens levels have decreased to approximately 50% of the premenopausal concentrations. Since the decrease in estrogen levels occurs in the fifth decade of life, this means that most women will spend more than 30 years in postmenopausal status. A good body of evidence suggests that changes in hormonal status, particularly the decline in estrogen, in the menopause years may have a detrimental effect on women's health (Table 2). Accordingly, it has been reported that the decrease in estrogen contributes to the decrease in bone mass density, the redistribution of subcutaneous fat to the visceral area, the increased risk of cardiovascular disease and the decrease in quality of life.

In addition, hormonal changes may also have a direct effect on muscle mass. The measurement of urinary estrogens metabolites could add new evidence as for the role of estrogens in sarcopenia. It remains certain, though, that the decline in muscle mass is associated with an increased risk of functional impairment and physical disability. Finally, further randomized controlled trials are needed to investigate the effects of physical activity as well as hormone and phytoestrogen supplementation on sarcopenia (Messier et al., 2011).

Hot flushes common in almost 85% of women, appear to result from a dysfunction of thermoregulatory centers in the hypothalamus and are correlated with pulses of circulating estrogen and gonadotropin secretion in menopausal women (López et al., 2000).

A recent review of literature from 1990 until 2010, compare oral and transdermal delivery systems for postmenopausal estrogen therapy in domains of lipid effects; cardiovascular, inflammatory, and thrombotic effects; effect on insulin-like growth factor, insulin resistance, and metabolic syndrome; sexual effects; metabolic effects including weight; and effects on target organs bone, breast, and uterus.

Significant differences appear to exist between oral and transdermal estrogens in terms of hormonal bioavailability and metabolism, with implications for clinical efficacy, potential side effects, and risk profile of different hormone therapy options, but as neither results nor study designs were uniform, not complete conclusions could be done. Weight gain appears to be slightly lower with a transdermal delivery system. Oral estrogen's significant increase in hepatic sex hormone binding globulin production lowers testosterone availability compared with transdermal delivery, with clinically relevant effects on sexual vigor (Goodman, 2012).

The relationship between menopause and cognitive decline has been the subject of intense research since a number of studies have shown that hormone replacement therapy could reduce the risk of developing Alzheimer's disease (AD) in women. In contrast, research into andropause has only recently begun. Furthermore, evidence now suggests that steroidogenesis is not restricted to the gonads and adrenals, and that the brain is capable of producing its own steroid hormones, including testosterone and estrogen (Bates et al., 2005). Male aging is associated with a variable but generally gradual decline in androgen activity, which can manifest as sexual dysfunction, lethargy, loss of muscle and bone mass, increased frailty, loss of balance, cognitive impairment and decreased general well-being, such as depression and irritability. Andropause is defined as the partial or relative deficiency of androgens and characteristic associated symptoms. These symptoms suggest that androgens may have an important modulatory role in cognition and mental health. Indeed memory loss was the third most common reported symptom of andropause, after erectile dysfunction and general weakness in a survey of elderly men (Bates et al., 2005).

Mild cognitive impairment (MCI) is becoming fashionable as a diagnosis, representing a state of cognitive decline associated with negligible functional loss. MCI is important as it often precedes Alzheimer disease (AD). Recognizing MCI may lead to preventive strategies that can delay the onset of AD. Many patients in transition into andropause report problems with their memory. There is strong evidence from basic sciences and epidemiological studies that both estrogens and androgens play a protective role in neurodegeneration. The evidence from small prospective clinical trials lends support to the role of hormones in improving cognitive function. Patients have reported memory improvements in both declarative and procedural domains after being on hormonal replacement. Authors have hypothesized androgens and perhaps selective androgen receptor modulators as future treatment options for MCI in aging males (Tan et al., 2003).

Moment	**Definition***	**Estradiol-E2 (effects, target tissues)**	**Progesterone-P4 (effects, target tissues)**	**Testosterone-T (effects, target tissues)**
Puberty	Acquisition of gonadotropin secretion, gametogenesis, gonadal steroids secretion, reproductive behaviour and secondary sex	Pituitary, Hypothalamus. Increase responsiveness to GnRH Increase of GH Increase of IGF-I		Genital enlargement Muscle strength Body composition Spermatogenesis
Fertilization	The process of combining the male gamete, or sperm, with the female gamete, or ovum. The product of fertilization is a cell called a zygote	Oocytes. Inhibits abnormalities Stimulates maturation Success of fertilization Acrosome reaction	Oocytes. Inhibits abnormalities Stimulates maturation Spermatozoa. Acrosome reaction	Oocytes. Inhibits abnormalities Stimulates maturation Success of fertilization
Gestation	Pregnancy. The period that a female is pregnant between conception and parturition		Myometrium, decreases contractions Endometrium, "maternal" secretions	
Placentation	The structural organization and physical relationship of the fetal membranes to the endometrium that	placenta Control of placental mass Inhibit 17a-hydroxylase expression in the placenta	Immunosuppressant of the placenta	Ovary. Cross talk with placental androgens

http://dx.doi.org/10.5772/52994

Moment	Definition*	Estradiol-E2 (effects, target tissues)	Progesterone-P4 (effects, target tissues)	Testosterone-T (effects, target tissues)
	provides the site of metabolic exchange between the dam and the fetus			
Parturition	To give birth	Ovary. Increases, OTR, production of PF2a Endometrium. Increases lubrication Myometrium. Increases ER, OTR, Increases contractions Hypothalamus. Increases OT secretion	Ovary. Converted to E2	
Postpartum or puerperium	The period between parturition and return to the normal cycling state of the ovaries and uterus	Brain. Male and female. Maternal and paternal behavior Endometrium. Myometrium.Contractions and placental membranes and loquia expulsion Ovary: cross-talk with P4	Ovary. Croos –talk with E2 Hypothalamus, Gn RH production control	Paternal behavior
Lactation	Formation and /or secretion of milk by the mammary glands	Mammary gland: development, mammogenesis Cross-talk with IGF-I and EGF: modulation of lactation and involution (autophagy)	Mammary gland: development, mammogenesis Cross-talk with IGF-I and EGF: modulation of lactation and involution (autophagy)	Mammary gland: development, mammogenesis Cross-talk with IGF-I and EGF: modulation of lactation and involution (autophagy)
Menopause	Permanent cessation of menses; termination of menstrual cycles brought about by depletion of ovarian follicles	Bone. Regulates bone mass Muscle. Regulates muscle mass Subcutaneous visceral fat Heart:cardiovascular desease Brain: hot flushes, depression,irritability		
Andropause	A variable complex of symptoms, including decreased Leydig cell numbers and androgen production, occurring in men after middle age			Bone. Mass loss Muscle. Mass loss Reprod. Tract.erectil dysfunction Brain. Memory loss, cognitive impairment

*modified from Senger, 2006

Table 2. Gonadal steroids regulation of clue reproductive moments. Definitions, target tissues and main sex steroids effects

4. Gonadal steroid hormones action on other systems

4.1. Energy homeostasis, sex hormones implications

Since the adipose tissue hormone leptin was discovered in 1996, its energy balance regulatory effects have been well investigated and accepted. The interaction of leptin and its membrane receptors within different systems were also the focus of interest of many researches making the protein and the receptor almost ubiquitous in mammals. Thus, it is of big interest the relationship of leptin with sex steroids. Early in this chapter, it was described how leptin regulates gonadal steroidogenesis (Montaño et al., 2009; Ruiz-Cortes et al., 2003; Ruiz-Cortes and Olivera, 2010). However, in 2000, Mystkowski and Schwartz postulated also that sex steroids and leptin regulate one another's production. Although gonadal steroids, unlike leptin, are clearly not critical to the maintenance of normal energy homeostasis, they do appear to function as physiologic modulators of this process. Gonadal steroids influence food intake and body weight. Although the specific mechanisms underlying these effects are not clear, a consideration of their effects in the context of current models of energy homeostasis may ultimately lead to the identification of these mechanisms. When compared with leptin, the prototypical humoral signal of energy balance, sex steroids share many common properties related to food intake and body weight. Specifically, gonadal steroids circulate in proportion to fat mass and current energy balance, and administration of these compounds influences food intake, energy expenditure, body weight, and body composition. Moreover, both estrogens and androgens modulate central nervous system effectors of energy homeostasis that are targets for the action of leptin, including pathways that contain neuropeptide Y, pro-opiomelanocortin, or melanin-concentrating hormone (Mystkowski and Schwartz, 2000).

Several studies have reported decreased circulating estradiol levels in type 1 and type 2 diabetic animal models. Women with type 1 diabetes experience decreased sexual arousal function and have significantly reduced E2 levels compared to control subjects. Limited data are available in type 2 diabetic women. It was proposed that diabetes disrupts estrogen signaling. This hypothesis was partially supported by studies showing that E2 supplementation in diabetic animals ameliorates some of the diabetic complications in several organs and tissues, including those that control anabolic and catabolic pathways (food intake and energy expenditure) such as melanocortin in the hypothalamic arcuate nucleus and neurons containing neuropeptide Y. No studies are available on the therapeutic effects of estradiol supplementation in type 2 diabetic animals in ameliorating the changes in sex steroid receptor expression and tissue localization and distribution. For these reasons, researchers undertook studies to investigate the effects of type 2 diabetes on the expression, localization and distribution of estrogen, androgen and P4 receptors and to determine if E2 treatment of diabetic animals normalizes these changes. They found decreased levels of plasma E2 and reduced ER expression in type 1 and type 2 diabetic animals suggesting that estrogen signaling is impaired in the diabetic state. They conclude specifically, in a vaginal model, that sex steroid hormone receptor signaling is important in female genital sexual arousal function. These findings further demonstrate that E2 supplementation provides a protective effect by up-regulating the expression of sex steroid receptor proteins (Cushman et al., 2009).

Important tissues implicated in homeostasis are fat mass and muscle mass. Effects of androgens in those systems are well known. As general information, males typically have less body fat than females. Recent results indicate that androgens inhibit the ability of some fat cells to store lipids by blocking a signal transduction pathway that normally supports adipocyte function. Also, androgens, but not estrogens, increase beta adrenergic receptors while decreasing alpha adrenergic receptors resulting in increased levels of epinephrine/ norepinephrine due to lack of alpha-2 receptor negative feedback and decreased fat accumulation due to epinephrine/ norepinephrine then acting on lipolysis-inducing beta receptors.

About androgens and muscle mass, it is clear that males typically have more skeletal muscle mass than females and this is because androgens promote the enlargement of skeletal muscle cells and probably act in a coordinated manner to function by acting on several cell types in skeletal muscle tissue. One type of cell that conveys hormone signals to generating muscle is the myoblast. Higher androgen levels lead to increased expression of androgen receptor. Fusion of myoblasts generates myotubes, in a process that is linked to androgen receptor levels much more expressed in males but also having effect in females (Figure 6).

Sex hormones play essential roles in the regulation of appetite, eating behaviour and energy metabolism and have been implicated in several major clinical disorders in women. Estrogen inhibits food intake, whereas progesterone and testosterone may stimulate appetite. Interactions between sex hormones and neuroendocrinological mechanisms in the control of appetite and eating in women have been recently reviewed. Hirschberg indicates that the roles played by sex hormones in the development of eating disorders and obesity are clearer now a days. For instance, androgens may promote bulimia by stimulating appetite and reducing impulse control, a proposal supported by the observation that antiandrogenic treatment attenuates bulimic behaviour. Androgens are also involved in the pathophysiology of abdominal obesity in women. On the other hand, hormone replacement therapy with estrogen counteracts the weight gain and accumulation of abdominal fat associated with the menopausal transition. The author conclude that sex hormones and/or agents that exhibit similar activities may provide novel strategies for the treatment of eating disorders and android obesity, two of the most serious health problems for women today (Hirschberg, 2012).

4.2. Cardiovascular system

Sex steroids effects, as reviewed in the sex steroids molecular pathways section, have "the long" pathway and the rapid one. In the case of the cardiovascular system in mammals, the rapid non-transcriptional is the mechanism that explains the implications of gonadal steroids.

Traish et al. have recently reviewed the topic of androgens modulation of the lipid profiles and contribution to development and progression of atherosclerosis. They found studies in animals and humans suggesting that androgen deficiency is associated with increased triglycerides (TGs), total cholesterol (TC), and low-density lipoprotein cholesterol (LDL-C). Although the effects of androgen deficiency on high-density lipoprotein cholesterol (HDL-C) remains controversial, recent data suggest that androgen therapy is associated with increased levels of HDL-C and may improve reverse cholesterol transport. Animal studies suggested that androgen deprivation adversely affect lipid profiles and this was reversed by androgen treatment. Furthermore, androgen treatment of hypogonadal men significantly improved lipid profiles. Emerging data indicate that androgens play an important role in lipid metabolism. Therefore androgens are critical in the prevention and progression of atherosclerosis (Traish et al., 2009a).

Androgen deficiency contributes to increased TGs, TC, LDL-C and reduced HDL-C while androgen treatment results in a favorable lipid profile, suggesting that androgens may provide a protective effect against the development and/or progression of atherosclerosis.

Until recently, it was thought that male gender contributes to the risk of atherosclerosis and this was attributed to androgens. Evidence is emerging that androgen deficiency is more likely to be associated with atherosclerosis than gender per se. T treatment of hypogonadal men resulted in reduced pro-inflammatory cytokines, total cholesterol, and triglyceride levels. In women,T use was reported for sexual dysfunction, abnormal uterine bleeding, dysmenorrhea, menopausal symptoms, chronic mastitis and lactation, and benign and malignant tumors of the breast, uterus, and ovaries (Traish et al., 2009b). However, these authors literally conclude: "health-care professionals engaged in the management of women's health issues have observed the benefits of androgen therapy throughout much of the 20th century. Despite this clinical use of testosterone in women for more than seven decades, contemporary testosterone therapy in women is hotly debated, misunderstood, and often misrepresented in the medical community"(Traish et al., 2009b).

New evidence suggests that androgen deficiency alters lipid profiles, which ultimately contribute to oxidative stress, endothelial dysfunction and increased production of pro-inflammatory factors, thus promoting the pathogenic process leading to atherosclerosis (Figure 6). Future research should focus on delineating the physiological or biochemical mechanisms and should focus on the molecular basis of androgen action in regulating lipid metabolism and endothelial function in order to have a better understanding of the role of androgens, deficiency and vascular diseases (Traish et al., 2009a).

4.3. Sex steroids, the brain and behavior

Almost all the sex steroids have something to do with the brain. It is maybe because of this part of the pathway that they are so important in the mammals general physiology (Figure 6).

Circulating levels of androgens can influence human behavior because some neurons are sensitive to steroid hormones. Androgen levels have been implicated in the regulation of human aggression and libido (Figure 6). Indeed, androgens are capable of altering the structure of the brain in several species, including mice, rats, and primates, producing sex differences. Numerous reports have outlined that androgens alone are capable of altering the structure of the brain; however, it is difficult to identify which alterations in neuro-anatomy stem from androgens or estrogens, because of their potential for conversion.

Estrogens are effective regulators of brain cell morphology and tissue organization through the regulation of the cytoskeleton. Many of these regulatory actions related to cell morphology are achieved through rapid, non-classical signaling of sex steroid receptors to kinase cascades, independently from nuclear alteration of gene expression or protein synthesis. Brain cell morphology is then reported to be controlled by estrogens that regulate the development of neuron/neuron interconnections and dendritic spine density.This is thought to be critical for gender-specific differences in brain function and dysfunction. The recent advancements in the characterization of the molecular basis of the extra-nuclear signaling of estrogen helps to understand the role of estrogen in the brain and central nervous system, and may in the future turn out to be of relevance for clinical purposes (Sanchez and Simoncini, 2010).

Studies in animals have made abundantly clear the important role played by gonadal steroids in the regulation of behavior. Given the importance of reproductive behavior in the survival of the species, the potency and range (e.g., learning and memory, appetite, aggression, affiliation) of these behavioral effects are not surprising. The role of gonadal steroids in human behavior is both more complex and more poorly delineated.

The role of gonadal steroids in behavior in men and women include the exquisite context dependency of responses to gonadal steroid signals and the role of both gonadal steroids and context in several reproductive endocrine-related mood disorders such as menstrual cycle-related mood disorders, perimenopausal and periandropause depression, postpartum depression, hormone replacement therapy-related dysphoria, androgen-anabolic replacement, use or abuse(Rubinow et al., 2002).

Depression is more common in women, and women appear to respond better to selective serotonin reuptake inhibitors (SSRIs) than men. In addition, SSRIs are an excellent treatment for premenstrual dysphoria disorder. Thus, a sex specific effect of E2 and P4 on function of the serotonin transporter is quite important. However, the effect is the opposite of what would be predicted from the clinical literature, further underscoring the complexity of understanding the interactions between ovarian hormones and serotonin systems. Perhaps these findings help to better understand the vulnerability to mood disorders at times when E2 and P4 are high, such as the luteal phase of the menstrual cycle. Of note is the fact that these changes in response to E2 and P4 were not observed in hippocampi of male (Young and Becker, 2009).

In domestic animals the reproductive bevavior can take place only if the neurons in the hypothalamus have been sensitized to respond to sensory signals. T in the male is aromatized to E2 in the brain and E2 promotes reproductive behavior. In the male there is a relatively constant supply of T (every 4 to 6 h) and thus E2, to the hypothalamus. This allows the male to initiate reproductive behavior at any time. In contrast the female experiences high E2 during follicular phase only and will display sexual receptivity during estrus only. Under E2 influence, sensory inputs such as olfaction, audition, vision, and tactility send neural messages to the hypothalamus and cause the release of behavior specific peptides or neurotransmitters. In the mid brain, those hypothalamic signals are translated into fast responses. Synapsis between neurons of the mid brain and neurons in the medulla transmit the signal to the spinal cord and then to motor neurons that innervate muscles as during the lordosis and mounting occurring in domestic animals (Senger, 2006)

4.4. Gonadal steroids on bone turnover

In a very complete and recent review paper, Karsenty proposed that the well recognized sex steroid hormones regulation of bone mass accrual, is essential for skeletal development and maintenance of bone health throughout adult. Testosterone and estrogen positively influence growth, maturation, and maintenance of the female and male skeleton. Their effects are mediated mainly by slow genomic mechanisms through nuclear hormonal receptors, and possibly through the fast nongenomic mechanisms by membrane associated receptors and signaling cascades. But, on the other hand, the authors exposes the hypothesis that bone may regulates the female fertility by osteocalcin and that osteocalcin signaling in Leydig cells of the testis as a novel mode of regulation of testosterone synthesis observed in males but not in females (Karsenty, 2012).

Sex steroids play an important role in bone growth and the attainment of peak bone mass. They are, at least in part, responsible for the gender differences in bone growth, which emerges during adolescence. The skeletal sexual dimorphism is mainly due to a stimulatory androgen action on periosteal bone formation in men, whereas an inhibitory estrogen-related action occurs in women (Karsenty, 2012 ; Venken et al., 2006). In addition to the sex steroid hormones, several studies have shown that other hormones negatively regulated by estrogen, such as growth hormone (GH) and insulin-like growth factor 1 (IGF1), may further contribute to the development of the skeletal sexual dimorphism. Sex steroid hormones maintain skeletal integrity.

Testosterone and estrogens are also crucial for maintaining bone mass accrual during adulthood in the female and male skeleton. The loss of ovarian function underlies the development of osteoporosis (Karsenty, 2012 ; Vanderschueren et al., 2004). Estrogen deficiency is a major pathogenic factor in the bone loss associated with menopause and the development of osteoporosis in postmenopausal women. This rapid bone loss can be prevented by estrogen administration, and characteristically results in an increase in bone mineral density during the first months of treatment. Additionally, the loss of testicular function also underlies bone loss in men. Although osteoporosis more commonly affects women, the loss of androgens in males following castration or a decrease in androgen levels related to aging, during andropause, has the same dramatic effect on the skeleton. Androgens favor periostal bone formation in men, and maintain trabecular bone mass and integrity (Karsenty, 2012 ; Vanderschueren et al., 2004)(Figure 6).

http://dx.doi.org/10.5772/52994

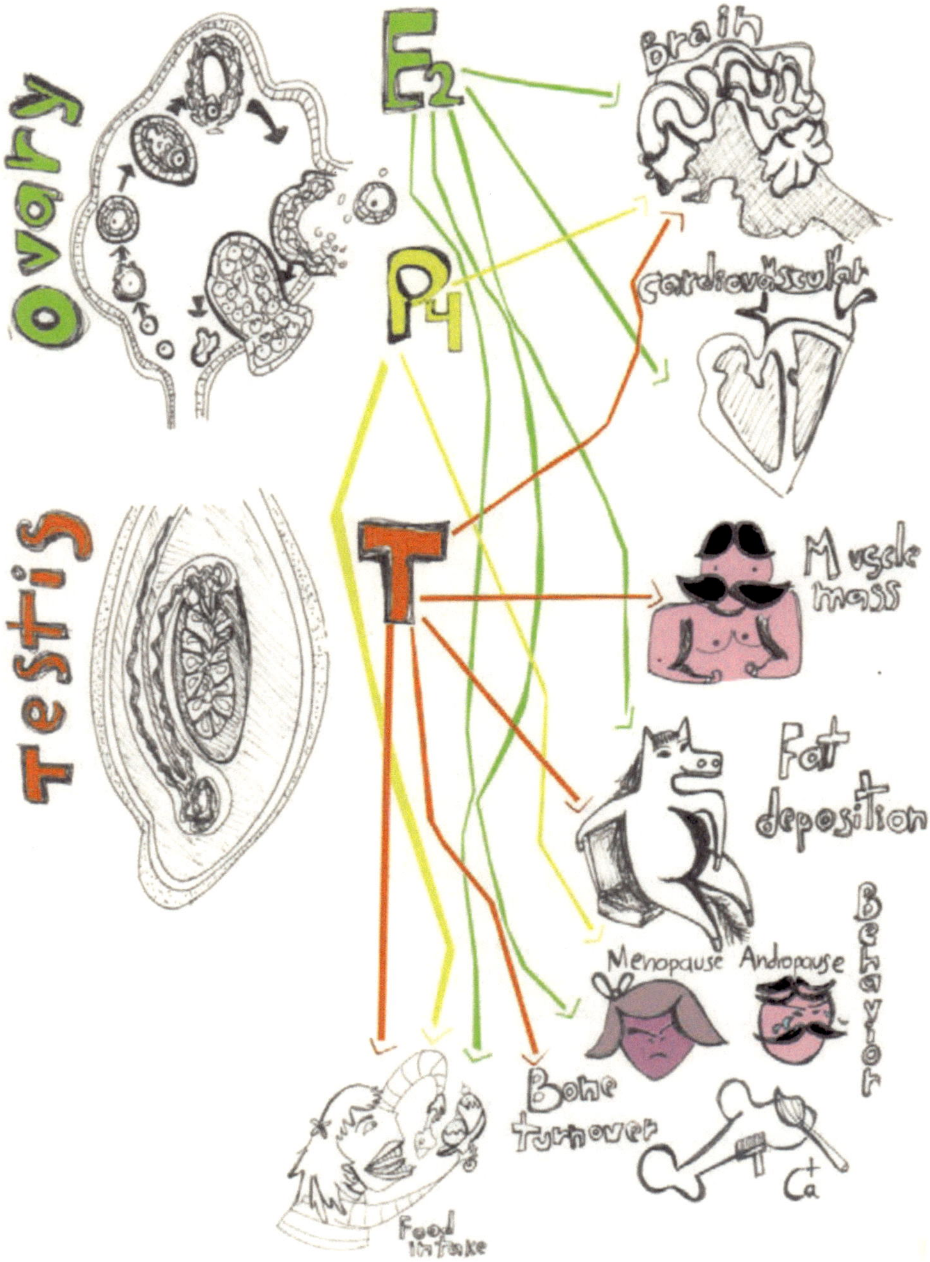

Figure 6. Sex steroids effects in different systems, a general view in mammals. Sex steroids produced in ovary and testis are regulating different organs and tissues in the brain (behavior,menopause,andropause), food intake and general homeostasis, cardiovascular system, muscle, fat and bone mass.

5. Conclusions and perspectives

Paraphrasing a paper first sentence: "Sex matters to every cell of the body" (Young and Becker, 2009) and gonadal steroids are mediating such a huge task. Since the discovery of those hormones (eighteen century), androgens, estrogens and progestogens, were classified more in a sex manner. It is well known now that males and females share the steroidogenesis pathways and sex steroids effects in many organs and systems such as the brain, muscle, fat, bone, reproductive system, cardiovascular system, homeostasis system (body weight-composition, food intake). The unraveling of this complex panorama of action and interaction of gonadal sex steroids indicates that almost no organ is left out of the sex hormones scope. One the most interesting feature of sex steroids action are the alternates pathways they are using to exert they modulating role by their membrane, cytoplasmic or nuclear receptor molecular activation (rapid and/or genomic mechanism) or in the very pertinent called "cross-talk" with other hormones, growth factors, transcription factors signaling pathways. Organism are integrated entities fulfilling their specific functions, and not as isolated group of distinct cell types (Karsenty, 2012) and it is amazing to realize how gonads via sex steroids are able to modulate and integrate such an intrincate orchestra. From a molecular point of view, the multiple signaling pathways already described for androgens and estrogens and their interactions are just the beginning of the understanding of the complex cross talk and interorgan connections. Some species can support gestation with just gonadal-corpus luteum P4 synthesis; other early during pregnancy can afford ovariectomy and the placenta would replace the steroid production. This turnover do not occur as an isolated event but more as unique interaction or cross-talk between placenta and ovaries (placental androgens aromatized in the ovary); similar interaction is happening between ovarian theca and granulosa cells and between Leydig and Sertoli testicular cells where androgens synthesis and aromatization to estradiol take place in a paracrine manner. Other amazing phenomenum is the autocrine dialogue in granulosa cells during luteinization, where granulosa producing high concentration of E2 switch their steroid production to P4 secretion. Again in this case the molecular machinery implicated in the sex steroid production is model of versatility and adaptation. Thus, the evolutionary aspect should be taken also in account for future studies about the cellular and molecular pathways of gonadal sex steroids action and interaction in mammals.

There are still several pieces of the puzzle that are to be found. Perspective to further research includes studies on the new class of steroid receptors (implicated in the rapid action signaling); the exact role of E2 and inhibin in male reproduction; the anabolic synthetic products:use and abuse; the therapy of replacement in menopause and andropause: what is worst the loss of sex steroids, or the "non-natural" replacement therapy with cancer risk? What is the matter, the delivery system, the doses, the compounds (what about phytotherapy?), the duration of the treatment, the human being individuality and conscience? In domestic animals, sex steroids therapies, to regulate cyclicity or even to make monovulatory animals to superovulate, are very common practice and collateral effects are rare or inexistent. Of course, they are not long treatment but instead they are performed very frequently with remarkable positive results. The ultimate purpose of this review was not to propose the

http://dx.doi.org/10.5772/52994

ideal steroid therapy or to give all the molecular factors implicated in the action and interaction of sex steroids in mammals. However, it could allow a better understanding of the panoply of effects in reproductive and other systems.

Acknowledgements

Verónica Bermúdez, MV(c), for figure design.

Author details

Zulma Tatiana Ruiz-Cortés*

Address all correspondence to: biogenesis1995@gmail.com

University of Antioquia, Faculty of Agrarian Sciences, Biogénesis Research Group, Medellín, Colombia

References

[1] Adams NR. Detection of the effects of phytoestrogens on sheep and cattle. J Anim Sci 1995; 73: 1509-1515.

[2] Azhar S, Leers-Sucheta S, and Reaven E. Cholesterol uptake in adrenal and gonadal tissues: The sr-bi and 'selective' pathway connection. Front Biosci 2003; 8: s998-1029.

[3] Bates KA, Harvey AR, Carruthers M, and Martins RN. Androgens, andropause and neurodegeneration: Exploring the link between steroidogenesis, androgens and alzheimer's disease. Cell Mol Life Sci 2005; 62: 281-292.

[4] Ben-Zimra M, Koler M, Melamed-Book N, Arensburg J, Payne AH, and Orly J. Uterine and placental expression of steroidogenic genes during rodent pregnancy. Mol Cell Endocrinol 2002; 187: 223-231.

[5] Cato AC, Nestl A, and Mink S. Rapid actions of steroid receptors in cellular signaling pathways. Sci STKE 2002; 2002: re9.

[6] Cushman T, Kim N, Hoyt R, and Traish AM. Estradiol restores diabetes-induced reductions in sex steroid receptor expression and distribution in the vagina of db/db mouse model. J Steroid Biochem Mol Biol 2009; 114: 186-194.

[7] Charitidi K, Meltser I, Tahera Y, and Canlon B. Functional responses of estrogen receptors in the male and female auditory system. Hear Res 2009; 252: 71-78.

[8] Davis PJ, Lin HY, Mousa SA, Luidens MK, Hercbergs AA, Wehling M, and Davis FB. Overlapping nongenomic and genomic actions of thyroid hormone and steroids. Steroids 2011; 76: 829-833.

[9] de Kretser DM, Loveland KL, Meehan T, O'Bryan MK, Phillips DJ, and Wreford NG. Inhibins, activins and follistatin: Actions on the testis. Mol Cell Endocrinol 2001; 180: 87-92.

[10] Dimitrakakis C, Zhou J, and Bondy CA. Androgens and mammary growth and neoplasia. Fertil Steril 2002; 77 Suppl 4: S26-33.

[11] Evans NA. Current concepts in anabolic-androgenic steroids. Am J Sports Med 2004; 32: 534-542.

[12] Fang X, Wong S, and Mitchell BF. Relationships among sex steroids, oxytocin, and their receptors in the rat uterus during late gestation and at parturition. Endocrinology 1996; 137: 3213-3219.

[13] Fertility Weekly. 2011. Correlation between fertilization and sex steroid levels in ff and granulosa cells. 5/16/2011, p8 (accessed 16 august 2012).

[14] Fishel SB, Edwards RG, and Walters DE. Follicular steroids as a prognosticator of successful fertilization of human oocytes in vitro. J Endocrinol 1983; 99: 335-344.

[15] Fite JE, and French JA. Pre- and postpartum sex steroids in female marmosets (callithrix kuhlii): Is there a link with infant survivorship and maternal behavior? Horm Behav 2000; 38: 1-12.

[16] Foster TC. Interaction of rapid signal transduction cascades and gene expression in mediating estrogen effects on memory over the life span. Front Neuroendocrinol 2005; 26: 51-64.

[17] Giraldo Echeverri C, Ruiz-Cortes ZT, Restrepo L, and Olivera Angel M. 2005. Interrupción temporal del amamantamiento (ita) vacas cebú y su efecto en la función ovárica (temporary suckling interruption (tsi) in zebu cows and effect in the ovary function) Revista Electrónica de Veterinaria - REDVET www.veterinaria.org/revistas/redvet No. VI. p 1-11.

[18] Goodman MP. Are all estrogens created equal? A review of oral vs. Transdermal therapy. J Womens Health (Larchmt) 2012; 21: 161-169.

[19] GyeongsangNationalUniversity. Natural synchronization processes. Http://nongae.Gsnu.Ac.Kr/~cspark/teaching/chap4.Html (accessed 1 august 2012).

[20] Hiort O. Androgens and puberty. Best Pract Res Clin Endocrinol Metab 2002; 16: 31-41.

[21] Hirschberg AL. Sex hormones, appetite and eating behaviour in women. Maturitas 2012; 71: 248-256.

[22] Hu J, Zhang Z, Shen WJ, and Azhar S. Cellular cholesterol delivery, intracellular processing and utilization for biosynthesis of steroid hormones. Nutr Metab (Lond) 2010; 7: 47.

[23] Illingworth PJ, Groome NP, Byrd W, Rainey WE, McNeilly AS, Mather JP, and Bremner WJ. Inhibin-b: A likely candidate for the physiologically important form of inhibin in men. J Clin Endocrinol Metab 1996; 81: 1321-1325.

[24] Karsenty G. The mutual dependence between bone and gonads. J Endocrinol 2012 213: 107-114.

[25] Lamb JD, Zamah AM, Shen S, McCulloch C, Cedars MI, and Rosen MP. Follicular fluid steroid hormone levels are associated with fertilization outcome after intracytoplasmic sperm injection. Fertil Steril 2010; 94: 952-957.

[26] Lamote I, Meyer E, Massart-Leen AM, and Burvenich C. Sex steroids and growth factors in the regulation of mammary gland proliferation, differentiation, and involution. Steroids 2004; 69: 145-159.

[27] Levin ER, and Pietras RJ. Estrogen receptors outside the nucleus in breast cancer. Breast Cancer Res Treat 2008; 108: 351-361.

[28] López A, Gomez L, Ruiz Cortes Z, Olivera M, and Giraldo A. Reconocimiento materno de la prenez e implantacion del embrión: Modelo bovino. Analecta Veterinaria 2008; 28: 42-47.

[29] López F, Finn P, Lawson M, Negro-Vilar A, Lobo R, Kelsey. J, and Marcus R. Chapter 3 - regulation of the hypothalamic-pituitary-gonadal axis: Role of gonadal steroids and implications for the menopause Menopause. Academic Press 2000. 33-60.

[30] Luconi M, Forti G, and Baldi E. Genomic and nongenomic effects of estrogens: Molecular mechanisms of action and clinical implications for male reproduction. J Steroid Biochem Mol Biol 2002; 80: 369-381.

[31] Luconi M, Muratori M, Forti G, and Baldi E. Identification and characterization of a novel functional estrogen receptor on human sperm membrane that interferes with progesterone effects. J Clin Endocrinol Metab 1999; 84: 1670-1678.

[32] Mahesh VB, and Nazian SJ. Role of sex steroids in the initiation of puberty. J Steroid Biochem 1979; 11: 587-591.

[33] Meinecke-Tillrnann S, Gips H, Meinecke B, and Finkenberg A. Concentrations of oestrone and oestradiol-l 7β in the peripheral plasma of the nanny goat during the oestrous cycle, gestation and puerperium. Reproduction in Domestic Animals 1983; 21: 207-213.

[34] Merlino AA, Welsh TN, Tan H, Yi LJ, Cannon V, Mercer BM, and Mesiano S. Nuclear progesterone receptors in the human pregnancy myometrium: Evidence that parturition involves functional progesterone withdrawal mediated by increased expression of progesterone receptor-a. J Clin Endocrinol Metab 2007; 92: 1927-1933.

[35] Mesiano S, and Welsh TN. Steroid hormone control of myometrial contractility and parturition. Semin Cell Dev Biol 2007; 18: 321-331.

[36] Messier V, Rabasa-Lhoret R, Barbat-Artigas S, Elisha B, Karelis AD, and Aubertin-Leheudre M. Menopause and sarcopenia: A potential role for sex hormones. Maturitas 2011; 68: 331-336.

[37] Michels G, and Hoppe UC. Rapid actions of androgens. Front Neuroendocrinol 2008; 29: 182-198.

[38] Montano E, Olivera M, and Ruiz-Cortes ZT. Association between leptin, lh and its receptor and luteinization and progesterone accumulation (p4) in bovine granulosa cell in vitro. Reprod Domest Anim 2009; 44: 699-704.

[39] Moor RM, Polge C, and Willadsen SM. Effect of follicular steroids on the maturation and fertilization of mammalian oocytes. J Embryol Exp Morphol 1980; 56: 319-335.

[40] Mystkowski P, and Schwartz MW. Gonadal steroids and energy homeostasis in the leptin era. Nutrition 2000; 16: 937-946.

[41] Nelson JF. Puberty, gonadal steroids and fertility: Potential reproductive markers of aging. Exp Gerontol 1988; 23: 359-367.

[42] Norris DO. Major human endocrine disorders related to reproduction.

[43] Vertebrate endocrinology. Elsevier 2007.

[44] Nunes S, Fite JE, and French JA. Variation in steroid hormones associated with infant care behaviour and experience in male marmosets (callithrix kuhlii). Anim Behav 2000; 60: 857-865.

[45] Pineda MH. Male reproductive system. In : Veterinary endocrinology and reproduction. 2003. Iowa state press In: Pineda, MH and Dooley, MP (eds.) 2003.

[46] Rochira V, Granata AR, Madeo B, Zirilli L, Rossi G, and Carani C. Estrogens in males: What have we learned in the last 10 years? Asian J Androl 2005; 7: 3-20.

[47] Rogol AD. Androgens and puberty. Mol Cell Endocrinol 2002; 198: 25-29.

[48] Rubinow DR, Schmidt PJ, Roca CA, Daly RC, Donald WP, Arthur PA, Susan EF, Anne M. Etgen and Robert T. RubinA2 - Donald W. Pfaff APASEFAME, and Robert TR. 84 - gonadal hormones and behavior in women: Concentrations versus context Hormones, brain and behavior. Academic Press 2002. 37-73.

[49] Ruiz-Cortes Z, and Olivera M. Association between leptin receptors in the testicle, leptin and testosterone levels in puber male calves. Revista MVZ Córdoba 2010; 15: 2204-2214.

[50] Ruiz-Cortes ZT, Kimmins S, Monaco L, Burns KH, Sassone-Corsi P, and Murphy BD. Estrogen mediates phosphorylation of histone h3 in ovarian follicle and mammary epithelial tumor cells via the mitotic kinase, aurora b. Mol Endocrinol 2005; 19: 2991-3000.

[51] Ruiz-Cortes ZT, Martel-Kennes Y, Gevry NY, Downey BR, Palin MF, and Murphy BD. Biphasic effects of leptin in porcine granulosa cells. Biol Reprod 2003; 68: 789-796.

[52] Ruiz-Cortes ZT, and Olivera-Angel M. Ovarian follicular dynamics in suckled zebu (bos indicus) cows monitored by real time ultrasonography. Anim Reprod Sci 1999; 54: 211-220.

[53] Sanchez AM, and Simoncini T. Extra-nuclear signaling of eralpha to the actin cytoskeleton in the central nervous system. Steroids 2010; 75: 528-532.

[54] Senger PL. 2006. Pathways to pregnancy and parturition. Second revised edition ed. Current Conceptions Inc., Pullman.

[55] Sevin G, Arun M, and Üstünes L. Androgens and anabolıc sterorıds

[56] Dahili Tıp Bilimleri Farmakoloji Dergisi 2005; 1.

[57] Simoncini T, Mannella P, Fornari L, Caruso A, Varone G, and Genazzani AR. Genomic and non-genomic effects of estrogens on endothelial cells. Steroids 2004; 69: 537-542.

[58] Sobolewska A, Gajewska M, Zarzynska J, Gajkowska B, and Motyl T. Igf-i, egf, and sex steroids regulate autophagy in bovine mammary epithelial cells via the mtor pathway. Eur J Cell Biol 2009; 88: 117-130.

[59] Stocco D, and McPhaul M. Physiology of testicular steroidogenesis. In: NeillJD (ed.) Physiology of reproduction. Elsevier 2006. 977-1016.

[60] Strauss JF, 3rd, Martinez F, and Kiriakidou M. Placental steroid hormone synthesis: Unique features and unanswered questions. Biol Reprod 1996; 54: 303-311.

[61] Svechnikov K, and Söder O. Ontogeny of gonadal sex steroids. Best Practice; Research Clinical Endocrinology; Metabolism 2008; 22: 95-106.

[62] Tan RS, Pu SJ, and Culberson JW. Role of androgens in mild cognitive impairment and possible interventions during andropause. Med Hypotheses 2003; 60: 448-452.

[63] Traish AM, Abdou R, and Kypreos KE. Androgen deficiency and atherosclerosis: The lipid link. Vascul Pharmacol 2009a; 51: 303-313.

[64] Traish AM, Feeley RJ, and Guay AT. Testosterone therapy in women with gynecological and sexual disorders: A triumph of clinical endocrinology from 1938 to 2008. J Sex Med 2009b; 6: 334-351.

[65] TulaneUniversity. History of androgens. Http://e.Hormone.Tulane.Edu/learning/androgens.Html (accessed, 1 august 2012).

[66] Vanderschueren D, Vandenput L, Boonen S, Lindberg MK, Bouillon R, and Ohlsson C. Androgens and bone. Endocr Rev 2004; 25: 389-425.

[67] Venken K, De Gendt K, Boonen S, Ophoff J, Bouillon R, Swinnen JV, Verhoeven G, and Vanderschueren D. Relative impact of androgen and estrogen receptor activa-

tion in the effects of androgens on trabecular and cortical bone in growing male mice: A study in the androgen receptor knockout mouse model. J Bone Miner Res 2006; 21: 576-585.

[68] Vicencio JM, Estrada M, Galvis D, Bravo R, Contreras AE, Rotter D, Szabadkai G, Hill JA, Rothermel BA, Jaimovich E, and Lavandero S. Anabolic androgenic steroids and intracellular calcium signaling: A mini review on mechanisms and physiological implications. Mini Rev Med Chem 2011; 11: 390-398.

[69] Wikipedia. Progesterone. Http://en.Wikipedia.Org/wiki/progesterone (accessed 9 august 2012).

[70] Wikipedia. Sex steroids. Http://en.Wikipedia.Org/wiki/sex_steroid (accessed 17 july 2012).

[71] Wood RI. Anabolic-androgenic steroid dependence? Insights from animals and humans. Front Neuroendocrinol 2008; 29: 490-506.

[72] World Health Organization International Programme on Chemical Safety. 2000. Toxicological evaluation of certain veterinary drug residues in food

[73] Fifty-second meeting of the Joint FAO/WHO. Expert Committee on Food Additives (JECFA).

[74] Young EA, and Becker JB. Perspective: Sex matters: Gonadal steroids and the brain. Neuropsychopharmacology 2009; 34: 537-538.

Chapter 2

The Biological Roles of Steroid Sulfonation

Paul Anthony Dawson

Additional information is available at the end of the chapter

http://dx.doi.org/10.5772/52714

1. Introduction

Although its role in mammalian physiology is currently underappreciated, sulfate is an obligate nutrient for numerous cellular and metabolic processes in human growth and development [1].The diet provides approximately one third of sulfate requirements in adults [2], although sulfate intake can vary greatly (1.5-16mmol/day) and is dependent on the source of drinking water (negligible to >500 mg/L) and types of food [3-5]. Brassica vegetables and commercial breads have a high sulfate content (>8.0umol/g) whereas low sulfate levels (<0.5umol/g) are found in some foods, including fresh onions, apples and oranges [5]. Once consumed, sulfate is absorbed through the intestinal epithelium into the blood, where it is maintained at approximately 0.3mM, making sulfate the fourth most abundant anion in human circulation [6, 7]. Blood sulfate levels are maintained by the kidneys, which filter sulfate in the glomerulus and then reabsorb the majority of sulfate back into circulation [8]. The process of sulfate reabsorption occurs in the proximal tubule of the kidney, and is mediated by two sulfate transporter proteins, SLC13A1 (aka NaS1, Sodium sulfate transporter 1) and SLC26A1 (aka SAT1, Sulfate anion transporter 1) [9]. The NaS1 protein is expressed on the apical membrane of epithelial cells in the proximal tubule where it mediates the first step of sulfate reabsorption [10], and SAT1 mediates the second step across the basolateral membrane [11] (Figure 1A). Mice lacking the NaS1 or SAT1 genes have sulfate wasting into the urine which leads to low blood sulfate levels (hyposulfataemia) [12, 13]. Humans with loss of function mutations (R12X and N174S) in the NaS1 gene also exhibit renal sulfate wasting and hyposulfataemia [14]. This depletion of sulfate from circulation reduces sulfate availability to cells throughout the body and leads to a reduced intracellular sulfate conjugation (sulfonation) capacity, as shown in the NaS1 and SAT1 null mice [12, 13, 15].

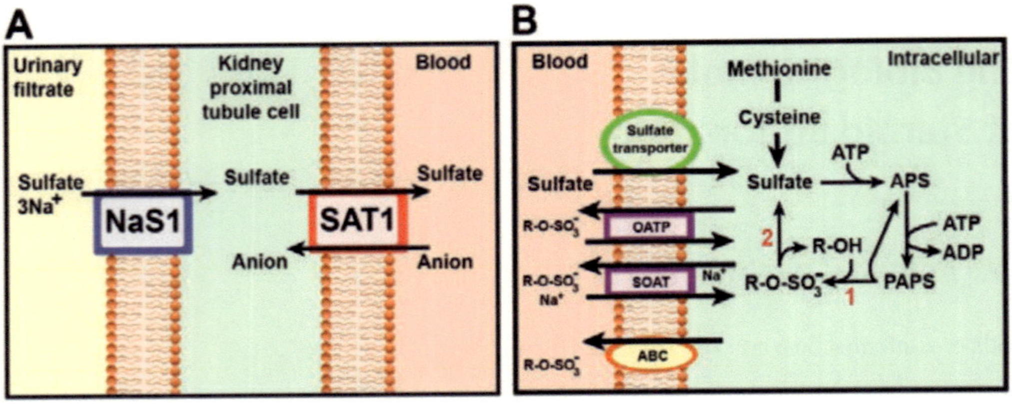

Figure 1. Sulfate levels need to be maintained for sulfonation reactions to function effectively. *(A)* In the kidneys, filtered sulfate is reabsorbed through epithelial cells in the proximal tubule via NaS1 on the apical membrane and then by SAT1 on the basolateral membrane. *(B)* Intracellular sulfate is obtained from extracellular sources via sulfate transporters, and is derived from the metabolism of methionine and cysteine. Sulfate and ATP are converted to the universal sulfonate donor, PAPS. Both (*1*) sulfonation and (*2*) de-sulfonation reactions are active within intracellular metabolism. Sulfonated molecules are transported across the plasma membrane of cells via ATP binding cassette (ABC) proteins, sodium-dependent organic anion transporter (SOAT) and organic anion transporter polypeptides (OATPs), where they provide a circulating reservoir for cellular uptake and intracellular de-sulfonation. R-O-SO_3 represents sulfonated substrates, including steroids.

Intracellular sulfate is derived from the uptake of sulfate across the plasma membrane via sulfate transporters, and from the intracellular metabolism of sulfur-containing amino acids and thiols, as well as the removal of sulfate from substrates via sulfatases (Figure 1B). Certain cell types in adults, including chondrocytes, endothelial cells and hepatocytes have a high requirement for intracellular sulfonation, and are more reliant on transport of extracellular sulfate into the cell [16, 17]. In addition, the placenta and developing fetus are reliant on sulfate from the maternal circulation bcause placental and fetal cells have a relatively low capacity to form sulfate from methionine and cysteine [1, 18, 19]. Sulfonation reactions in all organisms require the conversion of sulfate to the universal sulfonate (SO_3^-) donor, 3′-phosphoadenosine 5′phosphosulfate (PAPS) [20]. The generation of PAPS is mediated by the bifunctional enzyme, PAPS synthetase, which sulfurylates ATP to form adenosine 5′-phosphosulfate (APS) followed by phosphorylation to form PAPS [21] (Figure 1B). The sulfonate group from PAPS is then transferred to the target substrate via sulfotransferase enzymes, which can be grouped into two classes: (i) membrane-bound in the golgi where they sulfonate glycosaminoglycans, proteins, peptides and lipids; and (ii) cytosolic sulfotransferases which sulfonate neurotransmitters, bile acids, xenobiotics and steroids [22].

Early studies described the presence of steroid sulfates in biological samples, including urine [23]. Biochemists had also described the chemical incorporation of sulfate (SO_4^{2-}) into steroids [24], a process which we refer to as sulfation and not to be confused with the metabolic process of sulfonation which is mediated by sulfotransferases with PAPS as the sulfonate (SO_3^{2-}) donor [20]. In 1955, De Meio and Lewycka provided initial evidence that DHEA could be enzymatically conjugated with sulfate using rat liver extracts [25]. These findings

http://dx.doi.org/10.5772/52714

were supported by subsequent studies showing that rabbit liver extracts could mediate sulfate conjugation of 14 steroids, including testosterone and deoxycorticosterone [26]. The landmark report of sulfate activiation to PAPS [27] and the subsequent identification of sulfotransferases [22, 27], has led to our current understanding of sulfonation, and the physiological importance of this process in modulating the biological activity of steroids [28, 29]. Over the past decade, interest in steroid sulfonation and links to mammalian pathophysiology has expanded (Figure 2).

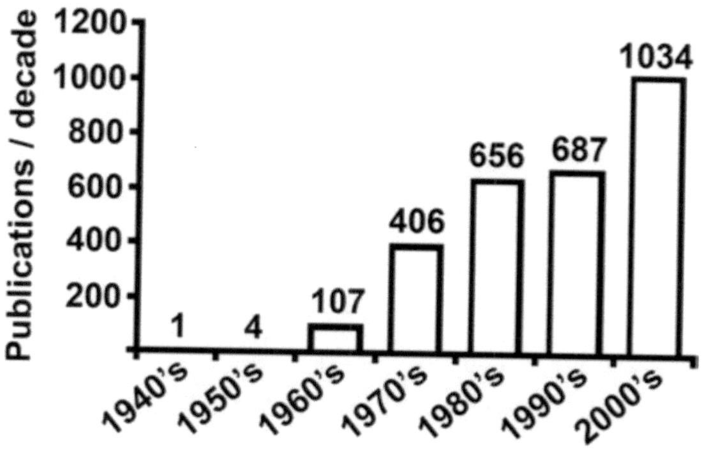

Figure 2. The number of articles published in the field of steroid sulfonation. Articles were identified in PubMed using the key words ((sulfonation or sulfation or sulfotransferase or sulfatase) and steroid). The increasing number of articles in recent years reflects the current interest in steroid sulfonation.

2. Steroid sulfotransferases

To date, five gene families of mammalian sulfotransferases (SULT1, SULT2, SULT3, SULT4 and SULT5) have been identified [22]. In humans, five subfamily members of SULT1 and SULT2 have been linked to steroid sulfonation (Table 1) with some overlap in the specificity of substrates (Figure 3).

Human SULT1A1 was initially cloned from liver where it mediates the sulfonation of numerous phenolic compounds [30]. SULT1A1 has since been found in several extrahepatic tissues, such as platlets which have been widely used for biochemcial phenotyping of six SULT1A1 alloenzymes, each with a different enzyme activity due to the presence of amino acid variants: SULT1A1*1, SULT1A1*2 (R213H), SULT1A1*3 (M223V), SULT1A*4 (R37G), SULT1A1*V (A147T + E181G + R213H), and SULT1A1*VI (P90L + V243A) [22, 31-33]. SULT1A1 exhibits high specific activity towards 17β-estradiol, 17β-estrone, DHEA and 2-methoxyestradiol at relatively high nonphysiological concentrations (i.e. micromolar) *in vitro* [33], suggesting that SULT1A1 may not play a major physiological role in steroid sulfonation.

SULT	Tissue expression	Steroid substrates	References
SULT1A1	liver, adrenal, bladder, platlets, bone,	17β-estradiol,	[31,34]
	brain, eye, intestine, kidney, lung,	17β-estrone, DHEA,	
	lymph, ovary, breast, spleen, pancreas,	2-methoxyestradiol	
	thyroid, testis, stomach, placenta,		
	salivary gland, prostate, uterus		
SULT1E1	adrenal, liver, heart, kidney, lung, eye,	17β-estradiol,	[22,35]
	muscle, pharynx, larynx, placenta,	17β-estrone, 17β-estriol	
	trachea, endometrium, stomach, brain	DHEA, pregnenolone	
SULT2A1	adrenal, liver, small intestine, muscle,	DHEA, pregnenolone	[28,32,36]
	brain, breast, placenta, stomach	androgens, 17β-estradiol	
SULT2B1a	ovary, lung, kidney, colon, skin, prostate	pregnenolone, DHEA	[37,38]
SULT2B1b	placenta, skin, prostate, colon	cholesterol, DHEA,	[39,40]
	lung, kidney, colon, stomach, spleen,	pregnenolone,	
	small intestine, thymus thyroid, liver	oxysterols	
	breast, platelets, ovary, brain		

Table 1. Human Sulfotransferases (SULTs), tissue expression and steroid specificity.

SULT1E1, also referred to as estrogen sulfotransferase, shows high affinity for 17β-estradiol, 17β-estrone and 17β-estriol, at physiological (nanomolar) concentrations, to form estrogen-3-sulfates (Figure 3). This enzyme also sulfonates DHEA and pregnenolone, as well as numerous synthetic estrogens, including diethylstilbestrol [33]. Human SULT1E1 is expressed in several tissues, with high levels detected in the liver and adrenal glands [22, 33]. Endometrial SULT1E1 levels are influenced by the stage of pregnancy and by the menstrual cycle [41, 42]. This most likely reflects the up-regulation of SULT1E1 gene expression by progesterone [43].

Originally named DHEA sulfotransferase [44], SULT2A1 is strongly expressed in the fetal adrenal gland (zona reticularis), as well as the adult liver, adrenal gland and duodenum, where it plays a major role in sulfonating DHEA [22, 33]. SULT2A1 also sulfonates other hydroxysteroids including pregnenolone, as well as 17β-estradiol and testosterone to form estradiol-17-sulfate and testosterone-17-sulfate, respectively [33].

The SULT2B1a and SULT2B1b proteins are encoded by the same gene but differ in the amino acid sequences at their amino-terminal ends, as a result of an alternative exon 1 [45]. SULT2B1a preferentially sulfonates pregnenolone [37, 38], whereas SULT2B1b plays a major role in cholesterol sulfonation, particularly in the skin [39, 40].

http://dx.doi.org/10.5772/52714

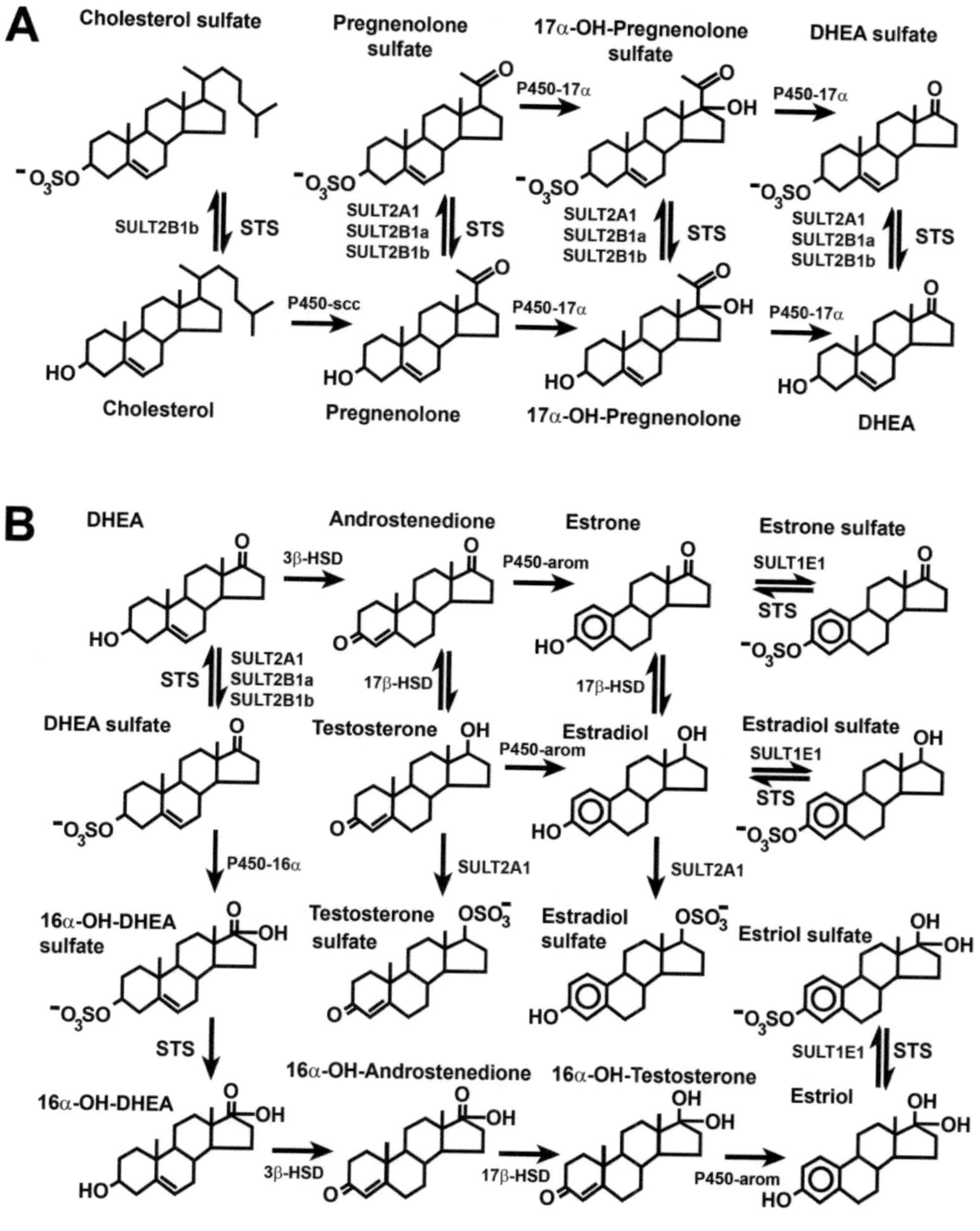

Figure 3. Steroid sulfonation and de-conjugation pathways play an important role in steroid metabolism, as well as regulating steroid half-life and activity. (*A*) Steroid sulfatase (STS) converts cholesterol sulfate to cholesterol, which is then transported into mitochondria for conversion to pregnenolone, and downstream adrenal products including DHEA and DHEA sulfate. (*B*) DHEA sulfate serves as the precursor molecule for synthesis of the non-adrenal steroid hormones, including testosterone and estrogens. In most cases, sulfonation decreases the biological activity of steroids by preventing binding to steroid receptors.

3. Steroid sulfatase

In humans, 17 sulfatases have been identified [46], of which steroid sulfatase (aka STS or aryl sulfatase C) mediates the hydrolysis of alkyl (e.g. DHEA-S, pregnenolone sulfate, deoxycorticosterone sulfate and cholesterol sulfate) and aryl (e.g. estrone sulfate, estradiol sulfate and estriol sulfate) steroid sulfates [47-49] (Figure 3). STS is a membrane-bound enzyme (EC 3.1.6.2), which has been detected in the rough endoplasmic reticulum, Golgi cisternae, trans-Golgi and plasma membrane, as well as in the coated pits, endosomes and multivesicular endosomes [50]. The STS gene is located on the short arm of the X chromosome, within a region (Xp22.3) that partially escapes X chromosome inactivation [51]. As a consequence, STS enzymatic activity in XX females is higher (by ≈1.6-fold) when compared to XY males. The human Y-chromosome contains an STS pseudogene that is most likely a gene duplication of STS on the X-chromosome, but it lacks the 5′-regulatory DNA sequences necessary for gene expression and hence does not express a functional STS protein [52]. STS is expressed in numerous fetal tissues, including brain, adrenal gland, small and large intestine, liver, thyroid, thymus, lung, heart and kidney [50]. In adults, STS expression is most abundant in testis, uterus, prostate, thyroid, lung, liver and skin. In addition, STS is strongly expressed in the placenta where it is responsible for desulfonating DHEA sulfate, which is derived from maternal circulation and the fetal adrenal glands. Placental STS also deconjugates 16α-hydroxy-DHEA sulfate (Figure 3), which is produced in the fetal liver [53]. Thus, STS plays an important step in the pathway for generating estriol, whcih is the most abundant estrogen during human pregnancy.

Deficiency of STS leads to X-linked ichthyosis (XLI, OMIM 308100), which affects approximately 1 in 6000 males [54, 55]. Most cases (≈80-90%) are caused by complete deletion of the STS gene, whereas small deletions or point mutations account for the remainder of cases [56]. Loss of STS leads to an accumulation (up to 20-fold increase) of its substrate, cholesterol sulfate, in plasma and red cell membranes, as well as the epidermis [57]. Excess cholesterol sulfate in the skin, delays desquamation which leads to hyperkeratosis that appears as large, polygonal, dark brown scales on the skin. Extracutaneous manifestations of this disorder include corneal opacity, cryptorchidism, epileptic seizures and reactive psychological disorders. Some isolated cases of X-linked ichthyosis have presented with pyloric hypertrophy, acute lymphoblastic lymphoma and congenital defect of the abdominal wall [57], however, the link between these clinical conditions and STS is not clear. The clinical manifestations of X-linked ichthyosis in STS deficient patients present after birth, indicating that loss of STS activity may not be essential for fetal development.

To function effectively, all sulfatases including STS, need to be post-translationally modified by the formylglycine generating enzyme (FGE), which is encoded by the sulfatase modifying factor 1 (SUMF1) gene [58]. Mutations in the SUMF1 gene, leads to multiple sulfatase deficiency (MSD, OMIM 272200), which is characterised by congenital growth retardation, skeletal abnormalities, neurological defects and early mortality. Similar phenotypes have been observed in Sumf1 knockout mice [59], confirming that other genes do not compensate for loss of SUMF1. These findings highlight the importance of maintaining the required balance of sulfonated substrates, including steroid sulfates, in mammalian physiology.

4. Physiological roles of sulfonated steroids

Steroid sulfates were initially thought to be end products of metabolism, with the sulfate merely increasing the water solubility of the steroid and enhancing its excretion into the urine [60]. More recent studies have revealed steroid sulfates to be important precursors for the formation of biologically active steroids, or to have physiological roles that are distinct from non-sulfonated steroids [28, 32].

The physicochemcial properties of steroids is markedly changed when conjugated to sulfate. In most cases, sulfonation decreases the biological activitiy of steroids by preventing their binding to steroid receptors [28]. For example, whilst estrogens bind to their genomic estrogen receptors, estrogen sulfates do not bind. This finding is supported by the over-expression of SULT1E1 in cultured human breast carcinoma-derived cells, as well as uterine endometrial Ishikawa cells, which abolish estrogen-stimulated cell proliferation [61, 62]. Conversely, increased expression of STS which increases unconjugated (active) steroid levels, leads to enhanced estrogen-stimulated cell proliferation [63]. Sulfate also contributes to the modulation of cholesterol function. In addition to serving as a substrate for adrenal and ovarian steroidogenesis, cholesterol sulfate has been linked to several biological processes, including: regulation of cholesterol synthesis; plasmin and thrombin activities; sperm capacitation; and activation of protein kinase C [50].

Sulfonation in the brain modulates the nongenomic actions of neurosteroids on $GABA_A$, *N*-methyl-D-aspartate, glutaminergic and σ-opioid receptors, usually in opposing ways [64]. For example, pregnenolone sulfate is a picrotoxin-like antagonist, whereas unconjugated pregnenolone is a barbiturate-like agonist. In addition, DHEA sulfate stimulates acetylcholine release from the hippocampus but unconjugated DHEA does not. These findings may be relevant to the association of prenenolone sulfate and DHEA sulfate with enhanced cognitive function in animals [64]. Furthermore, reduced circulating DHEA sulfate and pregnenolone sulfate levels have been linked with decreased cognitive function in humans. Studies have also reported reduced circulating DHEA sulfate levels in patients with Alzheimer's disease and multi-infarct dementia [65, 66]. These findings, together with the detection of SULT1A1, SULT1E1, SULT2A1, SULT2B1 and STS in the fetal and adult brain, suggests that sulfonation and deconjugation of neurosteroids contributes to neurodevelopment and maintenance of brain function. Of great interest is the detection of SULT4A1 in brain [67], however, its substrate and physiological role is yet unknown.

Steroid sulfates avidly bind to serum proteins, particularly albumin as well as corticosteroid binding globulin (aka CBG, transcortin) and sex hormone binding globulin (aka SHBG, androgen-binding protein, testosterone-binding β-globulin) [28, 68-71]. Binding of steroid sulfates to serum proteins slows their urinary clearance by approximately 2 orders of magnitude, when compared to unconjugated steroids [72]. Accordingly, circulating steroid sulfate levels are higher when compared to their non-sulfonated forms. For example, the ratio of estrogen sulfate to estrogen is approximately several-fold [28, 32]. The high level of albumin-bound steroid sulfates in circulation is proposed to provide a pool of inactive steroids which can be taken up by peripheral target tissues, where deconjugation via STS generates active steroids. Animal studies have provided evidence linking reduced sulfonation capacity with decreased plasma steroid sulfate levels and increased urinary steroid secretion [73]. The NaS1 knockout mouse, which exhibits hyposulfataemia and reduced sulfonation capacity [12, 15], has decreased (by ≈40-50%) circulating levels of DHEA, DHEA-S and corticosterone, whereas urinary levels of corticosterone and DHEA were increased (up to 40%) [73]. This study implied that the reduced sulfonation of steroids, led to the observed increased urinary steroid secretion which lowered circulating steroid levels. This proposal is supported by an earlier study, which reported reduced circulating DHEA-S levels in mice with low *Sult2a1* and sulfate donor 3′-phosphoadenosine 5′-phosphosulfate synthase 2 (*PAPSS2*) mRNA levels [74]. These findings highlight the functional consequences of steroid sulfonation in maintaining a circulating reservoir of steroids that can be drawn upon by target cells in the body.

Sulfonated steroids are moved through the plasma membrane of cells by several different transporter proteins, including the sodium-dependent organic anion transporter (aka SOAT) [75], the sodium-independent organic anion transporting polypeptides (aka OATPs) [76] and the ATP binding cassette (ABC) proteins [77] (Figure 1). ABC transporters are ubiquitously expressed and are mostly considered responsible for the efflux of steroid substrates, whereas SOAT and OATPs mediate tissue-specific bi-directional transport of steroid sulfates across the plasma membrane of cells. Initially identified in rat adrenal glands, SOAT has since been detected in human adrenal glands, as well as numerous additional tissues in rodents, including kidney, lung, mammary gland, liver, uterus, brain and testis. SOAT shares homolgy with the apical sodium-dependent bile acid transporter (aka ASBT, SLC10A2) but is not a bile acid transporter. Rather, SOAT transports steroid sulfates, including estrone-3-sulfate, pregnenolone sulfate and DHEA sulfate. Four families of OATP (OATP1, OATP2, OATP3 and OATP4) have been shown to transport DHEA sulfate and estrone-3-sulfate. The OATP1 genes are expressed throughout the body, with highest expression levels for sub-family members: OATP1A2 in the brain, liver, lung, kidney and testis; OATP1B1 and OATP1B3 specifically expressed in the liver; and OATP1C1 in the brain and testis. The OATP2 sub-family member OATP2B1 is expressed in numerous tissues, including liver, syncytiotrophoblasts of the placenta, mammary gland, heart, skeletal muscle and endothelial cells of the blood-brain barrier. The OATP3A1_v1 transporter is expressed in the germ cells of the testis, as well as in the choroid plexus and frontal cortex. Two OATP4 sub-family members have been identifed in the following tissues: OATP4A1 in heart, lung, liver, skeletal muscle, kidney, pancreas and syncytiotrophoblasts in the placenta; whereas OATP4C1 is localised to the basolateral membranes of renal proximal tubules. Whilst certain sulfonated steroids (i.e. DHEA sulfate and estrone-3-sulfate) have been used to test the substrate specificity of the above ABC, SOAT and OATPs, further studies are required to investigate all known naturally occuring (as well as synthetic) steroid sulfate substrates.

Together, these studies demonstrate that sulfate plays important but unappreciated roles in modulating circulating steroid levels and cellular efflux and uptake of steroids, as well as biotransforming the biological activity of steroids.

4.1. Steroid sulfates in pregnancy

Sulfonation of cholesterol in maternal and placental tissues provides an essential precursor for the synthesis of steroid sulfates, including DHEA sulfate. Whilst the steroid biosynthetic pathway is limited in the fetus, DHEA sulfate is produced in the fetal adrenal gland (zona reticularis) and then circulated to the placenta where it provides the major supply of DHEA sulfate (≈90%) for production of estrone, estradiol and other fetal steroids [1]. DHEA sulfate is also converted to 16α-hydroxy DHEA sulfate in the fetal liver, via 16α-hydroxylase, and subsequently converted to estriol (>60mg/day during the third trimester of human gestation) in the placenta (Figure 3). Whilst decreased levels of estriol in maternal circulation have been used as a marker for Down and trisomy 18 syndromes, pregnancy loss, as well as gross neural tube defects such as anencephaly [78], the role of perturbed DHEA and estriol sulfonation in modifying maternal estriol levels and possibly human fetal development, awaits further investigation.

Steroid sulfates are the major form of steroids supplied to fetal tissues. For example, placental estradiol-3-sulfate is taken up by the fetal brain where it is de-sulfonated by STS to estradiol (Figure 4), which acts as a potent stimulator of fetal adrenocorticotropin (ACTH) secretion and hypothalamus-pituitary-adrenal (HPA) axis [79]. Accordingly, the ratio of sulfonated (inactive) to unconjugated (active) steroids plays an important role in may of the steroid-responsive molecular events that regulate placental and fetal growth and development [28]. This is relevant to the mid-gestational fetal loss and placental thrombosis that was observed in mice lacking the Sult1e1 estrogen sulfotransferase [80]. Sult1e1 is highly expressed in the placenta where it is essential for generating estrone sulfate, estradiol-3-sulfate and estriol sulfate (Figure 3). In addition, Sult1e1 is abundantly expressed in the testis. Male Sult1e1 knockout mice develop Leydig cell hypertrophy/hyperplasia, seminiferous tubule damage, reduced sperm motility and sire smaller litters when compared to age-matched control males. These studies highlight the importance of estrogen sulfonation in maintaining mammalian pregnancy and normal male reproductive function.

A sufficient supply of intracellular sulfate needs to be maintained for sulfonation reactions to function effectively [60, 81]. During human and rodent pregnancy, maternal circulating sulfate levels increase approximately 2-fold, with levels peaking in the second and third trimesters [82-85]. This increase is associated with elevated kidney NaS1 and Sat1 gene expression [83, 86] and renal sulfate reabsorption [87] in the pregnant mother (Figure 4). The increased circulating sulfate level in pregnant humans (from ≈ 0.26 to 0.59 mM) [82, 88, 89] and mice (from ≈ 1.0 to 2.3 mM) [83] enhances sulfate availability to the placenta and fetus, and is remarkable since most circulating ions usually decrease slightly due to haemodilution [90]. Since the placenta and fetus have a relatively low capacity to generate sulfate from methionine and cysteine [18, 19], most of the sulfate in these tissues must come from the maternal circulation (Figure 4). This is consistent with fetal hyposulfatemia and negligible amniotic fluid sulfate levels in fetuses from pregnant hyposulfataemic NaS1 null mice [83]. Of great interest is the reduced fecundity of female NaS1 null mice [12], as a result of fetal death in late gestation (from embryonic day 12.5) [83] which is a similar gestational age when fetal death occurs in the Sult1e1 null mice [80]. These studies highlight the importance of maintaining a sufficient supply of sulfate to placental and fetal cells in mammalian gestation.

Recently, the relative abundance and cellular expression of all known placental sulfate transporters was described [91]. That study identified Slc13a4 (aka NaS2, Sodium sulfate transporter-2) to be the most abundant placental sulfate transporter, which was localised to the syncytiotrophoblasts of mouse placenta, where it is proposed to supply sulfate into the placenta from maternal circulation. The role of placental NaS2, as well as kidney NaS1 (Figure 4), in modulating placental endocrine function awaits further investigation.

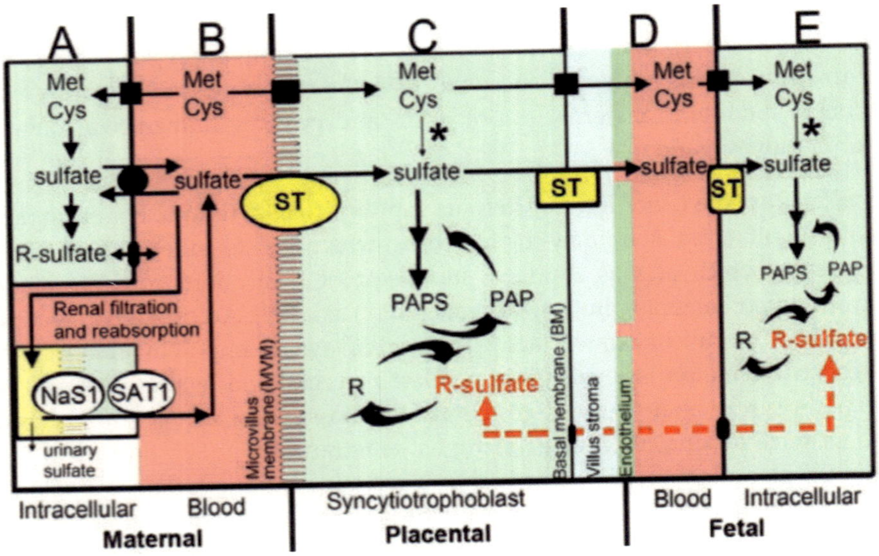

Figure 4. Sulfate supply from mother to placental and fetal tissues is essential for sulfonation reactions to function effectively. R-sulfate represents sulfonated substrates, including steroids such as estrogens and DHEA. During pregnancy: (*A*).Increased kidney NaS1 and SAT1 expression from early gestation (in mice from E4.5) enhances renal sulfate reabsorption, which leads to (*B*) ≈2-fold increased maternal blood sulfate levels. (*C*) NaS2 expression in syncytiotrophoblasts mediates sulfate transport (ST) for generation of the universal sulfate donor PAPS (3'-phosphoadenosine 5'-phosphosulfate). Both sulfonation and de-sulfonation are active within placental and fetal metabolism. (*D*) Sulfate is moved through the villus stroma and inter-endothelial clefts into fetal circulation. (*E*) Fetal intracellular sulfate levels are maintained by sulfate transporters (ST). *Negligible sulfate is derived from Methionine (Met) and Cysteine (Cys) in fetal and placental cells.

4.2. Role of steroid sulfotransferases and sulfatase in cancer

Over the past decade, interest in steroid sulfonation/de-sulfonation and cancer has expanded following our knowledge of sulfonated (inactive) and unconjugated (active) steroids and the requirement for unconjugated steroids (particularly 17 ▪ -estradiol) for maintaining growth of some carcinoma cells [28, 32]. STS is upregulated in many hormone-dependent neoplasms, including breast, endometrial, ovarian and prostate cancers [50, 64]. Increased STS causes the conversion of: (i) estrone sulfate to estrone which is then reduced to estradiol; and (ii) estradiol-3-sulfate to estradiol (Figure 3). Excess estradiol then binds to the estrogen receptor and causes cell proliferation [92]. In addition, upregulation of STS causes the conversion of DHEA sulfate to DHEA, which is then further metabolised to the active androgens: androstenediol, testosterone and dihydrotestosterone that bind the androgen receptor, leading to cell proliferation. STS is detected in most cases of: (i) malignant prostate cancer tissue (85%) but not in the non-neoplastic peripheral tissues; breast tumours (90%) and may be a predictor of recurrence of breast cancer in ER positive tumours; and (iii) ovarian cancer (97%) with low STS activity linked to increased survival time [92]. The link between STS, unconjugated estradiol, active androgens and tumour cell proliferation has led to the development of STS inhibitors [92]. Clinical trials with sulfatase inhibitors in patients with estrogen- and androgen-driven malignancies are in progress and we await outcomes.

The potential roles of steroid sulfotransferases in the induction and maintenance of hormone-dependent cancers has also gained attention. SULT1E1 activity is more abundant in normal breast cells lines when compared to cancer cells lines. In cultured carcinoma cells, transfection of SULT1E1 led to effective reductions in estrogen-mediated cell proliferation [61, 62]. This can be relevant to polymorphisms in the SULT1E1 gene which have been associated with increased risk of breast cancer and reduced disease free survival [93]. Additional studies have linked human sulfotransferase polymorphisms with numerous neoplasias, including endometrial, breast, prostate, lung, mouth, gastric, colorectal and bladder cancers [73, 93-95]. In addition, reduced SULT2A1 expression has been found in hepatocellular carcinoma cells (HCC), and the lowest level of SULT2A1 expression correlates with a higher grade and stage of HCC [96].

Animal studies have demonstrated the link between reduced sulfonation capacity and increased tumour cell growth [97]. The hyposulfataemic NaS1 null mouse, which has reduced circulating DHEA sulfate levels [73], was injected with tumour cells (TC-1) derived from lung epithelium. After 14 days, tumour weights from the NaS1 null mice were increased ≈12-fold when compared to the control mice with normal sulfonation capacity [97]. The tumours grown in NaS1 null mice also showed an increased abundance of vessels, indicating that reduced sulfate supply exacerbates angiogenesis in tumour cell growth. That study highlighted the importance of blood sulfate levels as a possible modulator of tumour growth.

4.3. Role of PAPS synthetase in steroid homeostasis

In addition to the requirement for intracellular sulfate levels, steroid sulfonation requires a sufficient supply of the PAPS sulfonate donor [20]. Generation of PAPS is the rate limiting step for all sulfonation reactions. PAPS is synthesized in two steps: (1) sulfurylation of ATP to form adenosine 5′-phosphosulfate (APS); (2) phosphorylation of APS to form PAPS. Both sulfurylation (EC 2.7.7.4) and kinase (EC 2.7.1.25) activities are mediated by the bifunctional enzyme, PAPS synthetase [21]. Two PAPS synthetase enzymes (PAPSS1 and PAPSS2) have been identified in rodents and humans [98-100]. PAPSS2 is the more abundant isoenzyme in tissues from adults such as the liver and adrenal glands that have a high sulfonation capacity, and its catalytic activity is approximately 10- to 15-fold higher when compared to PAPSS1 [32]. A number of gene variants have been found in the PAPSS1 gene [101] but their effect on sulfonation capacity is not yet known. Since PAPSS1 is the predominant PAPS syntthetase in the developing central nervous system and bone marrow, its loss is proposed to be embryologically lethal [32]. Mutations in the PAPSS2 gene have been linked to developmental dwarfism disorders, including spondyloepimetaphyseal dysplasia in humans, and brachymorphism in mice [98].

In one case, inactivating mutations in the PAPSS2 gene were linked to premature pubarche, hyperandrogenic anovulation and increased androgen levels in a young female patient [102]. Her endocrine profile showed androstenedione and testosterone levels at 2-fold above the upper limit of normal ranges, a DHEA level at the upper limit of the normal range, and DHEA sulfate level at one order of magnitude below the normal range. The clincial presentations of this patient were proposed to be a consequence of reduced DHEA sulfonation, which led to increased circulating levels of unconjugated DHEA that were converted to androgens. A more recent study showed a trend (P=0.06) for a lower ratio of circulating DHEA sulfate to DHEA, in a cohort (n=33) of children with premature adrenarche, and harbouring a polymorphism (rs182420) in the SULT2A1 gene [103]. SULT2A1 genetic variants have also been associated wtih reduced DHEA sulfate and inherited andrenal androgen excess in some women with polycystic ovary syndrome [104]. These findings identify a link between PAPSS2, SULT2A1, reduced sulfonation of DHEA and androgen excess disorders.

In addition, studies have linked reduced gene expression of both PAPSS2 and Sult2A1 to reduced circulating DHEA sulfate levels in mice with lipopolysaccaride-induced acute-phase response [74]. These findings suggest that perturbed steroid sulfonation may be a mechanism for decreased DHEA sulfate levels found in patients with infection, inflammation and trauma that induces metabolic changes in the liver as part of the acute-phase response.

In summary, there is growing body of evidence that disruption of the steroid sufonation pathway, via sulfate/PAPS supply and sulfotransferase activity, leads to perturbed endocrine homeostasis and associated clinical manifestations.

5. Conclusion

Sufficient intracellular sulfate levels and its sulfonate donor PAPS, as well as sulfotransferases (see Table 1), are required for maintaining steroid sulfonation capacity. Furthermore, sulfatases are needed to generate unconjugated active steroids. Together, sulfate transporters, PAPS synthetases, sulfotransferases and sulfatases are essential for maintaining a balance of steroid sulfates and unconjugated steroids, which play different biological roles in humans and animals. Whilst the field of steroid sulfonation is largely unappreciated, its significance is being realised with experimental findings from animal models of reduced sulfate supply (i.e. NaS1 null mouse) and loss of sulfotransferase activity (i.e. Sult1e1 null mouse), as well as links to certain cancers and increased androgen levels.

Acknowledgements

This work was financially supported by The Mater Foundation and the Mater Medical Research Institute. The author would like to acknowledge family support from his wife and children.

Author details

Paul Anthony Dawson

Address all correspondence to: paul.dawson@mmri.mater.org.au

Mater Medical Research Institute, South Brisbane, Queensland, Australia

References

[1] Dawson PA. Sulfate in fetal development. Semin Cell Dev Biol 2011;22(6) 653-9.

[2] Dietary Reference Intakes for Water Potassium Sodium Chloride and Sulfate. Sulfate. 2004[cited; Available from: http:www.nap.edu/openbook/0309091691/html/424.htm

[3] Allen HE, Halley-Henderson MA, Hass CN. Chemical composition of bottled mineral water. Arch Environ Health 1989;44(2) 102-16.

[4] Florin T, Neale G, Gibson GR, Christl SU, Cummings JH. Metabolism of dietary sulphate: absorption and excretion in humans. Gut 1991;32 766-73.

[5] Florin THJ, Neale G, Goretski S, Cummings JH. The sulfate content of foods and beverages. J Food Compos Anal 1993;6 140-51.

[6] Cole DE, Evrovski J. Quantitation of sulfate and thiosulfate in clinical samples by ion chromatography. J Chromatogr A 1997;789(1-2) 221-32.

[7] Murer H, Manganel M, Roch-Ramel F. Tubular transport of monocarboxylates, Krebs cycle intermediates and inorganic sulphate. In: Winhager E, ed. *Handbook of Physiology*: Oxford University Press 1992:2165-88.

[8] Ullrich KJ, Murer H. Sulphate and phosphate transport in the renal proximal tubule. Philos Trans R Soc Lond Biol 1982;299 549-58.

[9] Lee A, Dawson PA, Markovich D. NaSi-1 and Sat-1: Structure, Function and Transcriptional Regulation of two Genes encoding Renal Proximal Tubular Sulfate Transporters. Int J Biochem Cell Biol 2005;37(7) 1350-6.

[10] Lotscher M, Custer M, Quabius ES, Kaissling B, Murer H, Biber J. Immunolocalization of Na/SO4-cotransport (NaSi-1) in rat kidney. Pflugers ArchivEuropean Journal of Physiology 1996;432(3) 373-8.

[11] Karniski LP, Lotscher M, Fucentese M, Hilfiker H, Biber J, Murer H. Immunolocalization of sat-1 sulfate/oxalate/bicarbonate anion exchanger in the rat kidney. Am J Physiol 1998;275(1 Pt 2) F79-87.

[12] Dawson PA, Beck L, Markovich D. Hyposulfatemia, growth retardation, reduced fertility and seizures in mice lacking a functional NaS_i-1 gene. Proc Natl Acad Sci USA 2003;100(23) 13704-9.

[13] Dawson PA, Russell CS, Lee S, McLeay SC, van Dongen JM, Cowley DM, Clarke LA, Markovich D. Urolithiasis and hepatotoxicity are linked to the anion transporter Sat1 in mice. J Clin Invest 2010;120(3) 702-12.

[14] Bowling FG, Heussler HS, McWhinney A, Dawson PA. Plasma and urinary sulfate determination in a cohort with autism. Biochem Genet 2012;in press.

[15] Lee S, Dawson PA, Hewavitharana AK, Shaw PN, Markovich D. Disruption of NaS1 sulfate transport function in mice leads to enhanced acetaminophen-induced hepatotoxicity. Hepatology 2006;43(6) 1241-7.

[16] Humphries DE, Silbert CK, Silbert JE. Sulfation by cultured cells. Cysteine, cysteinesulphinic acid and sulphate as sources for proteoglycan sulfate. Biochem J 1988;252 305-8.

[17] Ito K, Kimata K, Sobue M, Suzuki S. Altered proteoglycan synthesis by epiphyseal cartilages in culture at low SO42- concentration. J Biol Chem 1982;257 917-23.

[18] Gaull G, Sturman JA, Raiha NC. Development of mammalian sulfur metabolism: absence of cystathionase in human fetal tissues. Pediatr Res 1972;6(6) 538-47.

[19] Loriette C, Chatagner F. Cysteine oxidase and cysteine sulfinic acid decarboxylase in developing rat liver. Experientia 1978;34(8) 981-2.

[20] Klassen CD, Boles J. The importance of 3'-phosphoadenosine 5'-phosphosulfate (PAPS) in the regulation of sulfation. FASEB J 1997;11 404-18.

[21] Venkatachalam KV. Human 3'-phosphoadenosine 5'-phosphosulfate (PAPS) synthase: biochemistry, molecular biology and genetic deficiency. IUBMB Life 2003;55(1) 1-11.

[22] Gamage N, Barnett A, Hempel N, Duggleby RG, Windmill KF, Martin JL, McManus ME. Human sulfotransferases and their role in chemical metabolism. Toxicol Sci 2006;90(1) 5-22.

[23] Klyne W, Schachter B, Marrian GF. The steroids of pregnant mares' urine. 1. A method for the extraction of steroid sulphates and the isolation of allopregn-16-en-3(beta)-ol-20-one sulphate. Biochem J 1948;43(2) 231-4.

[24] Yoder L, THomas BH. Antirachitic sulfonation of some steroids. JBiolChem 1948;178(1) 363-72.

[25] De Meio RH, Lewycka C. In vitro synthesis of dehydroepiandrosterone sulfate. Endocrinology 1955;56(4) 489-90.

[26] Lewbart ML, Schneider JJ. Enzymatic synthesis of steroid sulfates. J Biol Chem 1956;222(2) 787-94.

[27] Lipmann F. Biological sulfate activation and transfer. Science 1958;128(3324) 575-80.

[28] Strott CA. Steroid sulfotransferases. Endocr Rev 1996;17(6) 670-97.

[29] Luu-The V, Bernier F, Dufort I, Labrie F. Molecular biology of steroid sulfotransferases. Ann NY Acad Sci 1996;784 137-48.

[30] Wilborn TW, Comer KA, Dooley TP, Reardon IM, Heinrikson RL, Falany CN. Sequence analysis and expression of the cDNA for the phenol-sulfating form of human liver phenol sulfotransferase. Mol Pharmacol 1993;43(1) 70-7.

[31] Kauffman FC. Sulfonation in pharmacology and toxicology. Drug Metab Rev 2004;36(3-4) 823-43.

[32] Strott CA. Sulfonation and molecular action. Endocr Rev 2002;23(5) 703-32.

[33] Glatt H, Meinl W. Pharmacogenetics of soluble sulfotransferases (SULTs). Naunyn Schmiedebergs Arch Pharmacol 2004;369(1) 55-68.

[34] Falany JL, Falany CN. Regulation of estrogen activity by sulfation in human MCF-7 breast cancer cells. Oncol Res 1997;9(11-12) 589-96.

[35] Falany CN, Krasnykh V, Falany JL. Bacterial expression and characterization of a cDNA for human liver estrogen sulfotransferase. J Steroid Biochem Mol Biol 1995;52(6) 529-39.

[36] Comer KA, Falany JL, Falany CN. Cloning and expression of human liver dehydroepiandrosterone sulphotransferase. Biochem J 1993;289(Pt 1) 233-40.

[37] Geese WJ, Raftogianis RB. Biochemical characterization and tissue distribution of human SULT2B1. Biochem Biophys Res Commun 2001;288(1) 280-9.

[38] Meloche CA, Falany CN. Expression and characterization of the human 3 beta-hydroxysteroid sulfotransferases (SULT2B1a and SULT2B1b). J Steroid Biochem Mol Biol 2001;77(4-5) 261-9.

[39] Fuda H, Lee YC, Shimizu C, Javitt NB, Strott CA. Mutational analysis of human hydroxysteroid sulfotransferase SULT2B1 isoforms reveals that exon 1B of the SULT2B1 gene produces cholesterol sulfotransferase, whereas exon 1A yields pregnenolone sulfotransferase. J Biol Chem 2002;277(39) 36161-6.

[40] Javitt NB, Lee YC, Shimizu C, Fuda H, Strott CA. Cholesterol and hydroxycholesterol sulfotransferases: identification, distinction from dehydroepiandrosterone sulfotransferase, and differential tissue expression. Endocrinology 2001;142(7) 2978-84.

[41] Falany JL, Azziz R, Falany CN. Identification and characterization of cytosolic sulfotransferases in normal human endometrium. Chem Biol Interact 1998;109(1-3) 329-39.

[42] Rubin GL, Harrold AJ, Mills JA, Falany CN, Coughtrie MW. Regulation of sulphotransferase expression in the endometrium during the menstrual cycle, by oral contraceptives and during early pregnancy. Mol Hum Reprod 1999;5(11) 995-1002.

[43] Falany JL, Falany CN. Regulation of estrogen sulfotransferase in human endometrial adenocarcinoma cells by progesterone. Endocrinology 1996;137(4) 1395-401.

[44] Otterness DM, Wieben ED, Wood TC, Watson WG, Madden BJ, McCormick DJ, Weinshilboum RM. Human liver dehydroepiandrosterone sulfotransferase: molecular cloning and expression of cDNA. Mol Pharmacol 1992;41(5) 865-72.

[45] Her C, Wood TC, Eichler EE, Mohrenweiser HW, Ramagli LS, Siciliano MJ, Weinshilboum RM. Human hydroxysteroid sulfotransferase SULT2B1: two enzymes encoded by a single chromosome 19 gene. Genomics 1998;53(3) 284-95.

[46] Sardiello M, Annunziata I, Roma G, Ballabio A. Sulfatases and sulfatase modifying factors: an exclusive and promiscuous relationship. Hum Mol Genet 2005;14(21) 3203-17.

[47] Egyed J, Oakey RE. Hydrolysis of deoxycorticosterone-21-yl sulphate and dehydroepiandrosterone sulphate by microsomal preparations of human placentae: evidence for a common enzyme. J Endocrinol 1985;106(3) 295-301.

[48] Dibbelt L, Kuss E. Human placental steroid-sulfatase. Kinetics of the in-vitro hydrolysis of dehydroepiandrosterone 3-sulfate and of 16 alpha-hydroxydehydroepiandrosterone 3-sulfate. Hoppe Seylers Z Physiol Chem 1983;364(2) 187-91.

[49] Kester MH, Kaptein E, Van Dijk CH, Roest TJ, Tibboel D, Coughtrie MW, Visser TJ. Characterization of iodothyronine sulfatase activities in human and rat liver and placenta. Endocrinology 2002;143(3) 814-9.

[50] Reed MJ, Purohit A, Woo LW, Newman SP, Potter BV. Steroid sulfatase: molecular biology, regulation, and inhibition. Endocr Rev 2005;26(2) 171-202.

[51] Shapiro LJ, Mohandas T, Weiss R, Romeo G. Non-inactivation of an x-chromosome locus in man. Science 1979;204(4398) 1224-6.

[52] Yen PH, Allen E, Marsh B, Mohandas T, Wang N, Taggart RT, Shapiro LJ. Cloning and expression of steroid sulfatase cDNA and the frequent occurrence of deletions in STS deficiency: implications for X-Y interchange. Cell 1987;49(4) 443-54.

[53] Miller KK, Cai J, Ripp SL, Pierce WMJ, Rushmore TH, Prough RA. Stereo- and regioselectivity account for the diversity of dehydroepiandrosterone (DHEA) metabolites

produced by liver microsomal cytochromes P450. Drug Metab Dispos 2004;32(3) 305-13.

[54] Shapiro LJ, Weiss R, Buxman MM, Vidgoff J, Dimond RL, Roller JA, Wells RS. Enzymatic basis of typical X-linked icthyosis. Lancet 1978;2(8093) 756-7.

[55] Wells RS, Kerr CB. Clinical features of autosomal dominant and sex-linked ichthyosis in an English population. Br Med J 1966;1(5493) 947-50.

[56] Shapiro LJ, Yen P, Pomerantz D, Martin E, Rolewic L, Mohandas T. Molecular studies of deletions at the human steroid sulfatase locus. Proc Natl Acad Sci USA 1989;86(21) 8477-81.

[57] Hernandez-Martin A, Gonzalez-Sarmiento R, De Unamuno P. X-linked ichthyosis: an update. Br J Dermatol 1999;141 617-27.

[58] Cosma MP, Pepe S, Annunziata I, Newbold RF, Grompe M, Parenti G, Ballabio A. The multiple sulfatase deficiency gene encodes an essential and limiting factor for the activity of sulfatases. Cell 2003;113(4) 445-56.

[59] Settembre C, Annunziata I, Spampanato C, Zarcone D, Cobellis G, Nusco E, Zito E, Tacchetti C, Cosma MP, Ballabio A. Systemic inflammation and neurodegeneration in a mouse model of multiple sulfatase deficiency. Proc Natl Acad Sci USA 2007;104(11) 4506-11.

[60] Mulder GJ, Jakoby WB. Sulfation. In: Mulder GJ, ed. Conjugation Reactions in Drug Metabolism: An Integrated Approach: Substrates, Co-substrates, Enzymes and Their Interactions In Vivo and In Vitro. London: Taylor and Francis 1990:107-61.

[61] Tanaka K, Kubushiro K, Iwamori Y, Okairi Y, Kiguchi K, Ishiwata I, Tsukazaki K, Nozawa S, Iwamori M. Estrogen sulfotransferase and sulfatase: Roles in the regulation of estrogen activity in human uterine endometrial carcinomas. Cancer Science 2003;94(10) 871-6.

[62] Falany JL, Macrina N, Falany CN. Regulation of MCF-7 breast cancer cell growth by beta-estradiol sulfation. Breast Cancer Res Treat 2002;74 167-76.

[63] Pasqualini JR, Schatz B, Varin C, Nguyen BL. Recent data on estrogen sulfatases and sulfotransferases activities in human breast cancer. J Steroid Biochem Mol Biol 1992;41(3-8) 323-9.

[64] Kríz L, Bicíková M, Hampl R. Roles of steroid sulfatase in brain and other tissues. Physiol Res 2008;57(5) 657-68.

[65] Sunderland T, Merril CR, Harrington MG, Lawlor BA, Molchan SE, Martinez R, Murphy DL. Reduced plasma dehydroepiandrosterone concentrations in Alzheimer's disease. Lancet 1989;2(8662) 570.

[66] Yanase T, Fukahori M, Taniguchi S, Nishi Y, Sakai Y, Takayanagi R, Haji M, Nawata H. Serum dehydroepiandrosterone (DHEA) and DHEA-sulfate (DHEA-S) in Alzheimer's disease and in cerebrovascular dementia. Endocr J 1996;43(1) 119-23.

[67] Liyou NE, Buller KM, Tresillian MJ, Elvin CM, Scott HL, Dodd PR, Tannenberg AE, McManus ME. Localization of a brain sulfotransferase, SULT4A1, in the human and rat brain: an immunohistochemical study. J Histochem Cytochem 2003;51(12) 1655-64.

[68] Chader GJ, Rust N, Burton RM, Westphal U. Steroid-protein interactions. XXVI. Studies on the polymeric nature of the corticosteroid-binding globulin of the rabbit. J Biol Chem 1972;247(20) 6581-8.

[69] Dunn JF, Nisula BC, Rodbard D. Transport of steroid hormones: binding of 21 endogenous steroids to both testosterone-binding globulin and corticosteroid-binding globulin in human plasma. J Clin Endocrinol Metab 1981;53 58-68.

[70] Puche RC, Nes WR. Binding of dehydroepiandrosterone sulfate to serum albumin. Endocrinology 1962;70 857-63.

[71] Weiser JN, Do YS, Feldman D. Synthesis and secretion of corticosteroid-binding globulin by rat liver. A source of heterogeneity of hepatic corticosteroid-binders. J Clin Invest 1979;63 461-7.

[72] Wang DY, Bulbrook RD, Ellis F, Coombs MM. Metabolic clearance rates of pregnenolone, 17-acetoxypregnenolone and their sulphate esters in man and in rabbit. J Endocrinol 1967;39(3) 395-403.

[73] Dawson PA, Gardiner B, Lee S, Grimmond S, Markovich D. Kidney transcriptome reveals altered steroid homeostasis in NaS1 sulfate transporter null mice. J Steroid Biochem Mol Biol 2008;112(1-3) 55-62.

[74] Kim MS, Shigenaga J, Moser A, Grunfeld C, Feingold KR. Suppression of DHEA sulfotransferase (Sult2A1) during the acute-phase response. Am J Physiol Endocrinol Metab 2004;287(4) E731-E8.

[75] Geyer J, Wilke T, Petzinger E. The solute carrier family SLC10: more than a family of bile acid transporters regarding function and phylogenetic relationships. Naunyn Schmiedebergs Arch Pharmacol 2006;372(6) 413-31.

[76] Roth M, Obaidat A, Hagenbuch B. OATPs, OATs and OCTs: the organic anion and cation transporters of the SLCO and SLC22A gene superfamilies. Br J Pharmacol 2012;165(5) 1260-87.

[77] Moitra K, Silverton L, Limpert K, Im K, Dean M. Moving out: from sterol transport to drug resistance - the ABCG subfamily of efflux pumps. Drug Metabol Drug Interact 2011;26(3) 105-11.

[78] Alldred SK, Deeks JJ, Guo B, Neilson JP, Alfirevic Z. Second trimester serum tests for Down's Syndrome screening. Cochrane Database Syst Rev 2012;6 CD009925.

[79] Wood CE. Estrogen/hypothalamus-pituitary-adrenal axis interactions in the fetus: The interplay between placenta and fetal brain. J Soc Gynecol Investig 2005;12(2) 67-76.

[80] Tong MH, Jiang H, Liu P, Lawson JA, Brass LF, Song WC. Spontaneous fetal loss caused by placental thrombosis in estrogen sulfotransferase-deficient mice. Nat Med 2005;11(2) 153-9.

[81] Mulder GJ. Sulfate availability in vivo. In: Mulder GJ, ed. Sulfation of Drugs and Related Compounds. Boca Raton, FL: CRC 1981:32-52.

[82] Cole DE, Baldwin LS, Stirk LJ. Increased inorganic sulfate in mother and fetus at parturition: evidence for a fetal-to-maternal gradient. Am J Obstet Gynecol 1984;148(5) 596-9.

[83] Dawson PA, Sim P, Simmons DG, Markovich D. Fetal loss and hyposulfataemia in pregnant NaS1 transporter null mice. J Reprod Dev 2011;57(4) 444-9.

[84] Morris ME, Levy G. Serum concentration and renal excretion by normal adults of inorganic sulfate after acetaminophen, ascorbic acid, or sodium sulfate. Clin Pharmacol Ther 1983;33(4) 529-36.

[85] Tallgren LG. Inorganic sulphate in relation to the serum thyroxine level and in renal failure. Acta Med Scand 1980;suppl 640 1-100.

[86] Lee HJ, Balasubramanian SV, Morris ME. Effect of pregnancy, postnatal growth, and gender on renal sulfate transport. Proc Soc Exp Biol Med 1999;221 336-44.

[87] Cole DE, Baldwin LS, Stirk LJ. Increased renal reabsorption of inorganic sulfate in third-trimester high-risk pregnancies. Obstet Gynecol 1985;66(4) 485-90.

[88] Cole DE, Baldwin LS, Stirk LJ. Increased serum sulfate in pregnancy: relationship to gestational age. Clin Chem 1985;31(6) 866-7.

[89] Cole DE, Oulton M, Stirk LJ, Magor B. Increased inorganic sulfate concentrations in amniotic fluid. J Perinat Med 1992;20(6) 443-7.

[90] Lind T. Clinical chemistry of pregnancy. Adv Clin Chem 1980;21 1-24.

[91] Dawson PA, Rakoczy J, Simmons DG. Placental, Renal, and Ileal Sulfate Transporter Gene Expression in Mouse Gestation. Biol Reprod 2012; 87(2):43.

[92] Purohit A, Foster PA. Steroid sulfatase inhibitors for estrogen- and androgen-dependent cancers. J Endocrinol 2012;212(2) 99-110.

[93] Choi JY, Lee KM, Park SK, Noh DY, Ahn SH, Chung HW, Han W, Kim JS, Shin SG, Jang IJ, Yoo KY, Hirvonen A, Kang D. Genetic polymorphisms of SULT1A1 and SULT1E1 and the risk and survival of breast cancer. Cancer Epidemiol Biomarkers Prev 2005;14(5) 1090-5.

[94] Hirata H, Hinoda Y, Okayama N, Suehiro Y, Kawamoto K, Kikuno N, Rabban JT, Chen LM, Dahiya R. CYP1A1, SULT1A1, and SULT1E1 polymorphisms are risk factors for endometrial cancer susceptibility. Cancer 2008;112(9) 1964-73.

[95] Wilborn TW, Lang NP, Smith M, Meleth S, Falany CN. Association of SULT2A1 allelic variants with plasma adrenal androgens and prostate cancer in African American men. J Steroid Biochem Mol Biol 2006;99(4-5) 209-14.

[96] Huang LR, Coughtrie MW, Hsu HC. Down-regulation of dehydroepiandrosterone sulfotransferase gene in human hepatocellular carcinoma. Mol Cell Endocrinol 2005;231(1-2) 87-94.

[97] Dawson PA, Choyce A, Chuang C, Whitelock J, Markovich D, Leggatt GR. Enhanced tumor growth in the NaS1 sulfate transporter null mouse. Cancer Sci 2010;101(2) 369-73.

[98] Faiyaz ul Haque M, King LM, Krakow D, Cantor RM, Rusiniak ME, Swank RT, Superti-Furga A, Haque S, Abbas H, Ahmad W, Ahmad M, Cohn DH. Mutations in orthologous genes in human spondyloepimetaphyseal dysplasia and the brachymorphic mouse. Nat Genet 1998;20(2) 157-62.

[99] Kurima K, Warman ML, Krishnan S, Domowicz M, Krueger RCJ, Deyrup A, Schwartz NB. A member of a family of sulfate-activating enzymes causes murine brachymorphism. Proc Natl Acad Sci USA 1998;95(15) 8681-5.

[100] Xu ZH, Otterness DM, Freimuth RR, Carlini EJ, Wood TC, Mitchell S, Moon E, Kim UJ, Xu JP, Siciliano MJ, Weinshilboum RM. Human 3'-phosphoadenosine 5'-phosphosulfate synthetase 1 (PAPSS1) and PAPSS2: gene cloning, characterization and chromosomal localization. Biochem Biophys Res Commun 2000;268(2) 437-44.

[101] Xu ZH, Thomae BA, Eckloff BW, Wieben ED, Weinshilboum RM. Pharmacogenetics of human 3'-phosphoadenosine 5'-phosphosulfate synthetase 1 (PAPSS1): gene resequencing, sequence variation, and functional genomics. Biochem Pharmacol 2003;65(11) 1787-96.

[102] Noordam C, Dhir V, McNelis JC, Schlereth F, Hanley NA, Krone N, Smeitink JA, Smeets R, Sweep FC, Claahsen-van der Grinten HL, Arlt W. Inactivating PAPSS2 mutations in a patient with premature pubarche. N Engl J Med 2009;360(22) 2310-8.

[103] Utriainen P, Laakso S, Jääskeläinen J, Voutilainen R. Polymorphisms of POR, SULT2A1 and HSD11B1 in children with premature adrenarche. Metabolism 2012;PMID: 22445027.

[104] Goodarzi MO, Antoine HJ, Azziz R. Genes for enzymes regulating dehydroepiandrosterone sulfonation are associated with levels of dehydroepiandrosterone sulfate in polycystic ovary syndrome. J Clin Endocrinol Metab 2007;92(7) 2659-64.

Chapter 3

Hippocampal Function and Gonadal Steroids

Dai Mitsushima

Additional information is available at the end of the chapter

http://dx.doi.org/10.5772/52713

1. Introduction

The hippocampus plays a central role to form new episodic memory in various species including humans (Scoville and Milner, 1959). The hippocampal neurons seem to process variety of information, such as spatial location (Wills et al., 2010), temporal information (Mitsushima et al., 2009), and emotional state (Chen et al., 2011) within specific episodes (Komorowski et al., 2009; Gelbard-Sagiv et al., 2008). However, the critical mechanism how to sustain a piece of specific memory and how to organize the memory fragment to form "episodes" is still largely unknown.

Since selective blockade of long-term potentiation (LTP) induction by NMDA receptor antagonist impairs hippocampal learning (Morris et al., 1986), LTP has been considered as a cellular model of hippocampal memory (Bliss and Lømo, 1973). In 2006, *in vivo* field EPSC recording study showed that hippocampal learning induces LTP in CA1 region of hippocampus (Whitlock et al., 2006). Further, we revealed that learning-dependent synaptic delivery of AMPA receptors into the CA3-CA1 synapses is required for hippocampal learning (Mitsushima et al., 2011). Since there is no tetanus electrode in brain, endogenous trigger and/or the mechanism inducing the learning-dependent LTP were still unknown.

As an endogenous trigger of LTP, we hypothesized acetylcholine (ACh) release in the hippocampus that increases during learning or exploration in freely moving animals. In fact, without electrode for tetanus stimulation, bath treatment of ACh agonist not only induces specific bursts (Fisahn et al., 1998) but also forms LTP in CA1 region of hippocampal slices (Auerbach and Segal 1996). Moreover, bilateral intra-hippocampal treatments of muscarinic receptors impair hippocampal learning (Herrera-Morales et al., 2007; Rogers and Kesner 2004). In this review, we focused on *in vivo*ACh release in the hippocampus in order to improve our understanding of sex specific and steroids-dependent mechanism of hippocampal function.

2. Role of ACh in the hippocampus

A number of studies suggest that AChplays an important role in orchestrating major hippocampal functions (Fig. 1). In behavioural studies, ACh release increases during learning (Ragozzino et al., 1996; Stancampiano et al., 1999; Hironaka et al., 2001) and is positively correlated with learning performance (Gold, 2003; Parent and Baxter, 2004). Bilateral injections of scopolamine into the dorsal hippocampus impair spatial learning ability (Herrera-Morales et al., 2007), suggesting that muscarinic ACh receptors mediate the formation of spatial memory. At the network level, ACh generates a theta rhythm (Lee et al., 1994) that modulates the induction of long-term potentiation (LTP) in hippocampal CA1 neurons (Hyman et al., 2003). Studies exploring a genetic deficiency of muscarinic ACh receptors (M_1or M_2) further show the impairment of LTP in the CA1 region (Seeger et al., 2004; Shinoe et al., 2005). At the cellular level, both pyramidal and non-pyramidal neurons in the hippocampal CA1 area receive direct cholinergic afferents mediated by muscarinic receptors (Cole and Nicoll, 1983; Markram and Segal, 1990; Widmer et al., 2006). *In vitro* studies showed that bath application of carbachol, a cholinergic agonist, induces LTP in CA1 pyramidal neurons without electrical stimulus, suggesting that ACh in the hippocampus plays a principal role in the synaptic plasticity of the CA1 pyramidal neurons (Auerbach and Segal, 1996). Furthermore, a recent study revealed an intracellular mechanism of ACh: focal activation of muscarinic ACh receptors in one CA1 pyramidal neuron induces Ca^{2+} release from inositol 1,4,5-trisphosphate-sensitive stores to induce LTP (Fernández de Sevilla, 2008).

Not only is ACh critically involved in synaptic plasticity, ACh release in the hippocampus is also responsible for neurogenesis in the dentate gyrus. Thus, neurotoxic lesions of forebrain cholinergic neurons or long-term scopolamine treatment significantly decreases the number of newborn cells in the dentate gyrus, approximately 90% of those were also positive for the neuron-specific marker NeuN (Mohapel et al., 2005; Kotani et al., 2006).

3. Monitoring of in vivoACh release

Cholinergic neurons within the basal forebrain provide the major projection to the neocortex and hippocampus (Mesulam, et al., 1983). Cortical regions receive cholinergic inputs mainly from the nucleus basalismagnocellularis(NBM) or the diagonal band of Broca, whereas the hippocampus receives cholinergic inputs mostly from the medial septum and horizontal limb of the diagonal band of Broca (Mesulam, et al., 1983). Because the cholinergic projections are necessary to maintain learning and memory (Perry et al., 1999, Sarterand Parikh, 2005), we hypothesized that *in vivo* monitoring of ACh release in the hippocampus is necessary to elucidate learning function. To measure ACh release, we have performed *in vivo* microdialysis studies in freely moving rats. Briefly, a microdialysis probe with a semi-permeable membrane (1.0 mm in length) was inserted into a specific brain area via a surgically pre-implanted guide cannula. We perfused the inside of the membrane with artificial cerebrospinal fluid, and assayed ACh in dialysates using a high-performance liquid

http://dx.doi.org/10.5772/52713

chromatography system. As a result, we were successful in determining an *in vivo* ACh release profile in selected brain areas in freely moving rats (Figure 2).

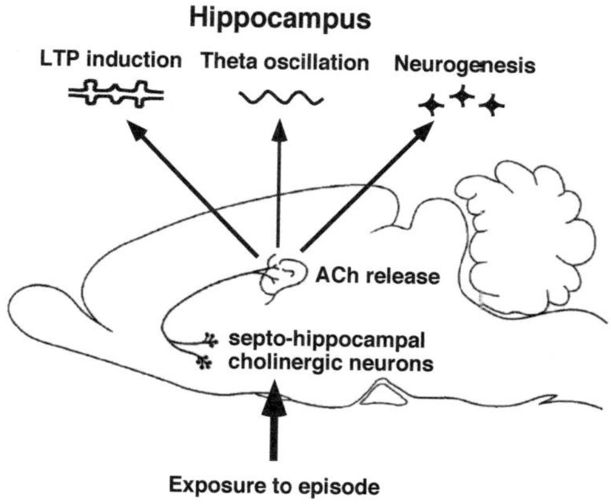

Figure 1. Schematic illustration of septo-hippocampal cholinergic neurons in rats. Exposure to episode induces ACh release in the hippocampus that activates hippocampal functions. Scopolamine induces amnesia in many mammalian species, including humans. For example, many people remember where they were and what they were doing when serious events occur. ACh, acetylcholine. LTP, long-term potentiation.

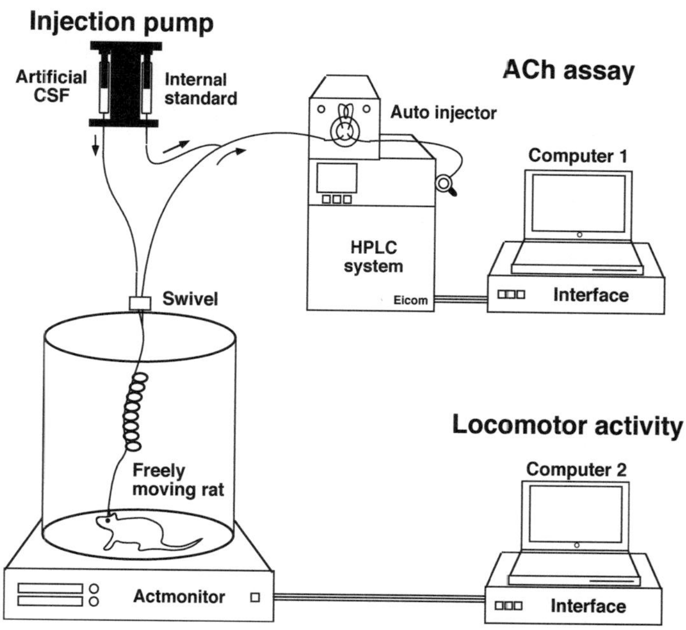

Figure 2. Experimental setup of *in vivo* microdialysis system. We examined *in vivo* ACh release and spontaneous locomotor activity in the same subject.

4. Sex differences inACh release

We first reported sex-specificACh release in the hippocampus in 2003 (Mitsushima et al., 2003). Gonadally intact male rats consistently show a greater ACh release in the hippocampus compared with diestrous or proestrous female rats, suggesting a sexually dimorphic septo-hippocampal cholinergic system. Moreover, we found that sex-dependent ACh release also shows a time-dependent 24-h profile: ACh release in the hippocampus was relatively similar in the light phase, but consistently lower in female compared with male rats in the dark phase (Masuda et al., 2005). Although ACh release clearly showed a daily rhythm in female rats, females exhibited smaller amplitude of daily change than males. However, it is necessary to rule out the possibility that the sex difference in ACh release reflects the differences in spontaneous locomotor activity levels. By simultaneous monitoring of ACh levels and spontaneous locomotor activity, we revealed a real sex difference in the "ACh release property" (Figure 3, Mitsushima et al., 2009): males showed higher ACh release than females while displaying similar levels of behavioural activity. Although female rats showed slightly higher overall spontaneous activity than intact male rats, male rats showed higher ACh release than female rats. Simple linear regression analysis was used to evaluate the relationship between ACh levels and spontaneous locomotor activity (Figure 3). Pearson's correlation coefficient (r) or slope of the best fit line was calculated for each rat, and sex difference was evaluated using ANOVA. We found that the data from intact males had a steeps lope of fit line, while the data from females had a gentle slope. These results suggest that sex-specific ACh release is not due to the change in spontaneous behavior, but due to actual differences in the ACh release property in gonadally intact rats (Mitsushima et al., 2009).

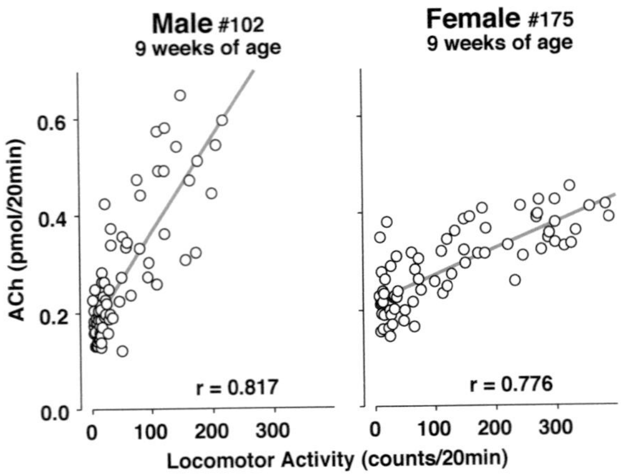

Figure 3. Sex specific ACh release property in behaving rats. Representative data from a male (#102) and a female (#175) rat were shown. Simple linear regression analysis revealed a sex-specific "ACh release property." Male rats showed higher ACh release than females undergoing similar behavioural activity levels. Although both sexes showed a high correlation, male rats showed a steeper slope than female rats in the hippocampus (see Mitsushima et al., 2009). Conversely, in neocortical area, females show higher ACh release and correlation than males (see Takase et al., 2009)

http://dx.doi.org/10.5772/52713

To evaluate neuroanatomical sex difference in the septo-hippocampal cholinergic neurons, we performed immunocytochemistry. Stereological analysis showed that no sex difference was observed in the number and the distribution of choline acetyltransferaseimmunoreactive(ChAT-ir) cells in the medial septum or horizontal limb of diagonal band (Takase et al., 2009). Since the number of septo-hippocampal cholinergic neurons does not appear to be involved in the sex difference in ACh release in the hippocampus, we hypothesized that sex-specific neural circuits or substance(s) may control the endogenous release.

5. Neural control of septo-hippocampal cholinergic neurons

Neurotransmitters may be involved in expression of the sex difference in ACh release. For instance, dopaminergic neurons in the ventral tegmental area (A10) have been shown to control septo-hippocampal cholinergic neurons through the A10-septal dopaminergic pathway in male rats(Swanson, 1982; Nilsson et al., 1992; Yanai etal., 1993). A neuroanatomical study suggested that dopamine D_2receptors rather than D_1 receptors mediate the dopaminergic control of septo-hippocampal cholinergic neurons (Weiner et al., 1991). It has been shown that opiatergic neurons also control septo-hippocampal cholinergic neurons in male rats (Mizuno and Kimura, 1996); the injection of naloxone, a μ opioid receptor antagonist, into the medial septum markedly increased ACh release in the hippocampus, while a μ opioid receptor agonist decreased its release (Mizuno and Kimura, 1996). In contrast, GABA seems to inhibit septo-hippocampal cholinergic neurons; the injection of muscimol, a GABA receptor agonist, into the medial septum decreased ACh release in the hippocampus, while the injection of bicuculline, a GABA receptor antagonist, increased it (Moor et al., 1998). Although the neural systems are still unknown for female rats, it seems likely that neural control of septo-hippocampal cholinergic neurons is involved in the expression of sex differences in ACh release. It will be important to investigate these neural systems in female rats in future studies.

6. Circulating sex steroids activate ACh release

Not only neurotransmitters, but also circulating sex steroids, may regulate cholinergic neurons. In fact, neuroanatomical studies have demonstrated that, in intact male and female rats, a number of dopaminergic neurons in the A10 region have androgen receptor immunoreactivity (Kritzer,1997) and 45-60% of cholinergic neurons in the medial septum have estrogen receptor α immunoreactivity (Miettinen et al.,2002; Mufson et al., 1999). Taken together with the fact that female rats show a greater circulating estrogen concentration than male rats (Shors et al., 2001; Mitsushima et al., 2003b) and male rats show a greater circulating androgen concentration than female rats (Falvo et al., 1974; Rush and Blake, 1982), it is possible that cholinergic neurons are affected by sex steroids differently in male and female rats.

The activational effects of sex steroids on cholinergic neurons have been suggested by previous neuroanatomical and neurochemical findings. For example, male gonadectomy decreases the density of cholinergic fibers in the dorsal hippocampus, while testosterone replacement in gonadectomized male rats maintains fibre density (Nakamura et al., 2002). Also, estradiol increases the induction of choline acetyltransferase in the basal forebrain in gonadectomized female rats (Luine et al., 1986; McEwen and Alves, 1999). A previous *in vitro* study demonstrated that estradiol treatment increases both high affinity choline uptake and ACh synthesis in basal forebrain neurons (Pongrac et al., 2004). Furthermore, we recently reported an activational effect of sex steroids on the maintenance of stress-induced ACh release in the dorsal hippocampus in immobilized rats (Mitsushima et al., 2008). These findings suggest the activational effect of sex steroids on ACh release in the dorsal hippocampus, and we presented conclusive evidence of activational effects on dynamic ACh changes in behaving animals. To analyze the precise effects of sex steroids on ACh release, we simultaneously analyzed ACh release and spontaneous locomotor activity to determine the precise effect of sex steroids. Simultaneous analysis revealed that gonadectomy severely impaired ACh release without affecting spontaneous locomotor activity levels. Moreover, the activational effect on ACh release was apparent, especially during the active period, ie the dark phase, but not during the rest period, the light phase (Figure 4 and Mitsushima et al., 2009). Our results provide the first evidence that the sex-specific 24-h profile of ACh release is highly dependent on the presence of sex steroids.

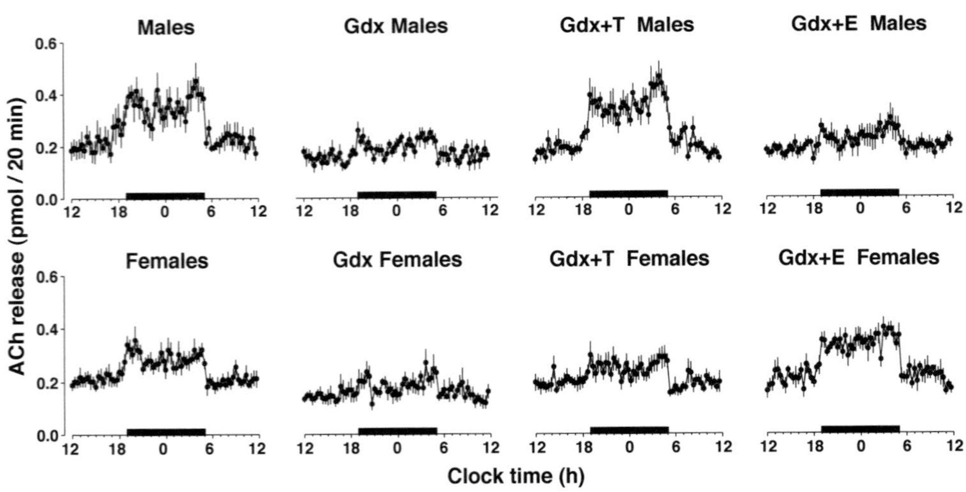

Figure 4. ACh release in the hippocampus is time-dependent, sex-specific, and hormone-dependent. Time-dependent ACh release may transmits the information such as time of day. Experiments were performed 2 weeks after gonadectomy or steroid replacement. Horizontal black bars indicate the dark phase. Gdx, gonadectomized. +T, testosterone-priming. +E, estradiol-priming. The number of animals was 6 to 8 in each group. 19h to 5h is the dark phase, shown as black bars on the x axes.(see Mitsushima et al., 2009)

Moreover, we found that after gonadectomy, the positive correlation between ACh release and locomotor activity levels was severely impaired, suggesting that hippocampal function

http://dx.doi.org/10.5772/52713

may not always be activated at low sex steroid levels (Mitsushima et al., 2009). This therefore suggests that learning impairment in gonadectomized rats (Gibbs and Pfaff, 1992; Daniel et al., 1997; Kritzer et al., 2001; Markowska et al., 2002; Luine et al., 2003) may be due to insufficient activation of hippocampus at the appropriate time. Because the replacement of sex-specific steroids restored the high positive correlation between ACh release and activity levels, the correlation appears to depend on the presence of sex steroids. These results suggest that circulating sex steroids strengthen the coupling between spontaneous behaviour and ACh release (Mitsushima et al., 2009).

7. Sexual differentiation produces the sex-specific activational effect

The activational effect of sex steroids was sex-specific (Figure 4). Testosterone replacement in gonadectomized female rats failed to increase ACh release to levels seen in gonadectomized testosterone-primed male rats. Similarly, estradiol replacement was unable to restore ACh release in gonadectomized male rats. Moreover, estradiol consistently increases N-methyl-D-aspartate receptor binding and spine density in the CA1 area of gonadectomized female rats, although the treatment fails to increase these same parameters in gonadectomized male rats (Romeo et al., 2005; Parducz et al., 2006). These results suggest that sex-specific steroids are important for maintaining hippocampal function. Based on our data, we hypothesized that the action of sex-specific steroids is due to neonatal sexual differentiation rather than the activational effects of sex steroids in adult rats. Moreover, in the latest study, we found that neonatal androgenization in females increased ACh release to resemble that of normal males without affecting spontaneous activity levels (Mitsushima et al., 2009). These results indicate an organizational effect on sex-specific ACh release in behaving rats, and support currently accepted theories of sexual differentiation.

Because testosterone can be aromatized to estradiol in the forebrain, neonatal sex steroids activate both estrogen and androgen receptors (McEwen, 1981). In our study, both testosterone and estradiol treatment in neonatal female pups masculinized ACh release profile in adults, suggesting an estrogen receptor-mediated masculinization of septo-hippocampal cholinergic systems (Mitsushima et al., 2009). These results are consistent with the previous finding that testosterone or estradiol treatment in neonatal female pups improves their adult spatial performance, whereas neonatal gonadectomy in male pups impairs the performance (Williams and Meck, 1991). In contrast, dihydrotestosterone treatment failed to masculinize the ACh release profile. Although dihydrotestosterone has been classically considered as a prototypical androgen receptor agonist, a metabolite of dihydrotestosterone, 3β-diol, has a higher affinity for estrogen receptor β (Lund et al., 2006). Therefore, dihydrotestosterone and its metabolites may stimulate both androgen receptor and estrogen receptor β, whereas estradiol stimulates estrogen receptor α and β. Considering the action of sex steroids and their metabolites, estrogen receptor α may mediate the organizational effect on the septo-hippocampal cholinergic system.

8. Interaction with environmental conditions

Various environmental conditions may interact with the activational effects of sex steroids. First, we reported an interaction between stress and sex steroids. Although sex steroids did not show activational effects on baseline levels of ACh release, sex steroids clearly activated the immobility stress-induced ACh release response. In addition, we found that the contributing sex hormone effect to maintain the ACh release response was sex-specific: testosterone enhanced the ACh release response in male rats, while estradiol maintained the response in females (Mitsushima et al., 2008). Second, we reported an interaction between the light/dark cycle and sex steroids. Although sex steroids slightly enhanced ACh release during the light phase, the activational effects were much stronger during the dark phase (Figure 4). Considering the fact that the time-dependent activational effect was also sex-specific and hormone-dependent, environmental conditions seem to have complicated interactions with sex steroids (Mitsushima et al., 2009).

Some other environmental effects may affect the basal forebrain cholinergic system. Environmental conditions, such as complex or restricted(Brown, 1968; Smith, 1972),enriched or impoverished (Greenough et al., 1972), social or isolated conditions (Hymovitch,1952; Juraska et al., 1984; Seymoure et al., 1996), seem to affect spatial learning ability in a sex-specific manner. For example, male rats exhibited superior performance in learning maze tests compared with female rats if they were housed socially (Einon, 1980). But if they were housed in isolation, female rats exhibited a performance superior to that of male rats (Einon, 1980). Although few studies were performed on the relationship between the sex-specific environmental effects and ACh release in the brain, we have reported that 4-day housing in a small cage attenuates the ACh release in the hippocampus in male rats (Mitsushima et al., 1998), but not in female rats (Masuda et al., 2005). Taken together, these results suggest that housing conditions contribute to the sex difference in ACh release and spatial learning ability.

Feeding conditions after weaning also affect spatial learning ability. If fed pelleted diet (i.e. standard laboratory diet), male rats show performance superior to that of female rats (Beatty, 1984; Williams and Meck, 1991). But when fed powdered diet, female rats, but not male rats, showed improved performance (Endo et al.,1994; Takase et al., 2005a). In our study, it was found that feedingwith powdered diet after weaning increased ACh release in the hippocampus in female rats, but not in male rats(Takase et al., 2005b). 24-HACh release in female rats fed powdered diet was as high as that in male rats fed either powdered or pelleted diet, showing no sex difference. Since feeding with powdered diet improved spatial learning ability in female rats (Endo et al., 1994), the increase in the ACh release in the hippocampus in female rats fed powdered diet may partly contribute to this effect. Our findings provide evidence that environmental conditions such as housing or feeding may play a role in sex-specific hippocampal function.

http://dx.doi.org/10.5772/52713

9. Aging and Alzheimer's disease

Activational effects of sex steroids are very important in humans, since circulating sex steroid levels decline with age. A reduction in ACh synthesis is known as a common feature of Alzheimer's disease (Coyle et al., 1983), afflicting more than 18 million people worldwide (Ferri et al., 2005; Mount and Downtown 2006). The disease is the most common form of dementia (Cummings 2004) and is frequently accompanied by insomnia, poor concentration, and day/night confusion (McCurry et al., 2004; Starkstein et al., 2005). The centrally active acetylcholinesterase inhibitor (donepezil) is effective in not only mild, but also moderate to severe cases (Petersen et al., 2005; Winblad et al., 2006), proving the importance of endogenous ACh in humans. In addition, women are twice as likely to develop the disease (Swaab and Hofman 1995), and estradiol seems to play a protective role (Zandi et al., 2002; Norbury et al., 2007). A recent study using single photon emission tomography showed that estrogen replacement therapy in healthy post-menopausal women increases muscarinic M_1/M_4 receptor binding in the hippocampus (Norbury et al., 2007). Conversely in men, testosterone but not estradiol seems to play a protective role (Moffat et al., 2004; Rosario et al., 2004) and testosterone supplementation clearly improved hippocampal-dependent learning deficits in men with Alzheimer's disease (Cherrier et al., 2005). These results suggest a sex-specific activational effect of gonadal steroids on the cholinergic system in humans. Thus, there are many similarities between the rat model and human studies, supporting the idea that gonadal steroid replacement therapy or an increase in bioavailability is beneficial when there is a subthreshold level of the hormone. Based on the neonatal sexual differentiation of the septo-hippocampal cholinergic system, we may have to search for sex-specific clinical strategies for Alzheimer's disease.

10. Conclusions

Gonadally intact male rats consistently show a greater ACh release in the hippocampus compared with diestrous or proestrous female rats. The activational effects of sex steroids are important for sex-specific ACh release in the hippocampus, since impaired ACh release in gonadectomized rats does not show sex-specific effects. Neonatal treatment with either testosterone or estradiol clearly increased ACh release in female rats, suggesting neonatal sex differentiation of septo-hippocampal cholinergic systems. Moreover, environmental effects on the basal forebrain cholinergic system seem to be sex-specific; housing in a small cage attenuated ACh release in male ratsonly, while feeding with powdered diet after sexual maturation increases ACh release in female ratsonly. These results indicate that: (i) sex-specific circulating sex steroids are necessary for sex-specific ACh release, (ii) neonatal activation of estrogen receptors is sufficient to mediate masculinization of the septo-hippocampal cholinergic system, and (iii) sex-specific effects of environmental conditions may suggest an interaction with the effect of sex hormones.

Understanding the importance of gonadal steroids and the sex-specific effects in cognitive disorders such as Alzheimer's disease is essential for real improvementsin therapy.

Author details

Dai Mitsushima

Address all correspondence to: mitsu@yamaguchi-u.ac.jp

Yamaguchi University Graduate School of Medicine, Ube Yamaguchi, Japan

References

[1] Auerbach JM, Segal M (1996) Muscarinic receptors mediating depression and long-term potentiation in rat hippocampus. J Physiol 492:479–493.

[2] Beatty WW (1984) Hormonal organization of sex differences in play fighting and spatial behavior.Prog Brain Res 61:315–330.

[3] Bliss TVP, Lømo T (1973) Long-lasting potentiation of synaptic transmission in the dentate area of the anaesthetized rabbit following stimulation of the perforant path. J Physiol232 :331-356.

[4] Boccia MM, Blake MG, Krawczyk MC, Baratti CM (2010) Hippocampal alpha7 nicotinic receptors modulate memory reconsolidation of an inhibitory avoidance task in mice. Neuroscience 171: 531-543.

[5] Brown RT (1968) Early experience and problem-solving ability. J Comp PhysiolPsychol 65:433–440.

[6] Buzsáki G, Bickford RG, Ponomareff G, Thal LJ, Mandel R, Gage FH (1988) Nucleus basalis and thalamic control of neocortical activity in the freely moving rat. J Neurosci 8:4007–4026.

[7] Chen G, Wang LP, Tsien JZ (2009) Neural population-level memory traces in the mouse hippocampus. PLoS ONE 4: e8256.

[8] Cherrier MM, Matsumoto AM, Amory JK, Asthana S, Bremner W, Peskind ER, Raskind MA, Craft S (2005) Testosterone improves spatial memory in men with Alzheimer disease and mild cognitive impairment. Neurology 64:2063-2068.

[9] Cole AE, Nicoll RA (1983) Acetylcholine mediates a slow synaptic potential in hippocampal pyramidal cells. Science 221:1299–1301.

[10] Coyle JT, Price DL, DeLong MR (1983) Alzheimer's disease: a disorder of cortical cholinergic innervation. Science 219:1184-1190.

[11] Cummings JL (2004) Alzheimer's disease. New Engl J Med 351:56-67.

[12] Daniel JM, Fader AJ, Spencer AL, Dohanich GP (1997) Estrogen enhances performance of female rats during acquisition of a radial arm maze. HormBehav 32:217–225.

[13] Day J, Damsma G, Fibiger HC (1991) Cholinergic activity in the rat hippocampus, cortex and striatum correlates with locomotor activity: an in vivo microdialysis study. PharmacolBiochemBehav38:723–729.

[14] Eckel-Mahan KL, Phan T, Han S, Wang H, Chan GC, Scheiner ZS, Storm DR (2008) Circadian oscillation of hippocampal MAPK activity and cAMP: implications for memory persistence.Nat Neurosci 11:1074-1082.

[15] Einon D (1980) Spatial memory and response strategies in rats: Age, sex and rearing differences in performance. Q J ExpPsychol 32:473–489.

[16] Endo Y, Mizuno T, Fujita K, Funabashi T, Kimura F (1994) Soft-diet feeding during development enhances later learning abilities in female rats. PhysiolBehav 56:629–633.

[17] Falvo RE, Buhl A, Nalbandov AV (1974) Testosterone concentrations in the peripheral plasma of androgenized female rats and in the estrous cycle of normal female rats. Endocrinology 95:26–29.

[18] Fernández de Sevilla D, Nu´n˜ ez A, Borde M, Malinow R, Bun˜o W (2008) Cholinergic-mediated IP3-receptor activation induces long-lasting synaptic enhancement in CA1 pyramidal neurons. J Neurosci 28:1469–1478.

[19] Ferri CP, Prince M, Brayne C, Brodaty H, Fratiglioni L, Ganguli M, Hall K, Hasegawa K, Hendrie H, Huang Y, Jorm A, Mathers C, Menezes PR, Rimmer E, Scazufca M (2005) Global prevalence of dementia: a Delphi consensus study. Lancet 366: 2112–2117.

[20] Fisahn A, Pike FG, Buhl EH, Paulsen O (1998) Cholinergic induction of networkoscillations at 40Hz in the hippocampus in vitro. Nature 394:186-189.

[21] Gelbard-Sagiv H, Mukamel R, Harel M, Malach R, Fried I (2008) Internally generated reactivation of single neurons in human hippocampus during free recall. Science 322: 96-101.

[22] Gibbs RB, Pfaff DW (1992) Effects of estrogen and fimbria / fornix transaction on p75NGFR and ChAT expression in the medial septum and diagonal band of Broca. ExpNeurol116:23–39.

[23] Gold PE (2003) Acetylcholine modulation of neural systems involved in learning and memory.Neurobiol Learn Mem 80:194–210.

[24] Greenough WT, Madden TC, Fleischmann TB (1972) Effects of isolation, daily handling, and enriched rearing on maze learning.PsychonSci 27:279–280.

[25] Herrera-Morales W, Mar I, Serrano B, Bermu´dez-Rattoni F (2007) Activation of hippocampal postsynaptic muscarinic receptors is involved in long-term spatial memory formation. Eur J Neurosci 25:1581–1588.

[26] Hironaka N, Tanaka K, Izaki Y, Hori K, Nomura M (2001) Memory-related acetylcholine efflux from the rat prefrontal cortex and hippocampus: a microdialysis study. Brain Res 901:143–150.

[27] Hyman JM, Wyble BP, Goyal V, Rossi CA, Hasselmo ME (2003) Stimulation in hippocampal region CA1 in behaving rats yields long-term potentiation when delivered to the peak of theta and long-term depression when delivered to the trough. J Neurosci 23:11725–11731.

[28] Hymovitch B (1952) The effects of experimental variations on problem solving in the rat. J Comp PhysiolPsychol 45:313–321.

[29] Juraska JM, Henderson C, Muller J (1984) Differential rearing experience, gender, and radial maze performance.DevPsychobiol 17:209–215.

[30] sychobiol 17:209–215.

[31] Komorowski RW, Manns JR, Eichenbaum H (2009) Robust conjunctive item-place coding by hippocampal neurons parallels learning what happens where. J Neurosci 29:9918-9929.

[32] Kotani S, Yamauchi T, Teramoto T, Ogura H (2006) Pharmacological evidence of cholinergic involvement in adult hippocampal neurogenesis in rats. Neuroscience 142:505–514.

[33] Kritzer MF (1997) Selective colocalization of immunoreactivity for intracellular gonadal hormone receptors and tyrosine hydroxylase in the ventral tegmental area, substantianigra, and retrorubral fields in the rat. J Comp Neurol 379:247–260.

[34] Kritzer MF, McLaughlin PJ, Smirlis T, Robinson JK (2001) Gonadectomy impairs T-maze acquisition in adult male rats. HormBehav 39:167–174.

[35] Lee MG, Chrobak JJ, Sik A, Wiley RG, Buzsáki G (1994) Hippocampal theta activity following selective lesion of the septal cholinergic system. Neuroscience 62:1033–1047.

[36] Luine V, Jacome LF, MacLusky NJ (2003) Rapid enhancement of visual and place memory by estrogens in rats. Endocrinology 144:2836–2844.

[37] Luine VN, Renner KJ, McEwen BS (1986) Sex-dependent differences in estrogen regulation of choline acetyltransferaseare altered by neonatal treatments. Endocrinology 119:874–878.

[38] Lund TD, Hinds LR, Handa RJ (2006) The androgen 5 ▪ -dihydrotestosterone and its metabolite 5 ▪ -androstan-3 ▪ ,17 ▪ -diol inhibit the hypothalamo-pituitary-adrenal response to stress by acting through estrogen receptor ▪ -expressing neurons in the hypothalamus. J Neurosci 26:1448–1456.

[39] Markowska AJ, Savonenko AV (2002) Effectiveness of estrogen replacement in restoration of cognitive function after long-term estrogen withdrawal in aging rats. J Neurosci 22:10985–10995.

[40] Markram H, Segal M (1990) Long-lasting facilitation of excitatory postsynaptic potentials in the rat hippocampus by acetylcholine. J Physiol 427:381–393.

[41] Masuda J, Mitsushima D, Funabashi T, Kimura F (2005) Sex and housing conditions affect the 24-h acetylcholine release profile in the hippocampus in rats. Neuroscience 132:537–542.

[42] McCurry SM, Logsdon RG, Vitiello MV, Teri L (2004) Treatment of sleep and nighttime disturbances in Alzheimer's disease: a behavior management approach. Sleep Med 5:373-377.

[43] McEwen BS (1981) Neural gonadal steroid actions. Science 211:1303–1311.

[44] McEwen BS, Alves SE (1999) Estrogen actions in the central nervous system. Endocr Rev 20:279–307.

[45] Mesulam MM, Mufson EJ, Wainer BH, Levey AI (1983) Central cholinergic pathways in the rat: an overview based on an alternative nomenclature (Ch1-Ch6). Neuroscience 10:1185–1201.

[46] Miettinen RA, Kalesnykas G, Koivisto EH (2002) Estimation of the total number of cholinergic neurons containing estrogen receptor-a in the rat basal forebrain. J HistochemCytochem 50:891–902.

[47] Mitsushima D, Mizuno T, Kimura F (1996) Age-related changes in diurnal acetylcholine release in the prefrontal cortex of male rats as measured by microdialysis. Neuroscience 72:429–434.

[48] Mitsushima D, Yamanoi C, Kimura F (1998) Restriction of environmental space attenuates locomotor activity and hippocampal acetylcholine release in male rats. Brain Res 805:207–212.

[49] Mitsushima D, Funabashi T, Shinohara K, Kimura F (2001) Impairment of maze learning in rats by restricting environmental space. NeurosciLett 297:73–76.

[50] Mitsushima D, Masuda J, Kimura F (2003a) Sex differences in the stress-induced release of acetylcholine in the hippocampus and corticosterone from the adrenal cortex in rats. Neuroendocrinology 78:234–240.

[51] Mitsushima D, Tin-Tin-Win-Shwe, Kimura F (2003b) Sexual dimorphism in the GABAergic control of gonadotropin release in intact rats.Neurosci Res 46:399–405.

[52] Mitsushima D, Takase K, Funabashi T, Kimura F (2008) Gonadal steroid hormones maintain the stress-induced acetylcholine release in the hippocampus: simultaneous measurements of the extracellular acetylcholine and serum corticosterone levels in the same subjects.Endocrinology 149:802–811.

[53] Mitsushima D, Takase K, Funabashi T, Kimura F (2009) Gonadal steroids maintain 24-h acetylcholine release in the hippocampus: organizational and activational effects in behaving rats. J Neurosci29:3808–3815.

[54] Mitsushima D, Ishihara K, Sano A, Kessels HW, Takahashi T (2011) Contextual learning requires synaptic AMPA receptor delivery in the hippocampus. ProcNatlAcadSci USA 108: 12503-12508.

[55] Mizuno T, Endo Y, Arita J, Kimura F (1991) Acetylcholine release in the rat hippocampus as measured by the microdialysis method correlates with motor activity and exhibits a diurnal variation. Neuroscience 44:607–612.

[56] Mizuno T, Kimura F (1996) Medial septal injection of naloxone elevates acetylcholine release in the hippocampus and induces behavioral seizures in rats. Brain Res 713:1–7.

[57] Moffat SD, Zonderman AB, Metter EJ, Kawas C, Blackman MR, Harman SM, Resnick SM (2004) Free testosterone and risk for Alzheimer disease in older men. Neurology 62:188-193.

[58] Mohapel P, Leanza G, Kokaia M, Lindvall O (2005) Forebrain acetylcholine regulates adult hippocampal neurogenesis and learning. Neurobiol Aging 26:939–946.

[59] Morris RGM, Anderson E, Lynch GS, Baudry M (1986) Selective impairment of learning and blockade of long-term potentiation by an N-methyl-D-aspartate receptor antagonist, AP5. Nature 319: 774-776.

[60] Mount C, Downtown D (2006) Alzheimer disease: progress or profit? Nat Med 12:780-784.

[61] Moor E, DeBoer P, Westerink BHC (1998) GABA receptors and benzodiazepine binding sites modulate hippocampal acetylcholine release in vivo. Eur J Pharmacol 359:119–126.

[62] Mufson EJ, Cai WJ, Jaffar S, Chen E, Stebbins G, Sendera T, Kordower JH (1999) Estrogen receptor immunoreactivity within subregions of the rat forebrain: neuronal distribution and association with perikarya containing choline acetyltransferase. Brain Res 849:253–274.

[63] Nakamura N, Fujita H, Kawata M (2002) Effects of gonadectomy on immunoreactivity for choline acetyltransferase in the cortex, hippocampus, and basal forebrain of adult male rats. Neuroscience 109:473–485.

[64] Nilsson OG, Leanza G, Bjorklund A (1992) Acetylcholine release in the hippocampus: regulation by monoaminergic afferents as assessed by in vivo microdialysis. Brain Res 584:132–140.

[65] Norbury R, Travis MJ, Erlandsson K, Waddington W, Ell PJ, Murphy DGM (2007) Estrogen therapy and brain muscarinic receptor density in healthy females: a SPET study. HormBehav 51:249-257.

[66] Parducz A, Hajszan T, Maclusky NJ, Hoyk Z, Csakvari E, Kurunczi A, Prange-Kiel J, Leranth C (2006) Synaptic remodeling induced by gonadal hormones: neuronal plasticity as a mediator of neuroendocrine and behavioral responses to steroids. Neuroscience 138: 977–985.

[67] Parent MB, Baxter MG (2004) Septohippocampal acetylcholine: involved in but not necessary for learning and memory? Learn Mem 11: 9–20.

[68] Perry E, Walker M, Grace J, Perry R (1999) Acetylcholine in mind: a neurotransmitter correlate of consciousness? Trend Neurosci 22:273–280.

[69] Petersen RC, Thomas RG, Grundman M, Bennett D, Doody R, Ferris S, Galasko D, Jin S, Kaye J, Levey A, Pfeiffer E, Sano M, van Dyck CH, Thal LJ (2005) Vitamin E and donepezil for the treatment of mild cognitive impairment. New Engl J Med 352: 2379-2388.

[70] Pongrac JL, Gibbs RB, Defranco DB (2004) Estrogen-mediated regulation of cholinergic expression in basal forebrain neurons requires extracellular signal-regulated kinase activity. Neuroscience 124:809–816.

[71] Ragozzino ME, Unick KE, Gold PE (1996) Hippocampal acetylcholine release during memory testing in rats: augmentation by glucose. ProcNatlAcadSci USA 93:4693–4698.

[72] Rogers JL, Kesner RP (2004) Cholinergic modulation of the hippocampus during encoding and retrieval of tone/shock-induced fear conditioning. Learning Mem 11: 102-107.

[73] Romeo RD, McCarthy JB, Wang A, Milner TA, McEwen BS (2005) Sex differences in hippocampal estradiol-induced N-methyl-D-aspartic acid binding and ultrastructural localization of estrogen receptor- ▪ . Neuroendocrinology 81:391–399.

[74] Rosario ER, Chang L, Stanczyk FZ, Pike CJ (2004) Age-related testosterone deplation and the development of Alzheimer disease. JAMA 292:1431-1432.

[75] Rush ME, Blake CA (1982) Serum testosterone concentrations during the 4-day estrous cycle in normal and adrenalectomized rats. ProcSocExpBiol Med 169:216–221.

[76] Sarter M, Parikh V (2005) Choline transporters, cholinergic transmission and cognition. Nat Neurosci 6:48–56.

[77] Scoville WB & Milner B (1957) Loss of recent memory after bilateral hippocampal lesions. J Neurology, Neurosurgery and Psychiatry 20:11-21.

[78] Seeger T, Fedorova I, Zheng F, Miyakawa T, Koustova E, Gomeza J, Basile AS, Alzheimer C, Wess J (2004) M2 muscarinic acetylcholine receptor knock-out mice show deficits in behavioral flexibility, working memory, and hippocampal plasticity. J Neurosci 24:10117–10127.

[79] Seymoure P, Dou H, JuraskaJMze performance: influence of rearing environment and room cues. Psychobiology 24:33–37.

[80] Shinoe T, Matsui M, Taketo MM, Manabe T (2005) Modulation of synaptic plasticity by physiological activation of M1 muscarinic acetylcholine receptors in the mouse hippocampus. J Neurosci 25:11194–11200.

[81] Shors TJ, Chua C, Falduto J (2001) Sex differences and opposite effects of stress on dendritic spine density in the male versus female hippocampus. J Neurosci 21:6292–6297.

[82] Smith HV (1972) Effects of environmental enrichment on open-field activity and Hebb–Williams problem solving in rats. J Comp PhysiolPsychol 80:163–168.

[83] Stancampiano R, Cocco S, Cugusi C, Sarais L, Fadda F (1999) Serotonin and acetylcholine release response in the rat hippocampus during a spatial memory task. Neuroscience 89:1135–1143.

[84] Starkstein SE, Jorge R, Mizrahi R, Robinson RG (2005) The construct of minor and major depression in Alzheimer's disease. Am J Psychiatry 162:2086-2093.

[85] Swaab DF, Hofman MA (1995) Sexual differentiation of the human hypothalamus in relation to gender and sexual orientation. Trend Neurosci 18:264-270.

[86] Swanson LW (1982) The projections of the ventral tegmental area and adjacent regions: A combined fluorescent retrograde tracer and immunofluorescence study in the rat. Brain Res Bull 9:321–353.

[87] Takase K, Funabashi T, Mogi K, Mitsushima D, Kimura F (2005a) Feeding with powdered diet after weaning increases visuospatial ability in association with increases in the expression of N-methyl-D-aspartate receptors in the hippocampus of female rats. Neurosci Res 53:169–175.

[88] Takase K, Mitsushima D, Masuda J, Mogi K, Funabashi T, Endo Y, Kimura F (2005b) Feeding with powdered diet after weaning affects sex difference in acetylcholine release in the hippocampus in rats. Neuroscience 136:593–599.

[89] Takase K, Kimura F, Yagami T, Mitsushima D (2009) Sex-specific 24-h acetylcholine release profile in the medial prefrontal cortex: simultaneous measurement of spontaneous locomotor activity in behaving rats. Neuroscience159:7–15.

[90] van Praag H, Christie BR, Sejnowski TJ, Gage FH (1999) Running enhances neurogenesis, learning and long-term potentiation in mice. ProcNatlAcadSci USA 96:13427–13431.

[91] Weiner DM, Levey AI, Sunahara RK, Niznik HB, O'Dowd BF, Seeman P, Brann MR (1991) D1 and D2 dopamine receptor mRNA in rat brain. ProcNatlAcadSci U S A 88:1859–1863.

[92] Widmer H, Ferrigan L, Davies CH, Cobb SR (2006) Evoked slow muscarinic acetylcholinergic synaptic potentials in rat hippocampal interneurons. Hippocampus 16:617–628.

[93] Whitlock JR, Heynen AJ, Shuler MG, Bear MF (2006) Learning induces long-term potentiation in the hippocampus. Science 313: 1093-1097.

[94] Williams CL, Meck WH (1991) The organizational effects of gonadal steroids on sexually dimorphic spatial ability. Psychoneuroendocrinology 16:155–176.

[95] Wills TJ, Cacucci F, Burgess N, O'Keefe J (2010) Development of the hippocampal cognitive map in preweanling rats. Science 328: 1573-1576.

[96] Winblad B, Kilander L, Eriksson S, Minthon L, Båtsman S, Wetterholm AL, Jansson-Blixt C, Haglund A (2006) Donepezil in patients with severe Alzheimer's disease: double-blind, parallel-group, placebo-controlled study. Lancet 367:1057-1065.

[97] Yanai J, Rogel-Fuchs Y, Pick CG, Slotkin T, Seidler FJ, Zahalka EA, Newman ME (1993) Septohippocampal cholinergic changes after destruction of the A10-septal dopaminergic pathways. Neuropharmacology 32:113–117.

[98] Zandi PP, Carlson MC, Plassman BL, Welsh-Bohmer KA, Mayer LS, Steffens DC, Breitner JCS (2002) Hormone replacement therapy and incidence of Alzheimer disease in older women. JAMA 288:2123-2129.

Chapter 4

11β-Hydroxysteroid Dehydrogenases in the Regulation of Tissue Glucocorticoid Availability

Cidália Pereira, Rosário Monteiro,
Miguel Constância and Maria João Martins

Additional information is available at the end of the chapter

http://dx.doi.org/10.5772/53645

1. Introduction

The regulation of tissue-specific actions of glucocorticoids (GCs) goes far beyond the effects of the fluctuation of their circulating levels and can be controlled by local intracellular enzymes. In the past few years, evidence is being gathered not only on the relevance of such enzymes to GC physiological actions but also on their involvement in the pathophysiology of certain chronic disease states, in which circulating GC levels are not necessarily altered. These enzymes are hydroxysteroid dehydrogenases (11β-HSDs; EC 1.1.1.146), which interconvert inactive GCs and the active GCs (Gathercole & Stewart, 2010; Seckl & Walker, 2004; Stewart, 2005; Tomlinson et al., 2004).

2. Regulation of glucocorticoid synthesis by the hypothalamus-pituitary-adrenal axis

GCs are part of the hypothalamus-pituitary-adrenal (HPA) axis, a tighly controlled endocrine component with essential roles in the regulation of physiological processes, such as stress responses, energy metabolism, electrolyte levels, blood pressure, immunity, cognitive functions and cell proliferation and differentiation (Atanasov & Odermatt, 2007; Papadimitriou & Priftis, 2009). Cortisol constitutes the main active hormone of the HPA axis and is released by the adrenal gland under the control of the remaining hormones of the axis. Corticotropin-releasing hormone (CRH), produced by hypothalamic neurons, is released onto the anterior pituitary where it stimulates the synthesis and secretion of the adenocorticotropic hormone (ACTH) into the blood. This occurs in a pulsatile manner and with circadian rhythmicity, with higher levels being secreted in early morning and lowering through the afternoon and night (Gathercole & Stewart, 2010; White, 2008b). ACTH acts on the melanocortin 2 receptor (MC2R) in the adrenal cortex and has only a half-life of 10 min. There, it acutely increases cortisol and androgen production as well as the expression of the enzymes involved in their biosynthetic pathways, having a trophic effect on the adrenal cortex. Enhanced production of cortisol negatively regulates the synthesis and release of both CRH and ACTH by the hypothalamus and the pituitary, respectively, despite the ability of the hypothalamus to change the "set point" for the HPA axis to a higher level during severe or chronic stress. Regulators of the HPA axis include neurogenic and systemic stress (White, 2008b).

The zona fasciculata of the adrenal cortex is where the synthesis of most cortisol occurs. Through the stimulating action of ACTH, cholesterol esters, stored in the cytoplasm of these cells, are unsterified by cholesterol ester hydrolase and converted sequentially to pregnenolone [by cytochrome P450 (CYP) 11A1], progesterone [by 3β-hydroxysteroid dehydrogenase (3β-HSD)], 17-hydroxyprogesterone (by CYP17, 17-hydroxylase function), 11-deoxycortisol (by CYP21A2, 21-hydroxylase function) and cortisol (by CYP11B1, 11-hydroxylase function). As a minor pathway in humans, progesterone is converted to 11-deoxycorticosterone (by CYP11B2, 11-hydroxylase function) and then to corticosterone (by CYP11B2, 18-hydroxylase function). Plasma cortisol has a half-life of 70-120 min where it circulates bound to corticosteroid-binding globulin (CBG or transcortin; 90%) and to albumin (5-7%). The remaining constitutes the free, active, fraction (Tomlinson et al., 2004; White, 2008a).

Most cortisol actions take place through binding to GC receptors (GR) and mineralocorticoid receptors (MR) (Dzyakanchuk et al., 2009), nuclear receptors that are members of the steroid hormone receptor family (Gathercole & Stewart, 2010). Cortisol as well as the main GC in rodents, corticosterone, are active steroids whereas cortisone and 11-dehydrocorticosterone, the latter in rodents, are inactive steroids (Tomlinson et al., 2004). Upon GC-binding, the GR moves into the nucleus where it binds specific GC response elements (GRE) and recruits co-activators and co-repressors, which, once bound, enhance or repress gene transcription (Gathercole & Stewart, 2010). Cortisol and corticosterone are secreted in high amounts [15 mg/d (Cope & Black, 1958; Esteban et al., 1991) and 2 mg/d (Peterson & Pierce, 1960), respectively]. Cortisol concentration in the adrenal vein is about 3.7 nmol/mL whereas cortisone level is 0.13 nmol/mL, contrasting with 0.18 nmol/mL and 0.03 nmol/mL, respectively, in the vena cava (Tortorella et al., 1999). However, free cortisone concentrations are similar to those of free cortisol because of the lower binding of the former to CBG (Tomlinson et al., 2004). Cortisol is inactivated in the liver through conjugation with glucuronide and sulfate and subsequently excreted in the urine (Tomlinson et al., 2004; White, 2008b). In the liver, 5α- and 5β-reductases also inactivate cortisol and cortisone, in conjunction with 3α-HSD, to tetrahydrometabolites: 5α-tetrahydrocortisol, 5β-tetrahydrocortisol and tetrahydrocortisone (Campino et al., 2010; Russell & Wilson, 1994).

3. Regulation of tissue glucocorticoid availability

3.1. 11β-Hydroxysteroid dehydrogenase type 2

Cortisol is inactivated to cortisone, in humans, or corticosterone to 11-dehydrocorticosterone, in rodents, in order to avoid deleterious actions of active GCs overstimulation of the MR. This occurs because cortisol and aldosterone have the same *in vitro* affinity for the MR (Arriza et al., 1987; Gathercole & Stewart, 2010). The enzyme responsible for the regulation of active GC availability to the MR is 11β-HSD2, a NAD^+ dependent dehydrogenase. Its tissue expression is related to the presence of the MR, the kidney (distal convoluted tubule) being the typical example and the main location of cortisone production (Cooper & Stewart, 2009; Edwards et al., 1988; Gathercole & Stewart, 2010; Walker, B. & Andrew, 2006). However, 11β-HSD2 is also present in other locations such as the colon, salivary and sweat glands, placenta and vascular wall (Anagnostis et al., 2009; Andrews et al., 2003; Edwards et al., 1988; Ferrari, 2010; Funder et al., 1988; Gathercole & Stewart, 2010; Palermo et al., 2004).

Congenital deficiency of 11β-HSD2 in humans (Dave-Sharma et al., 1998; Gathercole & Stewart, 2010; Stewart et al., 1996), transgenic deletion in mice (Kotelevtsev et al., 1999) or pharmacological inhibition of 11β-HSD2 results in a clinical condition termed apparent mineralocorticoid excess (AME) syndrome (Sundbom et al., 2008). Affected subjects, despite having normal circulating levels of cortisol and no disturbances of the HPA axis, present with sodium retention, hypertension and hypokalemia (Anagnostis et al., 2009; Andrews et al., 2003; Edwards et al., 1988; Gathercole & Stewart, 2010; Monder et al., 1986; Mune et al., 1995; Palermo et al., 2004; Quinkler & Stewart, 2003; Stewart et al., 1996; Walker, B. & Andrew, 2006). These alterations arise from the activity of GCs on MR-expressing cells since the lack of GC inactivation allows their mineralocorticoid action. In this sense, AME has been considered a 'Cushing's disease of the kidney' (Stewart, 2005).

3.2. 11β-Hydroxysteroid dehydrogenase type 1

Opposite to 11β-HSD2, 11β-HSD1 reactivates inactive cortisone in humans (11-dehydrocorticosterone in rodents) back into cortisol (corticosterone in rodents) within cells expressing the enzyme (Anagnostis et al., 2009; Chapman et al., 2006; Espindola-Antunes & Kater, 2007; Stewart & Krozowski, 1999). This enzyme is in higher amounts in the liver, adipose tissue (AT), lung and the central nervous system. However, pancreas, kidney cortex, adrenal cortex, cardiac myocytes, bone, placenta, uterus, testis, oocytes and luteinized granulosa cells of the ovary, eye, pituitary, fibroblasts and immune, skeletal and smooth muscle cells are also sites of 11β-HSD1 expression (Anagnostis et al., 2009; Bujalska et al., 1997; Cooper & Stewart, 2009; Espindola-Antunes & Kater, 2007; Stewart & Krozowski, 1999; Tomlinson et al., 2004; Whorwood et al., 2001). In these locations, it is associated with GR rather than with MR (Walker, B. & Andrew, 2006). Acting as a reductase, it assures that GCs have access to GR since GR affinity for cortisol is relatively low, what becomes particularly relevant when cortisol levels are at their lowest due to their circadian variation (while cortisone levels remain constant) (Walker, B. & Andrew, 2006; Walker, B. et al., 1995).

Both 11β-HSD1 and 11β-HSD2 are located in the endoplasmic reticulum (ER). However, 11β-HSD1 is facing the lumen (Gathercole & Stewart, 2010; Ozols, 1995) where hexose-6-phosphate dehydrogenase (H6PDH) coexists and converts glucose-6-phosphate to 6-phosphogluconolactone in a reaction that regenerates NADPH from $NADP^+$ (Atanasov et al., 2008; Bujalska et al., 2005; Draper et al., 2003; Dzyakanchuk et al., 2009). The resulting high concentration of NADPH provides the reducing equivalents necessary for 11β-HSD1 activity. Another advantage of this cellular location is the maintenance of important intra-chain disulfide bonds within the 11β-HSD1 protein (Ozols, 1995; Tomlinson et al., 2004). Human 11β-HSD1 has three putative glycosylation sites: asparagine-X-serine sites at positions 123–125, 162–164 and 207–209 of the protein. However, it seems that, although not required for enzyme activity (Walker, E. et al., 2001) nor correct protein folding, glycosylation of 11β-HSD1 may be necessary for preventing protein aggregation and for stabilizing its structure within the ER (Tomlinson et al., 2004).

11β-HSD1 in intact cells such as hepatocytes (Jamieson et al., 1995) and adipocytes (Bujalska et al., 2002a; Bujalska et al., 2002b) [as well as in myocytes (Whorwood et al., 2001)] works mainly as a reductase, which is revealed by the higher affinity of the enzyme derived from these locations for cortisone than for cortisol (Stewart et al., 1994). However, *in vitro* when deprived of NADPH regeneration (Seckl & Walker, 2001; Walker, B. & Andrew, 2006) or in certain physiological or developmental states, it may work as a dehydrogenase, meaning that the enzyme is bidirectional (Cooper & Stewart, 2009; Tomlinson et al., 2004). This becomes evident when 11β-HSD1 switches from a dehydrogenase to a reductase functioning in human omental adipose stromal cells upon differentiation (Bujalska et al., 2002a; Bujalska et al., 2002b) or when it acts mainly as a dehydrogenase in the liver or AT of the *H6PDH* null mouse (Bujalska et al., 2008; Lavery et al., 2006).

The human *HSD11B1* gene is located in the chromosome 1 (1q32.2–41) and consists of six exons (182, 130, 111, 185, 143 and 617 bp, respectively) and five introns (776, 767, 120, 25,300 and 1,700 bp, respectively) with a total gene size of 30 kb (Draper et al., 2002; Tomlinson et al., 2004). 11β-HSD1 belongs to the short chain dehydrogenase/reductase (SDR) superfamily, a well-established enzyme family of oxido-reductases. Members of this family have a conserved N-terminal cofactor-binding domain, which confers specificity to NADPH, and a centrally located active site (Jornvall et al., 1995), containing invariant tyrosine, lysine and serine residues that consisted of the catalytic triad to which the essential presence of asparagine at 111 position has been added to form a tetrad (Filling et al., 2002; Oppermann et al., 2003; Tomlinson et al., 2004). The rat *HSD11B1* promoter has been cloned from genomic DNA (Moisan et al., 1992) and several transcription factor-binding sites were identified including several GRE consensus half-sites as well as hepatocyte nuclear factor 1, hepatocyte nuclear factor 3 and CCAAT/enhancer-binding proteins (C/EBP) sites (Williams et al., 2000). The importance of C/EBP-α has been highlighted in the regulation of *HSD11B1* transcription (Seckl & Walker, 2001; Wang et al., 1995). In human cell lines, there is evidence that promoter usage in expression of human *HSD11B1* is specific for tissue and differentiation status (Staab et al., 2011).

As with 11β-HSD2, congenital deficiency of 11β-HSD1 has been described in humans and gives rise to the apparent cortisone reductase deficiency syndrome (Phillipov et al., 1996). In this case, the lack of regeneration of cortisol in peripheral tissues results in the compensatory activation of the HPA axis translation into increased secretion of androgens by the adrenals, which, in affected females, originates hirsutism and oligomenorrhea. 11β-HSD1 congenital deficiency does not appear to protect against obesity. Curiously, the co-inheritance of inactivating mutations in both *HSD11B1* and *H6PDH* (Draper et al., 2003), decreasing NADPH supply and switching 11β-HSD1 to the dehydrogenase activity (Lavery et al., 2006), may also be in the origin of the syndrome.

3.3. Glucocorticoid deficiency

GC deficiency, seen in Addison's disease or ACTH deficiency, presents with weight loss and hypoglycemia as clinical features, that seem opposite to those of Cushing's syndrome (Walker, B., 2007). Some of these features of GC deficiency may be recapitulated in animals with type 2 diabetes mellitus (T2DM) and obesity after treatment with the GR antagonist RU38486 (mifepristone), which present with normalized blood glucose and ameliorated insulin resistance (IR) (Bitar, 2001; Gettys et al., 1997; Havel et al., 1996; Jacobson et al., 2005; Kusunoki et al., 1995; Walker, B., 2007; Watts et al., 2005). However, RU38486 may induce compensation from the HPA axis since it blocks GR involved in the HPA axis negative feedback control. Furthermore, progesterone receptor actions of the drug may also influence energy homeostasis (Picard et al., 2002). These effects of GC deficiency are in favor of the usefulness of strategies of reducing GCs action in the management of blood glucose levels and insulin sensitivity and, possibly, body weight.

3.4. Glucocorticoid excess

Although the elevation of GC levels in situations of stress is essential for survival, their chronic augmentation is associated with deleterious health outcomes. Opposite to their deficit, chronically elevated GC levels cause obesity, T2DM, heart disease, mood disorders and memory impairments (Wamil & Seckl, 2007). Elevated GC levels occur in Cushing's syndrome due to increased pathological secretion from the adrenal cortex (endogenous) or from prolonged anti-inflammatory GC treatment (iatrogenic) (Newell-Price et al., 2006). Cushing 's disease, a specific type of ACTH-dependent Cushing's syndrome, is characterized by increased ACTH secretion from a pituitary adenoma that in turn results in higher cortisol secretion from the adrenals (Cushing, 1932). Cushing's syndrome features include hypertension, rapidly accumulating visceral AT, IR (50% develop T2DM or impaired glucose tolerance) and hepatic steatosis (Stewart, 2005); muscle weakness, dyslipidemia, mood disturbances and infertility (Carroll & Findling, 2010; Newell-Price et al., 2006) are also frequently found. Although many of the clinical components (central weight gain, glucose intolerance and hypertension) are seen in other common conditions, identifying features unusual for the patient's age (e.g. early onset osteoporosis or hypertension), features more specific to Cushing's syndrome (e.g. easy bruising, facial plethora and violaceous striae) and patients with incidental adrenal mass or polycystic ovary syndrome should be helpful for the diagnosis (Carroll & Findling, 2010).

In effect, Cushing's syndrome represents a secondary cause of metabolic syndrome (MetSyn) (Stewart, 2005). Circulating cortisol concentrations are higher in patients with the MetSyn, hypertension or impaired glucose tolerance compared with healthy subjects, both in basal conditions and during dynamic stimulation (Anagnostis et al., 2009; Duclos et al., 2005; Misra et al., 2008; Phillips et al., 1998; Sen et al., 2008; Weigensberg et al., 2008), despite being within the normal range (Sen et al., 2008; Walker, B., 2006). This suggests increased activity of cortisol in the periphery and dysregulation of the HPA axis (Sen et al., 2008; Walker, B., 2006). However, it has also been proposed that variations in tissue cortisol concentrations could occur without any changes in plasma cortisol levels, provided that the latter are maintained by normal feedback regulation of the HPA axis (Walker, B. & Andrew, 2006). In regard to the visceral AT, this effect has been termed 'Cushing's disease of the omentum' (Bujalska et al., 1997; Stewart, 2005). Increased 11β-HSD1 activity in visceral AT may generate increased cortisol levels within both the AT and the liver and, thereby promotes features of the MetSyn (Walker, B. & Andrew, 2006). The rate of regeneration of cortisol in the visceral AT has been estimated to be sufficient to increase the concentration of cortisol in the portal vein (from about 120 nmol/L in the systemic circulation to about 155 nmol/L in the portal vein) and this has been confirmed in mice overexpressing 11β-HSD1 in the AT (Masuzaki et al., 2001; Walker, B. & Andrew, 2006).

In agreement, transgenic mice overexpressing 11β-HSD1 selectively in the AT or in the liver faithfully recapitulate MetSyn features and *HSD11B1* knockout mice or humans and rodents treated with 11β-HSD1 inhibitors seem to be protected from the cardiometabolic risks of obesity, T2DM and/or MetSyn. Very recently, we have reviewed the involvement of 11β-HSD1 in the pathophysiology of the MetSyn, obesity and T2DM, where a description not only of these animal models [also together with the animal model overexpressing 11β-HSD2 in the AT (phenotypically similar to the *HSD11B1* knockout animals)] but also of the nutritional and pharmacological modulation of 11β-HSD1 is provided (Pereira et al., 2011; 2012).

4. Epigenetics and 11β-hydroxysteroid dehydrogenase type 2

4.1. Epigenetic regulation of gene expression

Epigenetics is not a new area of investigation, as it was first described in the early 1940s (Jablonka & Lamb, 2002), but it is a hot topic of research today, since it became evident that genetic information alone is not sufficient to understand phenotypic manifestations. The way that the DNA code is translated into function depends not only on its sequence but also on the interaction with environmental factors (Ammerpoht & Siebert, 2011; Martin-Subero, 2011).

The word "epigenetic" was first described by Conrad Waddington, in 1942, as "the branch of biology which studies the causal interactions between genes and their products, which bring the phenotype into being" (Jablonka & Lamb, 2002; Waddington, 1942). Epigenetics may be seen as the link between genotype and phenotype, a phenomenon that changes the final outcome of a locus or chromosome without changing the underlying DNA sequence. In other words, epigenetics studies any potentially stable and, ideally, heritable change in gene expression or cellular phenotype that occurs without changes in Watson-Crick base-pairing of DNA (Goldberg et al., 2007; Jablonka & Lamb, 2002). By controlling gene activity and, therefore, the availability of the final gene product in the cell, epigenetic alterations can have similar effects as classical genetic mutations (Ammerpoht & Siebert, 2011).

Today's epigenetic research is converging in the study of covalent and noncovalent modifications of DNA and histone proteins and the mechanisms by which such modifications influence overall chromatin structure. DNA methylation is perhaps the best characterized chemical modification of chromatin. In mammals, nearly all DNA methylation occurs on cytosine residues of guanidine/cytosine (CpG) dinucleotides. In genome, there are some regions especially rich in CpG in what is called CpG islands, and DNA methylation of these islands correlates with transcriptional repression. DNA methylation plays a role in many cellular processes including X chromosome inactivation in female mammals and mammalian imprinting, which can be both stably maintained (Alikhani-Koopaei et al., 2004; Drake et al., 2012; Goldberg et al., 2007).

Covalent histone modification is another epigenetic mechanism as it changes chromatin conformation, probably because charge-altering modifications, such as acetylation and phosphorylation, which can directly alter the physical properties of the chromatin fiber, lead to changes in higher-order structures. Noncovalent mechanisms such as chromatin remodeling and the incorporation of specialized histone variants provide the cell with additional tools for introducing variation into the chromatin template. Collectively, covalent modifications, nucleosome remodeling and histone variants can work together and introduce meaningful variation into the chromatin fiber. Their collective contribution to epigenetics is being explored (Drake et al., 2012; Goldberg et al., 2007).

4.2. Epigenetic mechanisms of 11β-hydroxysteroid dehydrogenase type 2 regulation

At the present moment, to our knowledge, there is no published research on epigenetic regulation of 11β-HSD1. Nevertheless, besides mutations and environmental factors (like corticosterone hormones, growth factors, shear stress, inflammatory cytokines and hypoxia) (Atanasov et al., 2003; Baserga et al., 2010; Hardy & Yang, 2002) also epigenetic phenomena can regulate 11β-HSD2 abundance and activity (please see below for references).

The *HSD11B2* promoter comprises a highly guanidine + cytosine (G+C)-rich core, containing more than 80% G+C, and two typical CpG islands, bringing the possibility that CpG dinucleotide methylation plays a role in the cell type-specific and, possibly, in the epigenetically determined inter-individual variable expression of *HSD11B2* (Alikhani-Koopaei et al., 2004; Baserga et al., 2010). In this regard, Alikhani-Koopaei *et al* provided *in vitro* and *in vivo* evidence that 11β-HSD2 expression and activity are inversely correlated with the presence of methylation at the *HSD11B2* promoter region. They have found that CpG islands covering the promoter and exon 1 of *HSD11B2* are densely methylated in human tissues and cell lines with low expression (or activity) [liver, skeletal muscle and renal proximal tubules; MCF-7 and JEG-3 cells (breast adenocarcinoma and placenta choriocarcinoma cell lines, respectively)] but not in those with high expression (or activity) of 11β-HSD2 [placenta and renal distal tubules; SW620 cells (colon carcinoma cell line)]. DNA methyltransferase inhibitors enhance the transcription of *HSD11B2* and the activity of 11β-HSD2 in different human cell types (above mentioned cell lines and primary kidney cells).

Additionally, these inhibitors increase mRNA abundance in various tissues (liver, kidney and lung) and decrease the urinary GC metabolite ratios [corticosterone (THB and 5α-THB)]/[11-dehydrocorticosterone (THA)] in Wistar rats, indicating higher 11β-HSD2 activity (Alikhani-Koopaei et al., 2004).

A decrease in 11β-HSD2 activity, by decreasing renal GC deactivation, is associated with hypertension (Baserga et al., 2010; Pereira et al., 2011; 2012). In order to explore the possible relevance of *HSD11B2* promoter methylation in human blood pressure control, Friso *et al* examined peripheral blood mononuclear cell DNA methylation and urinary tetrahydrocortisol- *versus* tetrahydrocortisone-metabolites (THFs/THE) shuttle as a biochemical indicator of 11β-HSD2 activity. They have found that elevated *HSD11B2* promoter methylation is associated with hypertension developing in GC-treated rheumatoid arthritis patients in parallel with a higher urinary THFs/THE ratio (as a consequence of lower 11β-HSD2 activity). Essential hypertensive patients with elevated urinary THFs/THE ratio also have higher *HSD11B2* promoter methylation (Friso et al., 2008).

So, from animal and human studies it can be hypothesized that changes in the *HSD11B2* gene methylation patterns might explain the inter-individual differences in the expression and activity of 11β-HSD2 in mineralocorticoid target tissues and, consequently, might modulate blood pressure.

4.3. Intrauterine growth restriction and glucocorticoid prenatal overexposure *versus* epigenetic regulation of 11β-hydroxysteroid dehydrogenase type 2

The adverse effects of GC exposure in the prenatal period are related to changes in the expression of the GR and in the intracellular availability and level of GCs, which are modulated by 11β-HSDs as described above. 11β-HSD2, due to its localization to the syncytiotrophoblast layer of the placenta (the site of maternal-fetal exchange), constitutes a functional barrier restricting the free transfer of cortisol (in humans) or corticosterone (in rodents) between the maternal and fetal compartments, by converting maternal active metabolites to the corresponding inactive forms (cortisone and 11-dehydrocorticosterone in humans and rodents, respectively). Thus, the placental 11β-HSD2 protects the fetus from exposure to high levels of maternal GCs, its enzymatic activity being positively correlated with birth weight (in humans and rats) (Albiston et al., 1994; Baserga et al., 2007; Baserga et al., 2010; Benediktsson et al., 1993; Harris & Seckl, 2011; Kajantie et al., 2003; Krozowski et al., 1995; Lesage et al., 2001; Murphy et al., 2002; Pepe et al., 1999; Ronco et al., 2010; Stewart et al., 1995; Wyrwoll et al., 2012).

In line with the above described information, in a well-characterized animal model of intra-uterine growth restriction (IUGR) and adult onset hypertension [after bilateral uterine artery ligation, preformed on day 19 of gestation in Sprague-Dawley rats, uteroplacental insufficiency (UPI) occurs], Baserga *et al* report persistently decreased kidney 11β-HSD2 mRNA and protein levels through day 21 of life (juvenile rat) (Baserga et al., 2007; Baserga et al., 2010). Further developing this study, Baserga *et al* report that IUGR (as a consequence of UPI after surgery on day 19.5 of gestation in Sprague-Dawley rats) a) alters key transcription factors binding to the renal *HSD11B2* promoter [decreases SP1 (specificity protein 1) and NF-kB (nuclear factor-kappaB, p65) binding in males (transcriptional enhancers), while increases Egr-1 (early growth response factor) binding in females and NF-kB (p50) binding in males (transcriptional repressors)]; b) increases CpG methylation status as well as modifies the methylation pattern in several CpG sites of *HSD11B2* promoter at (post-birth) day 0, also in a sex-specific manner; and c) decreases trimethylation of H3K36 in exon 5 of *HSD11B2* at (post-birth) day 0 and day 21 in both genders (which is associated with decreased transcriptional elongation). The authors speculated that alterations in transcription factor binding and chromatin structure may play a role in *in utero* reprogramming (Baserga et al., 2010). In a recent paper, Marsit *et al* demonstrate an inverse association between measures of intrauterine growth, including birth weight and ponderal index, with the extent of DNA methylation of the *HSD11B2* gene promoter region, in the placenta of 185 healthy newborn infants. Growth restricted infants, and particularly those with clinically diagnosed IUGR, show greater methylation than their grown counterparts. An inverse relationship between the extent of *HSD11B2* methylation and infant quality of movement as well as a trend towards a positive correlation between *HSD11B2* methylation and infant attention have been identified. The authors suggested that an adverse intrauterine environment leading to growth restriction may enhance infant cortisol exposure and its downstream effects both by reducing *HSD11B2* expression and by allowing GR expression by maintaining low levels of methylation at that promoter. The enhanced levels of active cortisol and potentially enhanced response may then be responsible for inappropriate programming of the HPA axis as well as altered neuromuscular development in the infant (Marsit et al., 2012).

Very recently, Wyrwoll *et al* reported that, in Wistar rats, prenatal dexamethasone [Dex; subcutaneous injection of 100 μg Dex/kg or vehicle (Veh) from embryonic day (E) 15 to 19] which is not metabolized by 11β-HSD2, has opposite effects on placental choline and folate transport at E20. The placental transport capacity of choline is reduced by Dex, such that the fetus receives less choline/gram of fetal weight. In contrast, Dex increases placental folate transport, such that the Dex-exposed fetuses receive more folate/gram of fetal weight. Placental methionine transport and maternal plasma methionine concentrations are unaffected by Dex exposure, although fetal plasma methionine levels are reduced. As the establishment of epigenetic modifications in the fetus depends on the availability of methyl donors during fetal development, the authors suggested that, altogether, those changes in key components of the methyl donor cycle may explain the impact of prenatal GC overexposure on metabolic programming and disease risk in the offspring (Wyrwoll et al., 2012).

Both syncytialization and Dex stimulate leptin secretion from both the apical and basal surfaces of human choriocarcinoma BeWo cells. Additionally, transport of exogenous leptin is also evident in both the apical to basal and reverse direction, suggesting maternal-fetal exchange of leptin across the human placenta (Wyrwoll et al., 2005). It is recognized that leptin, besides being a proinflammatory cytokine and a regulator of appetite, body fat and bone metabolism, lung development and function, immune and thyroid functions, stress response, metabolic activity by peripheral tissues and energy balance, is also important for the establishment of pregnancy (D'Ippolito et al., 2012; Denver et al., 2011; Malik et al., 2001; Mantzoros et al., 2011; Wyrwoll et al., 2005), being positively associated with fetal (Tsai et al., 2004; Vatten et al., 2002; Wyrwoll et al., 2005) and placental (Jakimiuk et al., 2003; Wyrwoll et al., 2005) growths.

5. Interplay between glucocorticoid availability, diet and fetal programming

Both fetal GC exposure and maternal nutrition contribute to fetal programming. Maternal undernutrition increases cortisol and corticosterone plasma levels (in humans or rats, respectively) in both mothers and growth-retarded fetuses (Lesage et al., 2001).

Exposing rats *in utero* to high levels of Dex also reduces fetal and birth weights, increases blood pressure and causes fasting hyperglycemia, reactive hyperglycemia and hyperinsulinemia on oral glucose loading in the adult offspring (Benediktsson et al., 1993; Lesage et al., 2001; Nyirenda et al., 1998; Wyrwoll et al., 2012; Wyrwoll et al., 2006). Postnatal diet may counteract some of the fetal programming effects (Waddell et al., 2010; Wyrwoll et al., 2006; Wyrwoll et al., 2008).

Accordingly, in pregnant Wistar rats a magnesium-deficient diet (0.003% magnesium *versus* 0.082% magnesium in the control diet) increases methylation of specific CpG dinucleotides in the hepatic *HSD11B2* promoter of neonatal offspring (without gender differences) (Takaya et al., 2011), what might increase hepatic intracellular GC levels [increased GC levels have been associated with IR and T2DM (Pereira et al., 2011; 2012)] and contribute to unravel the mechanisms of the metabolic adverse effects associated to a low magnesium intake (Lecube et al., 2012; Lima et al., 2009; Takaya et al., 2011; Volpe, 2008).

Alterations of *HSD11B2* methylation have been recently reported by Drake *et al* on buffy coat DNA of adult individuals whose mothers ate an unbalanced diet in pregnancy: methylation at specific CpGs in the *HSD11B2* promoter correlates with neonatal anthropometric variables [birth weight (positively) and neonatal ponderal index (negatively)] and CpG methylation within *HSD11B2* and *GR* associates with increased adiposity and blood pressure in adulthood. The authors suggested that these results indicate a persisting epigenetic link between early life maternal diet and/or fetal growth and cardiovascular disease risk in humans (Drake et al., 2012).

Recent studies have identified programming effects of leptin that influence postnatal phenotype (Granado et al., 2012). Wyrwoll *et al* demonstrated that programmed hyperleptinemia and hypertension, also induced by Dex overexposure *in utero*, in Wistar rats [Dex administered in the drinking water (0.75 μg/mL) from day 13 of pregnancy until birth], are completely blocked in the offspring by a postnatal diet enriched with ω-3 fatty acids (the majority being long chain). In the absence of the ω-3 fatty acid supplementation, programmed hyperleptinemia is totally apparent by 6 months of age (in both sexes), being accompanied by an elevation of leptin mRNA expression in the AT (that is also completely abolished by the dietary supplementation). Programmed hypertension is evident in male offspring by 2 months and in female offspring by 6 months of age. Maternal Dex delays the onset of puberty in the offspring. These results demonstrated, for the first time, that modifications in the postnatal diet can prevent major adverse fetal programming outcomes (by increased GC exposure *in utero*) (Wyrwoll et al., 2006). In the same animal protocol, ω-3 fatty acid supplementation is also effective in preventing the increased plasma fasting insulin and interleukin-1β in the adult offspring exposed to GC excess *in utero*. However, raising animals from birth on a high ω-3 fatty acids diet do not prevent the programmed increase in plasma tumour necrosis factor-α and do not correct disturbances in skeletal muscle expression of SLC2A4 (formerly known as glucose transporter 4, GLUT4), PPAR-δ and uncoupling protein 3 mRNAs (Wyrwoll et al., 2008). However, the protective effects of the high ω-3 fatty acids diet are not mediated by changes in the adrenal function. Waddell *et al* reported that, in the just above mentioned animal protocol, prenatal Dex exposure also increases, in the adult offspring, stimulated urinary corticosterone and aldosterone (after overnight isolation) and plasma corticosterone levels (under anesthesia), what suggests heightened adrenal responsiveness to stress. These effects are not prevented by ω-3 fatty acids supplementation. Key steroidogenic genes expression levels and (adrenal weight)/(body weight) ratio are unaltered by prenatal Dex treatment or postnatal diet. Interestingly, adrenal mRNA expression of both *HSD11B2* and *MC2R* genes increases with Dex treatment. High ω-3 fatty acids diet partially attenuates the Dex-effect on *MC2R* mRNA expression but increases *HSD11B2* mRNA expression (Waddell et al., 2010).

6. Environmental pollutants *versus* epigenetic regulation of 11β-hydroxysteroid dehydrogenase type 2

Cadmium (Cd^{2+}) has been classified as a human carcinogen and has been identified as a new class of endocrine disruptor (Byrne et al., 2009; Henson & Chedrese, 2004; Ronco et al., 2010; Waisberg et al., 2003; Yang et al., 2006). Neonates delivered from mothers who smoked during pregnancy have reduced birth weight, compared to those neonates from non-smoking mothers, what is correlated to placental Cd^{2+} concentration (Ronco et al., 2005; Ronco et al., 2010). Placentas of mothers delivering low birth weight newborns show significantly higher Cd^{2+} concentrations than placentas associated to normal birth weight neonates, what suggests that placental accumulation of heavy metals is related to altered fetal growth mechanisms (Llanos & Ronco, 2009; Ronco et al., 2010). Epigenetic alterations mediate some toxic effects of environmental chemicals like Cd^{2+} (Baccarelli & Bollati, 2009; Ronco et al., 2010), with paradoxical effects on DNA methylation during Cd^{2+}-induced cellular transformation (Ronco et al., 2010; Takiguchi et al., 2003).

Using primary cultured human trophoblast cells as a model system Yang *et al*, reported that Cd^{2+} exposure results in a time- and concentration-dependent decrease in 11β-HSD2 activity, such that an 80% reduction is observed after 24 h of treatment at 1 μM (with a similar decrease in 11β-HSD2 protein and mRNA levels), suggesting that Cd^{2+} reduces 11β-HSD2 enzyme expression. Furthermore, Cd^{2+} diminishes *HSD11B2* promoter activity, indicative of repression of *HSD11B2* gene transcription. Overall, these results could represent one of the mechanisms involved in the Cd^{2+}-induced reduction in birth weight of smoker's newborns (Ronco et al., 2010; Yang et al., 2006). In line with this, Ronco *et al* observed that a 24 h exposure of JEG-3 cells to 1 μM of Cd^{2+} induces an increase in 11β-HSD2 activity and mRNA expression as well as a reduction in the methylation index of the *HSD11B2* gene. These results suggest that Cd^{2+}-induced endocrine disruptor effects on JEG-3 cells could be mediated by changes in the methylation status of some target genes (Ronco et al., 2010).

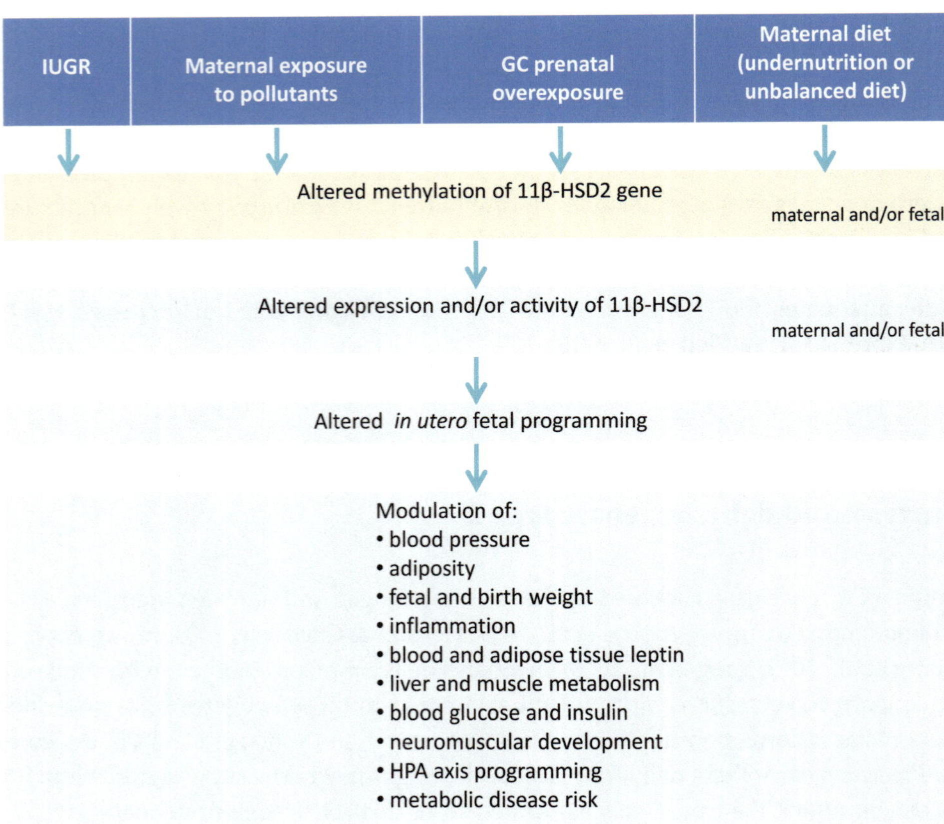

Figure 1. Possible factors of epigenetic 11β-HSD2 regulation. 11β-HSD2 - 11β-hydroxysteroid dehydrogenase type 2; GC - glucocorticoids; HPA - hypothalamus-pituitary-adrenal; IUGR - intrauterine growth restriction.

7. Conclusion

The present review highlights the importance of 11β-HSDs for the modulation of tissue CG availability. As depicted above, defects on expression and/or activity of these enzymes can affect physiology and result in clinical conditions related with impaired metabolic or blood pressure control. In this regard, knowing that these enzymes can be differentially modulated within different tissues and that nutritional cues or environmental factors, like pollutants, can modify their activity opens avenues for possible interventions at the level of treatment or prevention of conditions related with dysregulated tissue GC levels.

Furthermore, the contribution of epigenetics to the demonstration that tissue GC levels or their actions can be modified through interference with the expression of *HSD11B1* and *HSD11B2* (data presented here for the 11β-HSD2 enzyme is summarized in Figure 1) or components of the HPA axis, underscores the importance of transgenerational influences of GC level modifiers for the establishment of pathologies of epidemic proportions like obesity, hypertension and MetSyn. This awareness will allow not only to comprehend the pathophysiological processes involved but also paves the way towards the design and implementation of interventions in order to hamper the increase of such pathologies.

Acknowledgements

This work has been supported by FCT (Fundação para a Ciência e Tecnologia, PEst-OE/SAU/UI0038/2011) through the *Centro de Farmacologia e Biopatalogia Química*, Faculty of Medicine, University of Porto, which integrates the Department of Biochemistry (U38/FCT), Faculty of Medicine, University of Porto. Additional funding has been provided by FCT through the *Fundo Social Europeu, Programa Operacional Potencial Humano da UE* (SFRH/BPD/40110/2007 and SFRH/BDE/33798/2009).

Author details

Cidália Pereira[1], Rosário Monteiro[1], Miguel Constância[2] and Maria João Martins[1]

1 Department of Biochemistry (U38/FCT), Faculty of Medicine, University of Porto, Porto, Portugal

2 Metabolic Research Laboratories, Department of Obstetrics and Gynaecology University of Cambridge, Cambridge, United Kingdom

References

[1] Albiston, A.; Obeyesekere, V.; Smith, R., et al. (1994). Cloning and tissue distribution of the human 11 beta-hydroxysteroid dehydrogenase type 2 enzyme. *Mol Cell Endocrinol,* Vol.105, No.2, (Nov), pp. R11-17, ISSN:0303-7207

[2] Alikhani-Koopaei, R.; Fouladkou, F.; Frey, F., et al. (2004). Epigenetic regulation of 11 beta-hydroxysteroid dehydrogenase type 2 expression. *J Clin Invest,* Vol.114, No.8, (Oct), pp. 1146-1157, ISSN:0021-9738

[3] Ammerpoht, O. & Siebert, R. (2011). How to analyse epigenetic marks? *Pediatr Endocrinol Rev,* Vol.9 Suppl 1, (Sep), pp. 511-514, ISSN:1565-4753

[4] Anagnostis, P.; Athyros, V.; Tziomalos, K., et al. (2009). Clinical review: The pathogenetic role of cortisol in the metabolic syndrome: a hypothesis. *J Clin Endocrinol Metab,* Vol.94, No.8, (Aug), pp. 2692-2701, ISSN:1945-7197

[5] Andrews, R.; Rooyackers, O. & Walker, B. (2003). Effects of the 11 beta-hydroxysteroid dehydrogenase inhibitor carbenoxolone on insulin sensitivity in men with type 2 diabetes. *J Clin Endocrinol Metab,* Vol.88, No.1, (Jan), pp. 285-291, ISSN:0021-972X

[6] Arriza, J.; Weinberger, C.; Cerelli, G., et al. (1987). Cloning of human mineralocorticoid receptor complementary DNA: structural and functional kinship with the glucocorticoid receptor. *Science,* Vol.237, No.4812, (Jul 17), pp. 268-275, ISSN:0036-8075

[7] Atanasov, A.; Nashev, L.; Gelman, L., et al. (2008). Direct protein-protein interaction of 11beta-hydroxysteroid dehydrogenase type 1 and hexose-6-phosphate dehydrogenase in the endoplasmic reticulum lumen. *Biochim Biophys Acta,* Vol.1783, No.8, (Aug), pp. 1536-1543, ISSN:0006-3002

[8] Atanasov, A. & Odermatt, A. (2007). Readjusting the glucocorticoid balance: an opportunity for modulators of 11beta-hydroxysteroid dehydrogenase type 1 activity? *Endocr Metab Immune Disord Drug Targets,* Vol.7, No.2, (Jun), pp. 125-140, ISSN: 1871-5303

[9] Atanasov, A.; Tam, S.; Rocken, J., et al. (2003). Inhibition of 11 beta-hydroxysteroid dehydrogenase type 2 by dithiocarbamates. *Biochem Biophys Res Commun,* Vol.308, No.2, (Aug 22), pp. 257-262, ISSN:0006-291X

[10] Baccarelli, A. & Bollati, V. (2009). Epigenetics and environmental chemicals. *Curr Opin Pediatr,* Vol.21, No.2, (Apr), pp. 243-251, ISSN:1531-698X

[11] Baserga, M.; Hale, M.; Wang, Z., et al. (2007). Uteroplacental insufficiency alters nephrogenesis and downregulates cyclooxygenase-2 expression in a model of IUGR with adult-onset hypertension. *Am J Physiol Regul Integr Comp Physiol,* Vol.292, No.5, (May), pp. R1943-1955, ISSN:0363-6119

[12] Baserga, M.; Kaur, R.; Hale, M., et al. (2010). Fetal growth restriction alters transcription factor binding and epigenetic mechanisms of renal 11beta-hydroxysteroid dehy-

drogenase type 2 in a sex-specific manner. *Am J Physiol Regul Integr Comp Physiol,* Vol.299, No.1, (Jul), pp. R334-342, ISSN:1522-1490

[13] Benediktsson, R.; Lindsay, R.; Noble, J., et al. (1993). Glucocorticoid exposure in utero: new model for adult hypertension. *Lancet,* Vol.341, No.8841, (Feb 6), pp. 339-341, ISSN:0140-6736

[14] Bitar, M. (2001). Co-administration of etomoxir and RU-486 mitigates insulin resistance in hepatic and muscular tissues of STZ-induced diabetic rats. *Horm Metab Res,* Vol.33, No.10, (Oct), pp. 577-584, ISSN:0018-5043

[15] Bujalska, I.; Draper, N.; Michailidou, Z., et al. (2005). Hexose-6-phosphate dehydrogenase confers oxo-reductase activity upon 11 beta-hydroxysteroid dehydrogenase type 1. *J Mol Endocrinol,* Vol.34, No.3, (Jun), pp. 675-684, ISSN:0952-5041

[16] Bujalska, I.; Hewitt, K.; Hauton, D., et al. (2008). Lack of hexose-6-phosphate dehydrogenase impairs lipid mobilization from mouse adipose tissue. *Endocrinology,* Vol. 149, No.5, (May), pp. 2584-2591, ISSN:0013-7227

[17] Bujalska, I.; Kumar, S. & Stewart, P. (1997). Does central obesity reflect "Cushing's disease of the omentum"? *Lancet,* Vol.349, No.9060, (Apr 26), pp. 1210-1213, ISSN: 0140-6736

[18] Bujalska, I.; Walker, E.; Hewison, M., et al. (2002a). A switch in dehydrogenase to reductase activity of 11 beta-hydroxysteroid dehydrogenase type 1 upon differentiation of human omental adipose stromal cells. *J Clin Endocrinol Metab,* Vol.87, No.3, (Mar), pp. 1205-1210, ISSN:0021-972X

[19] Bujalska, I.; Walker, E.; Tomlinson, J., et al. (2002b). 11Beta-hydroxysteroid dehydrogenase type 1 in differentiating omental human preadipocytes: from de-activation to generation of cortisol. *Endocr Res,* Vol.28, No.4, (Nov), pp. 449-461, ISSN:0743-5800

[20] Byrne, C.; Divekar, S.; Storchan, G., et al. (2009). Cadmium--a metallohormone? *Toxicol Appl Pharmacol,* Vol.238, No.3, (Aug 1), pp. 266-271, ISSN:1096-0333

[21] Campino, C.; Carvajal, C.; Cornejo, J., et al. (2010). 11beta-Hydroxysteroid dehydrogenase type-2 and type-1 (11beta-HSD2 and 11beta-HSD1) and 5beta-reductase activities in the pathogenia of essential hypertension. *Endocrine,* Vol.37, No.1, (Feb), pp. 106-114, ISSN:1559-0100

[22] Carroll, T. & Findling, J. (2010). The diagnosis of Cushing's syndrome. *Rev Endocr Metab Disord,* Vol.11, No.2, (Jun), pp. 147-153, ISSN:1573-2606

[23] Chapman, K.; Coutinho, A.; Gray, M., et al. (2006). Local amplification of glucocorticoids by 11beta-hydroxysteroid dehydrogenase type 1 and its role in the inflammatory response. *Ann N Y Acad Sci,* Vol.1088, (Nov), pp. 265-273, ISSN:0077-8923

[24] Cooper, M. & Stewart, P. (2009). 11Beta-hydroxysteroid dehydrogenase type 1 and its role in the hypothalamus-pituitary-adrenal axis, metabolic syndrome, and inflammation. *J Clin Endocrinol Metab,* Vol.94, No.12, (Dec), pp. 4645-4654, ISSN:1945-7197

[25] Cope, C. & Black, E. (1958). The production rate of cortisol in man. *Br Med J*, Vol.1, No.5078, (May 3), pp. 1020-1024, ISSN:0007-1447

[26] Cushing, H. (1932). The basophil adenomas of the pituitary body and their clinical manifestations (pituitary basophilism). *Bull Johns Hopkins Hospital*, Vol.50, pp. 137-195, ISSN:0097-1383

[27] D'Ippolito, S.; Tersigni, C.; Scambia, G., et al. (2012). Adipokines, an adipose tissue and placental product with biological functions during pregnancy. *Biofactors*, Vol.38, No.1, (Jan), pp. 14-23, ISSN:1872-8081

[28] Dave-Sharma, S.; Wilson, R.; Harbison, M., et al. (1998). Examination of genotype and phenotype relationships in 14 patients with apparent mineralocorticoid excess. *J Clin Endocrinol Metab*, Vol.83, No.7, (Jul), pp. 2244-2254, ISSN:0021-972X

[29] Denver, R.; Bonett, R. & Boorse, G. (2011). Evolution of leptin structure and function. *Neuroendocrinology*, Vol.94, No.1, pp. 21-38, ISSN:1423-0194

[30] Drake, A.; McPherson, R.; Godfrey, K., et al. (2012). An unbalanced maternal diet in pregnancy associates with offspring epigenetic changes in genes controlling glucocorticoid action and fetal growth. *Clin Endocrinol (Oxf)*, Vol.(May 29), pp. ISSN: 1365-2265

[31] Draper, N.; Echwald, S.; Lavery, G., et al. (2002). Association studies between microsatellite markers within the gene encoding human 11beta-hydroxysteroid dehydrogenase type 1 and body mass index, waist to hip ratio, and glucocorticoid metabolism. *J Clin Endocrinol Metab*, Vol.87, No.11, (Nov), pp. 4984-4990, ISSN: 0021-972X

[32] Draper, N.; Walker, E.; Bujalska, I., et al. (2003). Mutations in the genes encoding 11beta-hydroxysteroid dehydrogenase type 1 and hexose-6-phosphate dehydrogenase interact to cause cortisone reductase deficiency. *Nat Genet*, Vol.34, No.4, (Aug), pp. 434-439, ISSN:1061-4036

[33] Duclos, M.; Marquez Pereira, P.; Barat, P., et al. (2005). Increased cortisol bioavailability, abdominal obesity, and the metabolic syndrome in obese women. *Obes Res*, Vol. 13, No.7, (Jul), pp. 1157-1166, ISSN:1071-7323

[34] Dzyakanchuk, A.; Balazs, Z.; Nashev, L., et al. (2009). 11beta-Hydroxysteroid dehydrogenase 1 reductase activity is dependent on a high ratio of NADPH/NADP(+) and is stimulated by extracellular glucose. *Mol Cell Endocrinol*, Vol.301, No.1-2, (Mar 25), pp. 137-141, ISSN:0303-7207

[35] Edwards, C.; Stewart, P.; Burt, D., et al. (1988). Localisation of 11 beta-hydroxysteroid dehydrogenase--tissue specific protector of the mineralocorticoid receptor. *Lancet*, Vol.2, No.8618, (Oct 29), pp. 986-989, ISSN:0140-6736

[36] Espindola-Antunes, D. & Kater, C. (2007). Adipose tissue expression of 11beta-hydroxysteroid dehydrogenase type 1 in Cushing's syndrome and in obesity. *Arq Bras Endocrinol Metabol*, Vol.51, No.8, (Nov), pp. 1397-1403, ISSN:0004-2730

[37] Esteban, N.; Loughlin, T.; Yergey, A., et al. (1991). Daily cortisol production rate in man determined by stable isotope dilution/mass spectrometry. *J Clin Endocrinol Metab,* Vol.72, No.1, (Jan), pp. 39-45, ISSN:0021-972X

[38] Ferrari, P. (2010). The role of 11beta-hydroxysteroid dehydrogenase type 2 in human hypertension. *Biochim Biophys Acta,* Vol.1802, No.12, (Dec), pp. 1178-1187, ISSN: 0006-3002

[39] Filling, C.; Berndt, K.; Benach, J., et al. (2002). Critical residues for structure and catalysis in short-chain dehydrogenases/reductases. *J Biol Chem,* Vol.277, No.28, (Jul 12), pp. 25677-25684, ISSN:0021-9258

[40] Friso, S.; Pizzolo, F.; Choi, S., et al. (2008). Epigenetic control of 11 beta-hydroxysteroid dehydrogenase 2 gene promoter is related to human hypertension. *Atherosclerosis,* Vol.199, No.2, (Aug), pp. 323-327, ISSN:1879-1484

[41] Funder, J.; Pearce, P.; Smith, R., et al. (1988). Mineralocorticoid action: target tissue specificity is enzyme, not receptor, mediated. *Science,* Vol.242, No.4878, (Oct 28), pp. 583-585, ISSN:0036-8075

[42] Gathercole, L. & Stewart, P. (2010). Targeting the pre-receptor metabolism of cortisol as a novel therapy in obesity and diabetes. *J Steroid Biochem Mol Biol,* Vol.122, No.1-3, (Oct), pp. 21-27, ISSN:1879-1220

[43] Gettys, T.; Watson, P.; Taylor, I., et al. (1997). RU-486 (Mifepristone) ameliorates diabetes but does not correct deficient beta-adrenergic signalling in adipocytes from mature C57BL/6J-ob/ob mice. *Int J Obes Relat Metab Disord,* Vol.21, No.10, (Oct), pp. 865-873, ISSN:0307-0565

[44] Goldberg, A.; Allis, C. & Bernstein, E. (2007). Epigenetics: a landscape takes shape. *Cell,* Vol.128, No.4, (Feb 23), pp. 635-638, ISSN:0092-8674

[45] Granado, M.; Fuente-Martin, E.; Garcia-Caceres, C., et al. (2012). Leptin in early life: a key factor for the development of the adult metabolic profile. *Obes Facts,* Vol.5, No.1, pp. 138-150, ISSN:1662-4033

[46] Hardy, D. & Yang, K. (2002). The expression of 11 beta-hydroxysteroid dehydrogenase type 2 is induced during trophoblast differentiation: effects of hypoxia. *J Clin Endocrinol Metab,* Vol.87, No.8, (Aug), pp. 3696-3701, ISSN:0021-972X

[47] Harris, A. & Seckl, J. (2011). Glucocorticoids, prenatal stress and the programming of disease. *Horm Behav,* Vol.59, No.3, (Mar), pp. 279-289, ISSN:1095-6867

[48] Havel, P.; Busch, B.; Curry, D., et al. (1996). Predominately glucocorticoid agonist actions of RU-486 in young specific-pathogen-free Zucker rats. *Am J Physiol,* Vol.271, No.3 Pt 2, (Sep), pp. R710-717, ISSN:0002-9513

[49] Henson, M. & Chedrese, P. (2004). Endocrine disruption by cadmium, a common environmental toxicant with paradoxical effects on reproduction. *Exp Biol Med (Maywood),* Vol.229, No.5, (May), pp. 383-392, ISSN:1535-3702

[50] Jablonka, E. & Lamb, M. (2002). The changing concept of epigenetics. *Ann N Y Acad Sci,* Vol.981, (Dec), pp. 82-96, ISSN:0077-8923

[51] Jacobson, P.; von Geldern, T.; Ohman, L., et al. (2005). Hepatic glucocorticoid receptor antagonism is sufficient to reduce elevated hepatic glucose output and improve glucose control in animal models of type 2 diabetes. *J Pharmacol Exp Ther,* Vol.314, No.1, (Jul), pp. 191-200, ISSN:0022-3565

[52] Jakimiuk, A.; Skalba, P.; Huterski, D., et al. (2003). Leptin messenger ribonucleic acid (mRNA) content in the human placenta at term: relationship to levels of leptin in cord blood and placental weight. *Gynecol Endocrinol,* Vol.17, No.4, (Aug), pp. 311-316, ISSN:0951-3590

[53] Jamieson, P.; Chapman, K.; Edwards, C., et al. (1995). 11 beta-hydroxysteroid dehydrogenase is an exclusive 11 beta- reductase in primary cultures of rat hepatocytes: effect of physicochemical and hormonal manipulations. *Endocrinology,* Vol.136, No. 11, (Nov), pp. 4754-4761, ISSN:0013-7227

[54] Jornvall, H.; Persson, B.; Krook, M., et al. (1995). Short-chain dehydrogenases/reductases (SDR). *Biochemistry,* Vol.34, No.18, (May 9), pp. 6003-6013, ISSN:0006-2960

[55] Kajantie, E.; Dunkel, L.; Turpeinen, U., et al. (2003). Placental 11 beta-hydroxysteroid dehydrogenase-2 and fetal cortisol/cortisone shuttle in small preterm infants. *J Clin Endocrinol Metab,* Vol.88, No.1, (Jan), pp. 493-500, ISSN:0021-972X

[56] Kotelevtsev, Y.; Brown, R.; Fleming, S., et al. (1999). Hypertension in mice lacking 11beta-hydroxysteroid dehydrogenase type 2. *J Clin Invest,* Vol.103, No.5, (Mar), pp. 683-689, ISSN:0021-9738

[57] Krozowski, Z.; MaGuire, J.; Stein-Oakley, A., et al. (1995). Immunohistochemical localization of the 11 beta-hydroxysteroid dehydrogenase type II enzyme in human kidney and placenta. *J Clin Endocrinol Metab,* Vol.80, No.7, (Jul), pp. 2203-2209, ISSN: 0021-972X

[58] Kusunoki, M.; Cooney, G.; Hara, T., et al. (1995). Amelioration of high-fat feeding-induced insulin resistance in skeletal muscle with the antiglucocorticoid RU486. *Diabetes,* Vol.44, No.6, (Jun), pp. 718-720, ISSN:0012-1797

[59] Lavery, G.; Walker, E.; Draper, N., et al. (2006). Hexose-6-phosphate dehydrogenase knock-out mice lack 11 beta-hydroxysteroid dehydrogenase type 1-mediated glucocorticoid generation. *J Biol Chem,* Vol.281, No.10, (Mar 10), pp. 6546-6551, ISSN: 0021-9258

[60] Lecube, A.; Baena-Fustegueras, J.; Fort, J., et al. (2012). Diabetes is the main factor accounting for hypomagnesemia in obese subjects. *PLoS One,* Vol.7, No.1, pp. e30599, ISSN:1932-6203

[61] Lesage, J.; Blondeau, B.; Grino, M., et al. (2001). Maternal undernutrition during late gestation induces fetal overexposure to glucocorticoids and intrauterine growth re-

tardation, and disturbs the hypothalamo-pituitary adrenal axis in the newborn rat. *Endocrinology,* Vol.142, No.5, (May), pp. 1692-1702, ISSN:0013-7227

[62] Lima, L.; Cruz, T.; Rodrigues, L., et al. (2009). Serum and intracellular magnesium deficiency in patients with metabolic syndrome--evidences for its relation to insulin resistance. *Diabetes Res Clin Pract,* Vol.83, No.2, (Feb), pp. 257-262, ISSN:1872-8227

[63] Llanos, M. & Ronco, A. (2009). Fetal growth restriction is related to placental levels of cadmium, lead and arsenic but not with antioxidant activities. *Reprod Toxicol,* Vol.27, No.1, (Jan), pp. 88-92, ISSN:0890-6238

[64] Malik, N.; Carter, N.; Murray, J., et al. (2001). Leptin requirement for conception, implantation, and gestation in the mouse. *Endocrinology,* Vol.142, No.12, (Dec), pp. 5198-5202, ISSN:0013-7227

[65] Mantzoros, C.; Magkos, F.; Brinkoetter, M., et al. (2011). Leptin in human physiology and pathophysiology. *Am J Physiol Endocrinol Metab,* Vol.301, No.4, (Oct), pp. E567-584, ISSN:1522-1555 (

[66] Marsit, C.; Maccani, M.; Padbury, J., et al. (2012). Placental 11-beta hydroxysteroid dehydrogenase methylation is associated with newborn growth and a measure of neurobehavioral outcome. *PLoS One,* Vol.7, No.3, pp. e33794, ISSN:1932-6203

[67] Martin-Subero, J. (2011). How epigenomics brings phenotype into being. *Pediatr Endocrinol Rev,* Vol.9 Suppl 1, (Sep), pp. 506-510, ISSN:1565-4753

[68] Masuzaki, H.; Paterson, J.; Shinyama, H., et al. (2001). A transgenic model of visceral obesity and the metabolic syndrome. *Science,* Vol.294, No.5549, (Dec 7), pp. 2166-2170, ISSN:0036-8075

[69] Misra, M.; Bredella, M.; Tsai, P., et al. (2008). Lower growth hormone and higher cortisol are associated with greater visceral adiposity, intramyocellular lipids, and insulin resistance in overweight girls. *Am J Physiol Endocrinol Metab,* Vol.295, No.2, (Aug), pp. E385-392, ISSN:0193-1849

[70] Moisan, M.; Edwards, C. & Seckl, J. (1992). Differential promoter usage by the rat 11 beta-hydroxysteroid dehydrogenase gene. *Mol Endocrinol,* Vol.6, No.7, (Jul), pp. 1082-1087, ISSN:0888-8809

[71] Monder, C.; Shackleton, C.; Bradlow, H., et al. (1986). The syndrome of apparent mineralocorticoid excess: its association with 11 beta-dehydrogenase and 5 beta-reductase deficiency and some consequences for corticosteroid metabolism. *J Clin Endocrinol Metab,* Vol.63, No.3, (Sep), pp. 550-557, ISSN:0021-972X

[72] Mune, T.; Rogerson, F.; Nikkila, H., et al. (1995). Human hypertension caused by mutations in the kidney isozyme of 11 beta-hydroxysteroid dehydrogenase. *Nat Genet,* Vol.10, No.4, (Aug), pp. 394-399, ISSN:1061-4036

[73] Murphy, V.; Zakar, T.; Smith, R., et al. (2002). Reduced 11beta-hydroxysteroid dehydrogenase type 2 activity is associated with decreased birth weight centile in preg-

nancies complicated by asthma. *J Clin Endocrinol Metab,* Vol.87, No.4, (Apr), pp. 1660-1668, ISSN:0021-972X

[74] Newell-Price, J.; Bertagna, X.; Grossman, A., et al. (2006). Cushing's syndrome. *Lancet,* Vol.367, No.9522, (May 13), pp. 1605-1617, ISSN:1474-547X

[75] Nyirenda, M.; Lindsay, R.; Kenyon, C., et al. (1998). Glucocorticoid exposure in late gestation permanently programs rat hepatic phosphoenolpyruvate carboxykinase and glucocorticoid receptor expression and causes glucose intolerance in adult offspring. *J Clin Invest,* Vol.101, No.10, (May 15), pp. 2174-2181, ISSN:0021-9738

[76] Oppermann, U.; Filling, C.; Hult, M., et al. (2003). Short-chain dehydrogenases/reductases (SDR): the 2002 update. *Chem Biol Interact,* Vol.143-144, (Feb 1), pp. 247-253, ISSN:0009-2797

[77] Ozols, J. (1995). Lumenal orientation and post-translational modifications of the liver microsomal 11 beta-hydroxysteroid dehydrogenase. *J Biol Chem,* Vol.270, No.17, (Apr 28), pp. 10360, ISSN:0021-9258

[78] Palermo, M.; Quinkler, M. & Stewart, P. (2004). Apparent mineralocorticoid excess syndrome: an overview. *Arq Bras Endocrinol Metabol,* Vol.48, No.5, (Oct), pp. 687-696, ISSN:0004-2730

[79] Papadimitriou, A. & Priftis, K. (2009). Regulation of the hypothalamic-pituitary-adrenal axis. *Neuroimmunomodulation,* Vol.16, No.5, pp. 265-271, ISSN:1423-0216

[80] Pepe, G.; Burch, M. & Albrecht, E. (1999). Expression of the 11beta-hydroxysteroid dehydrogenase types 1 and 2 proteins in human and baboon placental syncytiotrophoblast. *Placenta,* Vol.20, No.7, (Sep), pp. 575-582, ISSN:0143-4004

[81] Pereira, C.; Azevedo, I.; Monteiro, R., et al. (2011). 11β-Hydroxysteroid Dehydrogenase Type 1 and the Metabolic Syndrome. *Steroids – Clinical Aspect*. Abduljabbar, H., In Tech.

[82] Pereira, C.; Azevedo, I.; Monteiro, R., et al. (2012). 11beta-Hydroxysteroid dehydrogenase type 1: relevance of its modulation in the pathophysiology of obesity, the metabolic syndrome and type 2 diabetes mellitus. *Diabetes Obes Metab,* Vol.(Feb 9), pp. ISSN:1463-1326

[83] Peterson, R. & Pierce, C. (1960). The metabolism of corticosterone in man. *J Clin Invest,* Vol.39, (May), pp. 741-757, ISSN:0021-9738

[84] Phillipov, G.; Palermo, M. & Shackleton, C. (1996). Apparent cortisone reductase deficiency: a unique form of hypercortisolism. *J Clin Endocrinol Metab,* Vol.81, No.11, (Nov), pp. 3855-3860, ISSN:0021-972X

[85] Phillips, D.; Barker, D.; Fall, C., et al. (1998). Elevated plasma cortisol concentrations: a link between low birth weight and the insulin resistance syndrome? *J Clin Endocrinol Metab,* Vol.83, No.3, (Mar), pp. 757-760, ISSN:0021-972X

[86] Picard, F.; Wanatabe, M.; Schoonjans, K., et al. (2002). Progesterone receptor knockout mice have an improved glucose homeostasis secondary to beta -cell proliferation. *Proc Natl Acad Sci U S A,* Vol.99, No.24, (Nov 26), pp. 15644-15648, ISSN:0027-8424

[87] Quinkler, M. & Stewart, P. (2003). Hypertension and the cortisol-cortisone shuttle. *J Clin Endocrinol Metab,* Vol.88, No.6, (Jun), pp. 2384-2392, ISSN:0021-972X

[88] Ronco, A.; Arguello, G.; Munoz, L., et al. (2005). Metals content in placentas from moderate cigarette consumers: correlation with newborn birth weight. *Biometals,* Vol. 18, No.3, (Jun), pp. 233-241, ISSN:0966-0844

[89] Ronco, A.; Llaguno, E.; Epunan, M., et al. (2010). Effect of cadmium on cortisol production and 11beta-hydroxysteroid dehydrogenase 2 expression by cultured human choriocarcinoma cells (JEG-3). *Toxicol In Vitro,* Vol.24, No.6, (Sep), pp. 1532-1537, ISSN:1879-3177

[90] Russell, D. & Wilson, J. (1994). Steroid 5 alpha-reductase: two genes/two enzymes. *Annu Rev Biochem,* Vol.63, pp. 25-61, ISSN:0066-4154

[91] Seckl J. & Walker, B. (2001). Minireview: 11beta-hydroxysteroid dehydrogenase type 1- a tissue-specific amplifier of glucocorticoid action. *Endocrinology,* Vol.142, No.4, (Apr), pp. 1371-1376, ISSN:0013-7227

[92] Seckl J. & Walker, B. (2004). 11beta-hydroxysteroid dehydrogenase type 1 as a modulator of glucocorticoid action: from metabolism to memory. *Trends Endocrinol Metab,* Vol.15, No.9, (Nov), pp. 418-424, ISSN:1043-2760

[93] Sen, Y.; Aygun, D.; Yilmaz, E., et al. (2008). Children and adolescents with obesity and the metabolic syndrome have high circulating cortisol levels. *Neuro Endocrinol Lett,* Vol.29, No.1, (Feb), pp. 141-145, ISSN:0172-780X

[94] Sjöstrand, M.; Jansson, P.; Palming, J., et al. (2010). Repeated measurements of 11beta-HSD-1 activity in subcutaneous adipose tissue from lean, abdominally obese, and type 2 diabetes subjects--no change following a mixed meal. *Horm Metab Res,* Vol.42, No.11, (Oct), pp. 798-802, ISSN:1439-4286

[95] Staab, C.; Stegk, J.; Haenisch, S., et al. (2011). Analysis of alternative promoter usage in expression of HSD11B1 including the development of a transcript-specific quantitative real-time PCR method. *Chem Biol Interact,* Vol.191, No.1-3, (May 30), pp. 104-112, ISSN:1872-7786

[96] Stewart, P. (2005). Tissue-specific Cushing's syndrome uncovers a new target in treating the metabolic syndrome--11beta-hydroxysteroid dehydrogenase type 1. *Clin Med,* Vol.5, No.2, (Mar-Apr), pp. 142-146, ISSN:1470-2118

[97] Stewart, P. & Krozowski, Z. (1999). 11 beta-Hydroxysteroid dehydrogenase. *Vitam Horm,* Vol.57, pp. 249-324, ISSN:0083-6729

[98] Stewart, P.; Krozowski, Z.; Gupta, A., et al. (1996). Hypertension in the syndrome of apparent mineralocorticoid excess due to mutation of the 11 beta-hydroxysteroid de-

hydrogenase type 2 gene. *Lancet,* Vol.347, No.8994, (Jan 13), pp. 88-91, ISSN: 0140-6736

[99] Stewart, P.; Murry, B. & Mason, J. (1994). Human kidney 11 beta-hydroxysteroid dehydrogenase is a high affinity nicotinamide adenine dinucleotide-dependent enzyme and differs from the cloned type I isoform. *J Clin Endocrinol Metab,* Vol.79, No.2, (Aug), pp. 480-484, ISSN:0021-972X

[100] Stewart, P.; Rogerson, F. & Mason, J. (1995). Type 2 11 beta-hydroxysteroid dehydrogenase messenger ribonucleic acid and activity in human placenta and fetal membranes: its relationship to birth weight and putative role in fetal adrenal steroidogenesis. *J Clin Endocrinol Metab,* Vol.80, No.3, (Mar), pp. 885-890, ISSN: 0021-972X

[101] Sundbom, M.; Kaiser, C.; Bjorkstrand, E., et al. (2008). Inhibition of 11betaHSD1 with the S-phenylethylaminothiazolone BVT116429 increases adiponectin concentrations and improves glucose homeostasis in diabetic KKAy mice. *BMC Pharmacol,* Vol.8, pp. 3, ISSN:1471-2210

[102] Takaya, J.; Iharada, A.; Okihana, H., et al. (2011). Magnesium deficiency in pregnant rats alters methylation of specific cytosines in the hepatic hydroxysteroid dehydrogenase-2 promoter of the offspring. *Epigenetics,* Vol.6, No.5, (May), pp. 573-578, ISSN: 1559-2308

[103] Takiguchi, M.; Achanzar, W.; Qu, W., et al. (2003). Effects of cadmium on DNA-(Cytosine-5) methyltransferase activity and DNA methylation status during cadmium-induced cellular transformation. *Exp Cell Res,* Vol.286, No.2, (Jun 10), pp. 355-365, ISSN:0014-4827

[104] Tomlinson, J.; Walker, E.; Bujalska, I., et al. (2004). 11beta-hydroxysteroid dehydrogenase type 1: a tissue-specific regulator of glucocorticoid response. *Endocr Rev,* Vol. 25, No.5, (Oct), pp. 831-866, ISSN:0163-769X

[105] Tortorella, C.; Aragona, F. & Nussdorfer, G. (1999). In vivo evidence that human adrenal glands possess 11 beta-hydroxysteroid dehydrogenase activity. *Life Sci,* Vol. 65, No.26, pp. 2823-2827, ISSN:0024-3205

[106] Tsai, P.; Yu, C.; Hsu, S., et al. (2004). Cord plasma concentrations of adiponectin and leptin in healthy term neonates: positive correlation with birthweight and neonatal adiposity. *Clin Endocrinol (Oxf),* Vol.61, No.1, (Jul), pp. 88-93, ISSN:0300-0664

[107] Vatten, L.; Nilsen, S.; Odegard, R., et al. (2002). Insulin-like growth factor I and leptin in umbilical cord plasma and infant birth size at term. *Pediatrics,* Vol.109, No.6, (Jun), pp. 1131-1135, ISSN:1098-4275

[108] Volpe, S. (2008). Magnesium, the metabolic syndrome, insulin resistance, and type 2 diabetes mellitus. *Crit Rev Food Sci Nutr,* Vol.48, No.3, (Mar), pp. 293-300, ISSN: 1040-8398

[109] Waddell, B.; Bollen, M.; Wyrwoll, C., et al. (2010). Developmental programming of adult adrenal structure and steroidogenesis: effects of fetal glucocorticoid excess and postnatal dietary omega-3 fatty acids. *J Endocrinol,* Vol.205, No.2, (May), pp. 171-178, ISSN:1479-6805

[110] Waddington, C. (1942). The epigenotype. *Endeavour,* Vol.1, pp. 18-20,

[111] Waisberg, M.; Joseph, P.; Hale, B., et al. (2003). Molecular and cellular mechanisms of cadmium carcinogenesis. *Toxicology,* Vol.192, No.2-3, (Nov 5), pp. 95-117, ISSN: 0300-483X

[112] Walker, B. (2006). Cortisol--cause and cure for metabolic syndrome? *Diabet Med,* Vol. 23, No.12, (Dec), pp. 1281-1288, ISSN:0742-3071

[113] Walker, B. (2007). Extra-adrenal regeneration of glucocorticoids by 11beta-hydroxysteroid dehydrogenase type 1: physiological regulator and pharmacological target for energy partitioning. *Proc Nutr Soc,* Vol.66, No.1, (Feb), pp. 1-8, ISSN:0029-6651

[114] Walker, B. & Andrew, R. (2006). Tissue production of cortisol by 11beta-hydroxysteroid dehydrogenase type 1 and metabolic disease. *Ann N Y Acad Sci,* Vol.1083, (Nov), pp. 165-184, ISSN:0077-8923

[115] Walker, B.; Connacher, A.; Lindsay, R., et al. (1995). Carbenoxolone increases hepatic insulin sensitivity in man: a novel role for 11-oxosteroid reductase in enhancing glucocorticoid receptor activation. *J Clin Endocrinol Metab,* Vol.80, No.11, (Nov), pp. 3155-3159, ISSN:0021-972X

[116] Walker, E.; Clark, A.; Hewison, M., et al. (2001). Functional expression, characterization, and purification of the catalytic domain of human 11-beta -hydroxysteroid dehydrogenase type 1. *J Biol Chem,* Vol.276, No.24, (Jun 15), pp. 21343-21350, ISSN: 0021-9258

[117] Wamil, M. & Seckl, J. (2007). Inhibition of 11beta-hydroxysteroid dehydrogenase type 1 as a promising therapeutic target. *Drug Discov Today,* Vol.12, No.13-14, (Jul), pp. 504-520, ISSN:1359-6446

[118] Wang, N.; Finegold, M.; Bradley, A., et al. (1995). Impaired energy homeostasis in C/EBP alpha knockout mice. *Science,* Vol.269, No.5227, (Aug 25), pp. 1108-1112, ISSN: 0036-8075

[119] Watts, L.; Manchem, V.; Leedom, T., et al. (2005). Reduction of hepatic and adipose tissue glucocorticoid receptor expression with antisense oligonucleotides improves hyperglycemia and hyperlipidemia in diabetic rodents without causing systemic glucocorticoid antagonism. *Diabetes,* Vol.54, No.6, (Jun), pp. 1846-1853, ISSN:0012-1797

[120] Weigensberg, M.; Toledo-Corral, C. & Goran, M. (2008). Association between the metabolic syndrome and serum cortisol in overweight Latino youth. *J Clin Endocrinol Metab,* Vol.93, No.4, (Apr), pp. 1372-1378, ISSN:0021-972X

[121] White B. (2008a). The endocrine and reproductive systems – The adrenal gland. Philadelphia, Mosby Elsevier.

[122] White B. (2008b). The endocrine and reproductive systems – The hypothalamus and the pituitary gland. Philadelphia, Mosby Elsevier.

[123] Whorwood, C.; Donovan, S.; Wood, P., et al. (2001). Regulation of glucocorticoid receptor alpha and beta isoforms and type I 11beta-hydroxysteroid dehydrogenase expression in human skeletal muscle cells: a key role in the pathogenesis of insulin resistance? *J Clin Endocrinol Metab,* Vol.86, No.5, (May), pp. 2296-2308, ISSN: 0021-972X

[124] Williams, L.; Lyons, V.; MacLeod, I., et al. (2000). C/EBP regulates hepatic transcription of 11beta -hydroxysteroid dehydrogenase type 1. A novel mechanism for cross-talk between the C/EBP and glucocorticoid signaling pathways. *J Biol Chem,* Vol.275, No.39, (Sep 29), pp. 30232-30239, ISSN:0021-9258

[125] Wyrwoll, C.; Kerrigan, D.; Holmes, M., et al. (2012). Altered placental methyl donor transport in the dexamethasone programmed rat. *Placenta,* Vol.33, No.3, (Mar), pp. 220-223, ISSN:1532-3102

[126] Wyrwoll, C.; Mark, P.; Mori, T., et al. (2006). Prevention of programmed hyperleptinemia and hypertension by postnatal dietary omega-3 fatty acids. *Endocrinology,* Vol. 147, No.1, (Jan), pp. 599-606, ISSN:0013-7227

[127] Wyrwoll, C.; Mark, P.; Mori, T., et al. (2008). Developmental programming of adult hyperinsulinemia, increased proinflammatory cytokine production, and altered skeletal muscle expression of SLC2A4 (GLUT4) and uncoupling protein 3. *J Endocrinol,* Vol.198, No.3, (Sep), pp. 571-579, ISSN:1479-6805

[128] Wyrwoll, C.; Mark, P. & Waddell, B. (2005). Directional secretion and transport of leptin and expression of leptin receptor isoforms in human placental BeWo cells. *Mol Cell Endocrinol,* Vol.241, No.1-2, (Sep 28), pp. 73-79, ISSN:0303-7207

[129] Yang, K.; Julan, L.; Rubio, F., et al. (2006). Cadmium reduces 11 beta-hydroxysteroid dehydrogenase type 2 activity and expression in human placental trophoblast cells. *Am J Physiol Endocrinol Metab,* Vol.290, No.1, (Jan), pp. E135-E142, ISSN:0193-1849

Section 2

Steroids: Clinical Application

Chapter 5

Sex Steroid Production from Cryopreserved and Reimplanted Ovarian Tissue

Sanghoon Lee and Seung-Yup Ku

Additional information is available at the end of the chapter

http://dx.doi.org/10.5772/53098

1. Introduction

Fertility preservation is an emerging discipline that now has a key place in the care of reproductive-aged women with cancer. Because of improvement in diagnostic and therapeutic strategies, an increasingly larger number of women are surviving with cancer. In the US, more than 11 million are living with cancer and approximately 450,000 cancer survivors are of reproductive age. In addition, 4-5% of new cancer patients are younger than 35 years [1]. As a result, quality-of-life issues, including those involving fertility preservation, have gained a significant importance in the care of women with cancer.

Ovarian tissue cryopreservation and reimplantation is a main option to preserve their fertility in cancer patients who need cancer treatments without delay or do not want to undergo ovarian stimulation. For prepubertal girls with cancer, ovarian tissue freezing is the only option for fertility preservation. The first case of human ovarian tissue cryopreservation and auto-transplantation was reported in the year 2000 [2]. To date, a total of 17 babies from 12 patients have been born worldwide from ovarian tissue cryopreservation and reimplantation [3].

Even with remarkable advances in technology and increasing enthusiasm for clinical applications, human ovarian tissue transplantation is still considered as an investigational method. There are many uncertainties and unanswered questions including the restoration of ovarian function after transplantation. Thus, in this chapter, we would like to review the concepts and methods of fertility preservation, and endocrine function after ovarian transplantation in terms of sex steroid production from the cryopreserved and reimplanted ovary.

2. Gonadal damage

Chemotherapy and radiotherapy can cause severe gonadal damages resulting in amenorrhea with ovarian follicle loss in female and azoospermia in male. Adjuvant chemotherapy particularly with alkylating agents such as cyclophosphamide is gonadotoxic and induces premature ovarian failure. The drugs are generally classified as high risk (e.g. cyclophosphamide, chlorambucil, melphalan, busulfan, nitrogen mustard, and procarbazine), intermediate risk (e.g. cisplatin, and adriamycin), and low risk (e.g. methotrexate, 5-fluorouracil, vincristine, bleomycin, and actinomycin D) [4]. (Table 1) The degree of chemotherapy-induced ovarian damage is dependent on the patient's age, the drug used, and the dosage of the drugs. Since most cancer patients are treated with multi-agent chemotherapy protocols, it is not easy to assess the degree of gonadal damage caused by a single specific agent. Radiotherapy-induced follicular damage resulting in a high risk of prolonged amenorrhea in women can occur when exposed by pelvic or whole abdominal radiation dose ≥6 Gy in adult women, ≥10 Gy in postpubertal girls, and ≥15 Gy in prepubertal girls [5-9]. The radiation dose of concurrent chemoradiation therapy (CCRT) for patients with advanced stage cervical cancer is usually about 50 Gy. Thus gynecologic oncologists should consider a possibility of post-treatment infertility in patients who undergo CCRT.

High risk	Intermediate risk	Low risk
Cyclophosphamide	Cisplatin	Methotrexate
Chlorambucil	Adriamycin	5-Fluorouracil
Melphalan		Vincristine
Busulfan		Bleomycin
Nitrogen mustard		Actinomycin D
Procarbazine		

Table 1. The degree of gonadal damage by chemotherapy [4]

3. Candidates for and determinants of access to fertility preservation

Candidates for fertility preservation include patients with childhood cancers, breast cancers, gynecologic cancers, hematologic cancers such as leukemia and lymphoma, those who need hematopoietic stem cell transplantation or pelvic irradiation for other diseases, and those with a high risk of premature ovarian failure (or primary ovarian insufficiency). Since numerous departments are involved in fertility preservation treatment, collaborating as a team with several specialists who take part in the initial cancer diagnosis and treatment, including a mental health provider, is necessary to manage cancer patients.

Although under ideal circumstances patients should be referred to fertility preservation specialists before chemotherapy; however, many of those who do not have this opportunity may develop infertility and may be referred for post-chemotherapy assisted reproduction [10]. Because the likelihood of the success of assisted reproductive techniques after chemotherapy is significantly diminished [11], it is extremely important to understand the factors that determine the access to fertility preservation and early referral. In a previous study, we evaluated the socioeconomic, demographic, and medical factors that influence early referral (before cancer treatment) to fertility preservation versus delayed referral to post-chemotherapy assisted reproduction in 314 women with breast cancer. Factors favoring referrals for fertility preservation were older age, early stage breast cancer, cancer care at an academic center, and family history of breast cancer [12]. This information has revealed the barriers against accessing early fertility preservation care.

4. Importance of early referral to fertility preservation

Oncologists should recognize the importance of fertility preservation and early referral to specialists. Both embryo and oocyte freezing for fertility preservation require ovarian stimulation with gonadotropins. Since ovarian stimulation must be started within the first four days of the menstrual cycle to be effective, and requires approximately two weeks for completion, early referral is crucial to avoid delay in chemotherapy. The author's previous study concluded that early referral prior to breast surgery enables women with breast cancer to initiate a fertility preservation cycle sooner and to undergo multiple cycles of oocyte or embryo freezing, when desired. Referral prior to breast surgery (n=35) results in the initiation of chemotherapy on average 3 weeks earlier in single fertility preservation cycles, as well as when the data from double cycles are included, compared to those referred after breast surgery (n=58). This additional time allows patients to undergo multiple cycles of fertility preservation (9/35 vs. 1/58). Women who can undergo multiple cycles are likely to be at an advantage for fertility preservation because of the additional number of eggs or embryos generated [13].

A recent study, however, indicated that still less than half of physicians routinely refer cancer patients of childbearing age to reproductive specialists [14]. Another recent study reported that while most oncologists recognize the importance of discussing infertility risks after cancer treatment, few actually discuss fertility preservation with their patients [15]. In addition, Armuand *et al.* [16] reported that there have been sex differences in access to fertility-related information and the use of fertility preservation treatment. Only half of the women had discussed fertility issues with a health care professional, although the majority of men had received information about fertility preservation such as sperm cryopreservation [16]. Potential explanations are that sperm banking for men is an easy and well established method, and that the delay is negligible compared to the required duration of ovarian stimulation for embryo or oocyte cryopreservation.

Oncologists play a key role in understanding patients' concerns regarding fertility. Fertility preservation specialists should make an effort to publicize the significance of fertility preservation for reproductive women with cancer and should provide appropriate education for both associated physicians and cancer patients who wish to preserve their fertility. As important as it is to encourage oncologists to refer young people with cancer to fertility preservation counseling, it is just as important to emphasize referral as early in the process as possible to maximize the likelihood of success.

5. Standard methods for fertility preservation

The American Society of Clinical Oncology (ASCO) has issued practice guidelines for fertility preservation options in cancer patients [17]. Several well established methods of fertility preservation have been introduced, including embryo cryopreservation, gonadal shielding during radiotherapy, trachelectomy, and ovarian transposition. (Table 2)

Standard methods	Experimental methods
Embryo cryopreservation	Oocyte cryopreservation
Gonadal shielding during radiation therapy	Ovarian cryopreservation and transplantation
Ovarian transposition (oophoropexy)	Ovarian suppression with GnRH analogs or antagonists
Trachelectomy	
Other conservative gynecologic surgery	

Table 2. Fertility preservation options in females [17]

Embryo cryopreservation is a well-established technique and the current live-birth rate per transfer using frozen thawed embryos is 35.6% in US women under 35-year-old (http://www.sart.org, 2008). Embryo freezing should initially be considered for fertility preservation treatment if there is adequate time for ovarian stimulation and a partner or donor sperm.

Gonadal shielding during radiotherapy should be considered if radiotherapy is required for cancer treatment. For example, radiation plays an important role in the management of breast cancer, which can be classified into four categories: 1) Primary radiotherapy in breast-conserving treatment for early breast cancer, 2) Adjuvant radiotherapy after mastectomy for high-risk patients, 3) Radiotherapy after neo-adjuvant chemotherapy in locally-advanced breast cancers, and 4) Palliative radiotherapy for metastatic disease [18].

Trachelectomy is also an accepted method for the surgical management of early stage cervical cancer in women who wish to preserve their fertility. Cervical cancer is one of the most common cancers in women younger than 40 along with breast cancer, non-Hodgkin's lymphoma, and leukemia [19]. Indications for trachelectomy are described in Table 3.

1. Women who desire to preserve fertility (age<40-45)
2. Stage Ia1[a] (with lymph vascular space involvement), Ia2, Ib1
3. Lesion size ≤2 cm
4. Histologically squamous, adeno-, or adenosquamous carcinoma
5. No upper cervical canal involvement of cancer
6. No evidence of lymph node metastasis
[a]Conization, Ia1 without lymph vascular space involvement

Table 3. Indications for trachelectomy in cervical cancer [20]

Plante *et al.* [20] reported their experience with 125 patients who underwent vaginal radical trachelectomy. The recurrence rate of cervical cancer after trachelectomy was less than 5% and the death rate was less than 2%. Having lesions sized >2 cm was a strong risk factor for recurrence. A total of 58 women out of 125 conceived a total of 106 pregnancies, and of those, 73% of pregnancies reached the third trimester, of which, in turn, 75% gave birth at term. Overall, 13.5% of patients were associated with fertility problems.

Ovarian transposition can be performed not only for preservation of fertility but also for prevention of premature ovarian failure in cervical cancer patients who require radiotherapy. It is necessary for gynecologic oncologists to understand the field of radiotherapy to prepare for ovarian transposition. Usually, standard fields are used with the upper field border on the fourth/fifth lumbar vertebra [21]. It is widely accepted that surgical transposition should be at least 3 cm above the upper border of the radiation field [22]. Hwang *et al.* [23] reported that a location for the transposed ovary higher than 1.5 cm above the iliac crest is recommended to avoid ovarian failure after primary or adjuvant pelvic radiotherapy in cervical cancer.

To date, the remaining methods are considered to be experimental, although the oocyte survival rate (81% vs. 68%) and live-birth rate per embryo transfer (34% vs. 14%) of oocyte cryopreservation with vitrification is significantly higher than with conventional slow freezing methods [24]. Noyes *et al.* [25] asked whether it is "time to remove the experimental label" of oocyte cryopreservation. Because of the improvements in advanced technologies including freezing-thawing methods, a new guideline is necessary to update fertility preservation specialists with the latest knowledge.

6. Ovarian cryopreservation and transplantation

The first ovarian transplant with cryopreserved ovarian tissue was performed by Dr. Kutluk Oktay in 1999 [25]. In 2004, Dr. Donnez reported the first successful birth from slow, or controlled rate, frozen ovarian tissue [26].In 1997, samples of ovarian cortex were taken from a woman with Hodgkin's lymphoma and cryo-preserved in a rate freezer and stored in liquid nitrogen. After chemotherapy the patient had premature ovarian failure. In 2003, after freeze-thawing, orthotopic autotransplantation of ovarian cortical tissue was done by laparoscopy and five months after reimplantation signs indicated recovery of regular ovulatory cycles. A viable intrauterine pregnancy was confirmed eleven months after reimplantation that resulted in a live birth.

The first case report of nonautologous orthotopic transplantation of fresh ovarian tissue was from one monozygotic twin sister to the other, who had suffered from premature ovarian failure [27]. The procedure resulted in a live birth. These investigators have repeated this procedure in 10 sets of monozygotic twins [28], and successfully transplanted an intact fresh ovary [29]. Others have reported a live birth after allografting of ovarian cortex between monozygotic twins with Turner mosaic and discordant ovarian function [30].

Human ovarian tissues have been xenotransplanted to immunodeficient mice, with subsequent ovulation [31-33]; however, aberrant microtubule organization and chromatin patterns observed during the maturation process are of significant concern [34,35]. The risk of contamination with trans-species retroviral infections also needs to be addressed prior to testing this experimental approach clinically.

Successful pregnancies after ovarian tissue cryopreservation followed by transplantation have been reported in some human studies [36-39]. Transplantation of cryopreserved ovarian tissue has shown to be a potential method for recovery of ovarian function [2]. Advantages of ovarian tissue transplantation are not only preservation of fertility but also restoration of endocrine function in young women after cancer treatment.

Ovarian tissue cryopreservation and reimplantation is a main option for preserving the fertility of cancer patients who need cancer treatments without delay or do not want to undergo ovarian stimulation. For prepubertal girls diagnosed with cancer, ovarian tissue freezing is the only option for fertility preservation. To date, a total of 17 babies from 12 patients have been born worldwide from ovarian tissue cryopreservation and reimplantation [3]. Based on the site of reimplantation of cryopreserved ovarian tissue, transplantation can be classified into two different types: orthotopic (e.g. to remaining ovarian tissue or pelvic peritoneum) and heterotopic(e.g. in the abdominal wall, forearm, and chest wall) transplantation.

7. Sex steroid production from cryopreserved and reimplanted ovary

7.1. Types of sex steroids

Sex steroids or gonadal steroids are steroid hormones that interact with androgen or estrogen receptors [40]. Their effects are mediated by slow genomic mechanisms through nuclear receptors as well as by fast nongenomic mechanisms through membrane-associated receptors and signaling cascades [41]. The non-steroid hormones such as luteinizing hormone (LH), follicle-stimulating hormone (FSH) and gonadotropin-releasing hormone (GnRH) are usually not considered as sex hormones, even though they mainly play sex-related roles.

Natural sex steroids are produced by the gonads, adrenal glands, or conversion from other sex steroids in other tissues such as the liver or fat [42].

Two main classes of sex steroids are androgens and estrogens and their human derivatives are testosterone and estradiol, respectively. Progestogen is also regarded as a third class of sex steroids. Progesterone is the most important and only naturally-occurring human progestogen. In general, androgens are considered "male sex hormones", while estrogens and progestagens are considered as "female sex hormones".

Androgens	**Estrogens**	**Progestogens**
Anabolic steroids	Estradiol	Progesterone
Androstenedione	Estriol	
Dehydroepiandrosterone	Estrone	
Dihydrotestosterone		
Testosterone		

Table 4. Types of sex steroids [40,41]

Transplantation of cryopreserved ovarian tissue has shown to be a potential method for recovery of ovarian function [2]. Advantages of ovarian tissue transplantation are not only preserving fertility but also restoring endocrine function in young women after cancer treatment. In a review of successful orthotopic frozen-thawed ovarian reimplantation, restoration of ovarian activity was shown to be between 3.5 and 6.5 months after transplantation [43]. Oktay *et al.* [2,44] reported the first case of laparoscopic transplantation of frozen-thawed ovarian tissue into the pelvic sidewall with subsequent ovulation and subcutaneous ovarian transplantation to the forearm, which resulted in preserved endocrine function and follicular development. Approximately 10 weeks after ovarian transplantation to the forearm, endocrine function was restored with decreased FSH and LH levels, and cyclical variation of peripheral estradiol levels [44]. Silber reported the recovery of ovarian function in terms of recovery of menstrual cycles and hormone levels (FSH) approximately 80 to 140 days after reimplantation from their fresh and frozen transplant cases [3].

7.2. The longevity of ovarian transplantation

Dr. Kim reported the longevity of ovarian grafts in five cancer patients who underwent heterotopic autotransplantation of frozen-thawed ovarian tissue between 2001 and 2011 [45]. The age of patients at the time of ovarian transplantation was between 30 and 40. Cryopreserved ovarian tissue (for 1–10 years) was rapidly thawed and transplanted into the space between the rectus sheath and muscle. Endocrine function was measured by monthly blood tests (FSH, LH, E_2, progesterone and testosterone) and ultrasound after transplantation. The monitoring was continued until the cessation of endocrine function had been confirmed by consecutive blood tests (E_2<20 pg/mL; FSH≥35 IU/L).

Endocrine function was restored in all patients between 12–20 weeks after ovarian tissue transplantation. Four patients required the second transplantation one to two years after the first transplantation. The duration of endocrine function after the second transplantation was much longer (9–84 months). The longest duration of endocrine function was observed in a patient who underwent ovarian transplantation in 2003 and 2004 after radiotherapy for cervical cancer. Even for more than seven years after transplantation, endocrine function had not ceased (FSH 9.5 IU/L, E_2 108 pg/mL). She underwent three IVF cycles which resulted in four embryos.

The longevity of grafted ovarian tissue has been debated for many years. The duration of endocrine function after frozen-thawed ovarian tissue transplantation is still uncertain. Dr. Kim described that the endocrine function lasting for seven years can be established with heterotopic transplantation of cryobanked human ovarian tissue. This information will benefit young cancer survivors with premature ovarian failure.

In the UK, researchers indicated that the duration of graft life is greater than 7 years [46].Undoubtedly, the length of time the grafts function will depend on several factors [45, 46].

1. Age at the time of cryopreservation
2. Baseline ovarian reserve
3. History of cancer treatment
4. Techniques of ovarian tissue preparation
5. Freezing-thawing protocols
6. Number of cortical tissue grafted
7. Techniques and sites of transplantation
8. Degree of ischemia after transplantation
9. Number of follicles in the ovarian grafts

Table 5. Factors associated with the longevity of grafted ovarian tissue [45,46]

One of the most important factors may be the number of eggs' survival during the freezing-thawing and revascularization process. If one makes an assumption that one third of an ovary is transplanted into the patient (the proportion quoted in the linked report), and that during revascularization two thirds of the immature eggs are lost,[47,48] then we can calculate how many immature eggs are likely to survive the freeze/thaw and revascularization process to ensure that >1000 non-growing follicles are successfully transplanted (the number present at the menopause) [49,50]. It has been estimated that at age 36.9 years insufficient non-growing follicles will remain after cryopreservation to sustain ovarian function in 40% of the healthy population. At age 40 years we estimate that 60% of healthy women will be unlikely to benefit from ovarian cryopreservation.

We need to assess the indications and risk-benefit analysis carefully for future patients. The value of ovarian cryopreservation to preserve fertility for young cancer survivors may be proven, however the indications for those who should be offered this new technology are not yet established.

7.3. Ovarian function after isotransplantation

Dr. Silber reported his novel experience about the nine identical twin pairs discordant for premature ovarian failure that underwent their orthotopic ovarian isotransplantation between 2004 and 2008 [27]. All of these fresh ovary transplants were successful, resulting in 11 healthy babies in 7 of the 9 recipients. The same surgical techniques were then applied to 3 frozen ovary tissue transplants, up to 14 years after the ovary had been frozen, resulting in 3 more healthy babies [28,29].

Silber *et al* reported that the first rise in estradiol was observed 71 days after implantation of fresh tissue [27]. In their published series, the time to first menses after transplantation ranged between 65 to 93 days [28]. Recipients routinely resumed ovulatory menstrual cycles and normal Day 3 serum FSH levels by 4.5 months. Most conceived naturally (three of them twice or three times from the same graft). The duration of function of fresh ovarian grafts indicated minimal oocyte loss from ischemia period. Grafts of just modest portions of ovarian tissue have lasted >7 years. *In vitro* studies suggest that vitrification of ovarian tissue may be an improvement over the 70% oocyte viability loss from slow freeze [29].

This newly favorable experience is not limited just to one center [43]. Equally robust results are being experienced in Brussels, Paris, Spain, Denmark and Israel. Frozen ovarian grafts with the slow freeze technique in Denmark are lasting over 5 years and many spontaneous pregnancies have been reported without IVF techniques or other adjuvant treatment. To date, 28 healthy babies have been born from ovarian tissue grafting including fresh/frozen ovarian tissue transplantation, and most involved no IVF, and resulted from just regular intercourse without any other treatment [2].

7.4. Ovarian function after allogenic transplantation

Recently, autologous orthotopic transplantation of cryopreserved ovarian tissue has resulted in live births. Dr. Donnez reported three cases of ovarian transplantation between two genetically non-identical sisters in 2010 [51]. The three recipient patients presented with iatrogenic premature ovarian failure due to chemotherapy and radiotherapy. The recipients had all received bone marrow and ovarian tissue from their HLA-compatible sisters in each case.

None of the recipients were on any steroid or immunosuppressive therapy and all presented with documented premature ovarian failure. Their ovaries were atrophic and serial sections of biopsies failed to demonstrate the presence of any follicles. Premature ovarian failure was confirmed by very high FSH and LH levels, very low estradiol concentrations and the absence of follicles in large biopsies removed from the patients' atrophic ovaries during transplantation. For the first time, successful restoration of ovarian function after transplantation of ovarian cortex between genetically different sisters was reported.

The time interval between implantation of ovarian tissue and follicular development was found to be between 3.5 and 6 months, consistent with the previous study by Silber *et al* [27]. The time interval of 6 months observed in patients 1 was associated with a low follicular reserve in the donor (aged 32 years), and a delay for the primordial follicles development. In Patients 2 and 3, the follicular density of the donor ovarian specimen was high and recovery of ovarian activity occurred 3.5 months after reimplantation, as observed in the series of Silber and Gosden [28], who also observed an interval of 3.5 months after reimplantation of fresh ovarian cortex between monozygotic twins. In addition, the ischemic period was recently estimated to be between 3 and 5 days by van Eyck *et al.* [52,53].

7.5. Endocrine function after upper extremity ovarian autotransplantation in girls

Upper-extremity ovarian autologoustransplantation was used in three girls (ages 5, 2, and 1 year) diagnosed with Wilms tumor undergoing abdominal/pelvic radiation therapy at the tertiary pediatric medical center in the US [54]. Data were availablefor follow-up for 20-25 years.

Patients presented with Wilms tumor underwent surgical resection. Each patient underwent ovarian autotransplantation to upper extremity in order to move ovarian tissue out of the radiation field. Subjects 1 and 2 had thin slices from 1 ovary placed in the arm and subject 3 had a free transfer of the entire ovary into the axilla. Subjects 1 and 2 showed spontaneous follicular development of the autotransplanted ovarian tissue. They had fluctuating gonadotropin and estradiol levels until age 29 and 26, respectively; spontaneous menses until age 29 and 26; and cessation of spontaneous menses with elevated gonadotropins and low estradiol levels at age 30 and 26. Subject 3 had severe monthly axillary pain, and the ovary was transferred back into the pelvis. She then had ovarian dysfunction with intermittent spontaneous ovarian activity until age 25.

Ovarian autotransplantation to the upper extremity resulted in long-term sex steroid production for spontaneous puberty, menarche, follicular development, and menses with fluctuating gonadotropin and ovarian sex steroid levels and follicular activity that lasted for 13-15 years.

8. Breast cancer and sex steroid hormone

Breast cancer is the most common cancer in women of reproductive age in the US [55]. Most women with breast cancer require adjuvant chemotherapy including cyclophosphamide. At an average age of 40, administration of cyclophosphamide, methotrexate, and 5-Fluorouracil (CMF) or Adriamycin, cyclophosphamide and Taxol (AC+T) resulted in amenorrhea in 20% to 100% or 37% to 77% of patients followed up for 1 year after adjuvant chemotherapy, respectively [56].

For fertility preservation, ovarian stimulation with gonadotropins for embryo or oocyte cryopreservation results in excessive levels of estrogen production. To reduce estrogen exposure during ovarian stimulation in hormone-dependent cancer, a novel protocol using letrozole (a third generation aromatase inhibitor) and gonadotropins was developed by Dr. Oktay [57]. (Figure 1) Use of aromatase inhibitors became increasingly common in the treatment of breast cancer [58]. They have also recently been introduced for ovulation induction. When compared to clomiphene cycles, they produce comparable peak estradiol levels or

http://dx.doi.org/10.5772/53098

those even lower than the natural cycle. Because of their dual effects, they can be used in breast and endometrial cancer patients for ovulation induction. Tamoxifen cannot be used in those women during ovarian stimulation as it is antagonistic to the endometrium. Based on our unpublished data, long-term follow-up for up to 7 years, the letrozole protocol showed safe, efficient, and age-appropriate pregnancy success rates.

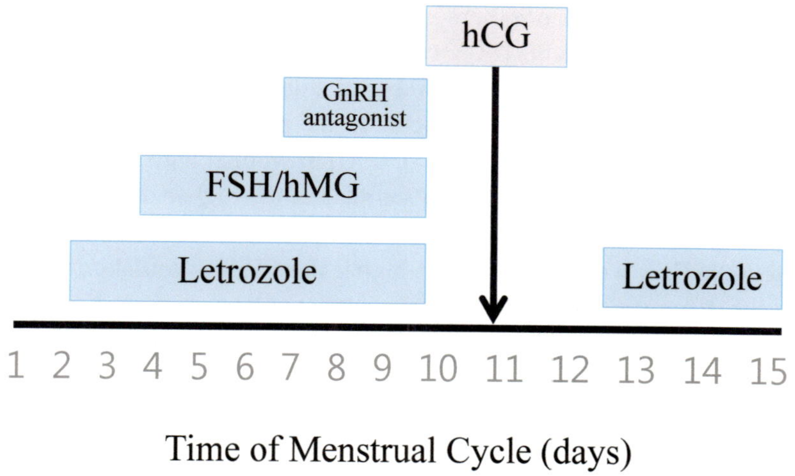

Figure 1. Protocol for ovarian stimulation with letrozole and gonadotropins in women with breast cancer [57]

In North America, Europe, and other parts of the world, aromatase inhibitors are available for the treatment of postmenopausal breast cancer, but not for ovulation induction. Letrozole and anastrozole are triazole (antifungal) derivatives that are potent, reversible, competitive, nonsteroidal aromatase inhibitors [59,60]. These drugs inhibit estrogen levels by 97 to 99 percent at doses of 1 to 5 mg/day which result in estrogen concentrations below the level detected by most sensitive immunoassays. Nonsteroidal aromatase inhibitors are completely absorbed after oral administration and cleared mainly by the liver. Mean terminal half-life is approximately 45 hours (range 30 to 60 hours). Exemestane is a steroidal aromatase inhibitor and its circulating half-life is approximately nine hours, but the inhibitory effect is potentially much longer because its effect on aromatase is irreversible [61].

Aromatase inhibitors are generally well tolerated and known side effects are hot flushes, nausea/vomiting, headache, back pain, and leg cramps [60,62,63]. These adverse effects were reported in older breast cancer patients who were given the drugs on a daily basis over several months in Phase III trials. Very few withdrew from the trials because of drug-related adverse effects [64,65]. In the clinical experience, using a short course of aromatase inhibitor for induction of ovulation in young healthy women had fewer side effects than with clomiphene citrate [57,66].

Ovarian stimulation for embryo or oocyte cryopreservation should be started within the first four days of the menstrual cycle. Depending on whether the referral is made before or after breast surgery, usually no more than one or two cycles of ovarian stimulation can be performed without delaying chemotherapy in women with breast cancer [13]. This delay is generally acceptable as multiple studies have shown no effect on survival or recurrence in breast cancer patients if chemotherapy had been initiated as late as 12 weeks after breast surgery [67,68].

In fertility preservation cycles, since there is limited time available prior to the onset of chemotherapy in breast cancer patients [13], ovarian stimulation is often performed with higher doses of gonadotropins to maximize the number of embryos or oocytes cryopreserved, and to increase the likelihood of future pregnancies. In the previous study, we compared a low dose FSH start (=150 IU) with a high dose (>150 IU) in women with breast cancer undergoing fertility preservation with letrozole and found that the higher dose FSH stimulation in letrozole cycles did not improve pregnancy outcomes, and may be associated with a lower live birth rate [69]. Thus we concluded that higher dose FSH stimulation with letrozole in women with breast cancer did not improve reproductive outcomes and may be associated with lower live birth rates. In addition, it may increase estrogen exposure as well as the costs of fertility preservation.

9. Ovarian suppression using GnRH agonist or antagonist to prevent gonadal damage

Given the current evidence, both the efficacy and safety of the use of GnRH agonists or antagonists during chemotherapy for prevention of gonadal damage are controversial. Several studies have suggested a decreased incidence of amenorrhea with the use of GnRH agonists throughout chemotherapy; however, most have been non-randomized or small sample sized studies. Only five randomized trials have been completed.

Badawy *et al.* [70] and Del Mastro *et al.* [71] demonstrated the positive effect of GnRH agonists on the resumption of menses and ovulation; however, Leonard *et al.* [72], Gerber *et al.* [73], and Munster *et al.* [74] revealed that there was no impact of GnRH agonists on the prevention of early menopause or ovarian function.

Recently, Partidge [75] reported that women who are interested in future fertility and the providers who are assisting them should not depend on GnRH agonist treatment during chemotherapy for preservation of menstrual and ovarian function or fertility. There is one randomized ongoing study by the Southwest Oncology Group, called the Prevention of Early Menopause Study, a large international multicenter trial. This study will provide additional complementary information including biomarkers of ovarian reserve and rates of long-term amenorrhea or premature ovarian failure in women with or without ovarian suppression throughout treatment period.

10. Conclusions

Based on our review, we believe that ovarian cryopreservation and reimplantation in women diagnosed with cancer before cancer treatments is an effective option to preserve their fertility and to restore gonadal endocrine function. Restoration of ovarian activity in terms of sex steroid production was observed in almost all cases of ovarian reimplantation. All pregnancies were reported from the orthotopic autotransplantation, but none from the heterotopic autotransplantation. Restoration of endocrine function has been demonstrated consistently in both methods, although heterotopic sites may not provide an optimal environment for pregnancy. Physicians should consider the life span and the time period for the initiation of sex steroid production of transplanted ovarian tissue in order to provide an exact data, especially when counseling and making a treatment plan for cancer survivors.

Author details

Sanghoon Lee[1] and Seung-Yup Ku[2*]

*Address all correspondence to: jyhsyk@snu.ac.kr

1 Department of Obstetrics and Gynecology, Korea University College of Medicine, Seoul, Korea

2 Department of Obstetrics and Gynecology, Seoul National University College of Medicine, Seoul, Korea

References

[1] Knapp CA, Quinn GP. Healthcare provider perspectives on fertilitypreservation for cancer patients. Cancer Treat Res. 2010;156:391–401.

[2] Oktay K, Karlikaya G. Ovarian function after transplantation of frozen, banked autologous ovarian tissue. NEngl J Med. 2000;342:1919.

[3] Sibler SJ. Ovarian cryopreservation and transplantation for fertility preservation.Mol Hum Reprod 2012;18:59-67.

[4] Rodriguez-Wallberg KA, Oktay K. Options on fertility preservation in female cancer patients. Cancer Treat Rev 2012;38:354-61.

[5] Sklar C. Maintenance of ovarian function and risk of premature menopause related to cancer treatment. J Natl Cancer InstMonogr 2005:25-7.

[6] Wallace WH, Thomson AB, Saran F, Kelsey TW. Predicting age of ovarian failure after radiation to a field that includes the ovaries.Int J RadiatOncolBiolPhys 2005;62:738-44.

[7] Wo JY, Viswanathan AN. Impact of radiotherapy on fertility, pregnancy, and neonatal outcomes in female cancer patients. Int J RadiatOncolBiolPhys 2009;73:1304-12.

[8] Green DM, Sklar CA, Boice JD Jr, Mulvihill JJ, Whitton JA, Stovall M, et al. Ovarian failure and reproductive outcomes after childhood cancer treatment: results from the Childhood Cancer Survivor Study. J ClinOncol 2009;27:2374-81.

[9] Chemaitilly W, Mertens AC, Mitby P, Whitton J, Stovall M, Yasui Y, et al. Acute ovarian failure in the childhood cancer survivor study. J ClinEndocrinolMetab 2006;91:1723-8.

[10] Oktem O, Oktay K. Fertility preservation for breast cancer patients. SeminReprod Med 2009;27:486-92.

[11] Azim A, Rauch ER, Ravich M, Witkin S, Oktay K. Ovarian reserve is impaired in cancer patients with normal baseline FSH who previously received chemotherapy as determined by response to controlled ovarian stimulation and anti-mullerian hormone measurements: a controlled study. FertilSteril 2006;86 (Suppl 2):S123-S4.

[12] Lee S, Heytens E, Moy F, Ozkavukcu S, Oktay K. Determinants of access to fertility preservation in women with breast cancer. FertilSteril 2011;95:1932-6.

[13] Lee S, Ozkavukcu S, Heytens E, Moy F, Oktay K. Value of early referral to fertility preservation in young women with breast cancer. J ClinOncol 2010;28:4683-6.

[14] Quinn GP, Vadaparampil ST, Lee JH, Jacobsen PB, Bepler G, Lancaster J, et al. Physician referral for fertility preservation in oncology patients: a national study of practice behaviors. J ClinOncol 2009;27:5952-7.

[15] Forman EJ, Anders CK, Behera MA. Pilot survey of oncologists regarding treatment-related infertility and fertility preservation in female cancer patients. J Reprod Med 2009;54:203-7.

[16] Armuand GM, Rodriguez-Wallberg KA, Wettergren L, Ahlgren J, Enblad G, Hoglund M, et al. Sex differences in fertility-related information received by young adult cancer survivors. J ClinOncol 2012;30:2147-53.

[17] Lee SJ, Schover LR, Partridge AH, Patrizio P, Wallace WH, Hagerty K, et al. American Society of Clinical Oncology recommendations on fertility preservation in cancer patients. J ClinOncol 2006;24:2917-31.

[18] Suh CO. Radiotherapy for breast cancer. J Korean Med Assoc 2003;46:503-11.

[19] Jemal A, Murray T, Ward E, Samuels A, Tiwari RC, Ghafoor A, et al. Cancer statistics, 2005. CA Cancer J Clin 2005;55:10-30.

[20] Plante M, Gregoire J, Renaud MC, Roy M. The vaginal radical trachelectomy: an update of a series of 125 cases and 106 pregnancies. GynecolOncol 2011;121:290-7.

[21] Marnitz S, Kohler C, Schneider A, Seiler F, Hinkelbein W. Interindividual variability of lymph drainages in patients with cervical cancer. Implication on irradiation planning.StrahlentherOnkol 2006;182:80-5.

[22] Martin JR, Kodaman P, Oktay K, Taylor HS. Ovarian cryopreservation with transposition of a contralateral ovary: a combined approach for fertility preservation in women receiving pelvic radiation. FertilSteril 2007;87:189 e5-7.

[23] Hwang JH, Yoo HJ, Park SH, Lim MC, Seo SS, Kang S, et al. Association between the location of transposed ovary and ovarian function in patients with uterine cervical cancer treated with (postoperative or primary) pelvic radiotherapy. FertilSteril 2012;97:1387-93 e2.

[24] Noyes N, Porcu E, Borini A. Over 900 oocyte cryopreservation babies born with no apparent increase in congenital anomalies.Reprod Biomed Online 2009;18:769-76.

[25] Oktay K, Oktem O. Ovarian cryopreservation and transplantation for fertility preservation for medical indications: report of an ongoing experience. Fertil.Steril. 2008;93(3): 762–8.

[26] Donnez J, Dolmans MM, Demylle D, et al. Livebirth after orthotopic transplantation of cryopreserved ovarian tissue. Lancet 2004;364:1405-10

[27] Silber SJ, Lenahan KM, Levine DJ, et al. Ovarian transplantation between monozygotic twins discordant for premature ovarian failure. N Engl J Med 2005; 353:58.

[28] Silber SJ, Gosden RG. Ovarian transplantation in a series of monozygotic twins discordant for ovarian failure. N Engl J Med 2007; 356:1382.

[29] Silber SJ, Grudzinskas G, Gosden RG. Successful pregnancy after microsurgical transplantation of an intact ovary. N Engl J Med 2008; 359:2617.

[30] Donnez J, Dolmans MM, Squifflet J, et al. Live birth after allografting of ovarian cortex between monozygotic twins with Turner syndrome (45,XO/46,XX mosaicism) and discordant ovarian function. FertilSteril 2011; 96:1407.

[31] Oktay K, Newton H, Mullan J, Gosden RG. Development of human primordial follicles to antral stages in SCID/hpg mice stimulated with follicle stimulating hormone. Hum Reprod 1998; 13:1133.

[32] Oktay K, Newton H, Gosden RG. Transplantation of cryopreserved human ovarian tissue results in follicle growth initiation in SCID mice. FertilSteril 2000;73:599.

[33] Gook DA, McCully BA, Edgar DH, McBain JC. Development of antral follicles in human cryopreserved ovarian tissue following xenografting. Hum Reprod 2001; 16:417.

[34] Lucifero D, Mertineit C, Clarke HJ, et al. Methylation dynamics of imprinted genes in mouse germ cells. Genomics 2002; 79:530.

[35] Kim SS, Kang HG, Kim NH, et al. Assessment of the integrity of human oocytes retrieved from cryopreserved ovarian tissue after xenotransplantation. Hum Reprod 2005; 20:2502.

[36] Donnez J, Dolmans MM, Demylle D, et al. Livebirth after orthotopic transplantation of cryopreserved ovarian tissue. Lancet 2004;364:1405-10

[37] Meirow D, Levron J, Eldar-Geva T, et al. Pregnancy after transplantation of cryopreserved ovarian tissue in a patient with ovarian failure after chemotherapy. N Engl J Med 2005;353:318-21

[38] Demeestere I, Simon P, Emiliani S, et al. Fertility preservation: successful transplantation of cryopreserved ovarian tissue in a young patient previously treated for Hodgkin's disease. Oncologist 2007;12:1437-42

[39] Andersen CY, Rosendahl M, Byskov AG, et al. Two successful pregnancies following autotransplantation of frozen/thawed ovarian tissue. Hum Reprod 2008;23:2266-72

[40] Guerriero G. Vertebrate sex steroid receptors: evolution, ligands, and neurodistribution. Ann N Y Acad Sci. 2009l;1163:154-68.

[41] Thakur MK, Paramanik V. Role of steroid hormone coregulators in health and disease. Horm Res. 2009;71(4):194-200.

[42] Brook CG. Mechanism of puberty.Horm Res. 1999;51Suppl 3:52-4.

[43] Donnez J, Silber S, Andersen CY, Demeestere I, Piver P, Meirow D, et al. Children born after autotransplantation of cryopreserved ovarian tissue. a review of 13 live births. Ann Med 2011;43:437-50.

[44] Oktay K, Economos K, Kan M, Rucinski J, Veeck L, Rosenwaks Z. Endocrine function and oocyte retrieval after autologous transplantation of ovarian cortical strips to the forearm. JAMA 2001;286:1490-3.

[45] Kim SS. Assessment of long term endocrine function after transplantation of frozen-thawed human ovarian tissue to the heterotopic site: 10 year longitudinal follow-up study. J Assist Reprod Genet. 2012;29:489-493

[46] Wallace WH, Kelsey TW, Anderson RA. Ovarian cryopreservation: experimental or established and a cure for the menopause? Reprod Biomed Online 2012;25:93-95

[47] Baird, D.T., Webb, R., Campbell, B.K., Harkness, L.M., Gosden,R.G. Long-term ovarian function in sheep after ovariectomyand transplantation of autografts stored at -196℃. Endocrinology 1999;140: 462–471.

[48] Demirci, B., Lornage, J., Salle, B., Frappart, L., Franck, M.,Guerin, J.F., 2001. Follicular viability and morphology ofsheep ovaries after exposure to cryoprotectant and cryopreservationwith different freezing protocols.Fertil.Steril.2001;75:754–762.

[49] Faddy, M.J., Gosden, R.G. A model conforming the decline infollicle numbers to the age of menopause in women. HumReprod. 1996;11:1484–1486.

[50] Wallace, W.H., Kelsey, T.W. Human ovarian reserve fromconception to the menopause. PLoS One 2010;5:e8772.

[51] Donnez J, Squifflet J, Pirard C, Jadoul P, Dolmans MM. Restroration of ovarian function after allografting of ovarian cortex between genetically non-identical sisters. Hum Reprod 2010;25:2489-2495

[52] Van Eyck AS, Jordan B, Gallez B, Heilier JF, Van Langendonckt A, Donnez J.Electron paramagnetic resonance as a tool to evaluate human ovariantissue reoxygenation after xenografting. FertilSteril 2009;92:374–381.

[53] Van Eyck AS, Bouzin C, Feron O, Romeu L, Van Langendonckt A,Donnez J, Dolmans MM. Both host and graft vessels contribute torevascularization of xenografted human ovarian tissue in a murinemodel. FertilSteril 2010;93:1676–1685.

[54] Laufer MR, Upton J, Schuster SR, Grier H, Emans SJ, Diller L. Ovarian tissue autologous transplantation to the upper extremity for girls receiving abdominal/pelvic radiation: 20-year follow-up of reproductive endocrine function. J PediatrAdolescGynecol 2010;23:107-110

[55] American Cancer Society: Cancer Facts & Figures 2009. [Internet]. Atlanta: American Cancer Society Inc.; c2009 [2012 Jun 27]. Available from: http://www.cancer.org/acs/groups/content/@nho/documents/document/500809webpdf.pdf.

[56] Sonmezer M, Oktay K. Fertility preservation in young women undergoing breast cancer therapy. Oncologist 2006;11:422-34.

[57] Azim AA, Costantini-Ferrando M, Oktay K. Safety of fertility preservation by ovarian stimulation with letrozole and gonadotropins in patients with breast cancer: a prospective controlled study. J ClinOncol 2008;26:2630-5

[58] Goss PE, Ingle JN, Martino S, Robert NJ, Muss HB, Piccart MJ, et al. A randomized trial of letrozole in postmenopausal women after five years of tamoxifen therapy for early-stage breast cancer. N Engl J Med 2003;349:1793-802.

[59] Buzdar A, Howell A. Advances in aromatase inhibition: clinical efficacy and tolerability in the treatment of breast cancer. Clin Cancer Res 2001; 7:2620-2635.

[60] Winer EP, Hudis C, Burstein HJ, et al. American Society of Clinical Oncology technology assessment on the use of aromatase inhibitors as adjuvant therapy for women with hormone receptor-positive breast cancer: status report 2002. J ClinOncol 2002; 20(15):3317-3327.

[61] Mauras N, Lima J, Patel D, et al. Pharmacokinetics and dose finding of a potent aromatase inhibitor, aromasin (exemestane), in young males. J ClinEndocrinolMetab 2003; 88:5951-5956.

[62] Buzdar A, Jonat W, Howell A, et al. Anastrozole, a potent and selective aromatase inhibitor, versus megestrol acetate in postmenopausal women with advanced breast

cancer: results of overview analysis of two phase III trials. Arimidex Study Group. J ClinOncol 1996; 14:2000-2011.

[63] Marty, M, Gershanovich, M, Campos, B, Romien, G, et al. Aromatase inhibitors, a new potent, selective aromatase inhibitor superior to aminoglutethimide in postmenopausal women with advanced breast cancer previously treated with antioestrogens. Proc Am SocClinOncol 1997; 16:156.

[64] Hamilton A, Piccart M. The third-generation non-steroidal aromatase inhibitors: a review of their clinical benefits in the second-line hormonal treatment of advanced breast cancer. Ann Oncol 1999; 10:377-384.

[65] Goss PE. Risks versus benefits in the clinical application of aromatase inhibitors.EndocrRelat Cancer 1999; 6:325-332.

[66] Oktay K. Further evidence on the safety and success of ovarian stimulation with letrozole and tamoxifen in breast cancer patients undergoing in vitro fertilization to cryopreserve their embryos for fertility preservation. J ClinOncol 2005;23:3858-3859

[67] Lohrisch C, Paltiel C, Gelmon K, Speers C, Taylor S, Barnett J, et al. Impact on survival of time from definitive surgery to initiation of adjuvant chemotherapy for early-stage breast cancer. J ClinOncol 2006;24:4888-94.

[68] Cold S, During M, Ewertz M, Knoop A, Moller S. Does timing of adjuvant chemotherapy influence the prognosis after early breast cancer? Results of the Danish Breast Cancer Cooperative Group (DBCG). Br J Cancer 2005;93:627-32

[69] Lee S, Oktay K. Does higher starting dose of FSH stimulation with letrozole improve fertility preservation outcomes in women with breast cancer.FertilSteril2012 Jul 6. [Epub ahead of print]

[70] Badawy A, Elnashar A, El-Ashry M, Shahat M. Gonadotropin-releasing hormone agonists for prevention of chemotherapy-induced ovarian damage: prospective randomized study. FertilSteril 2009;91:694-7.

[71] Del Mastro L, Boni L, Michelotti A, Gamucci T, Olmeo N, Gori S, et al. Effect of the gonadotropin-releasing hormone analogue triptorelin on the occurrence of chemotherapy-induced early menopause in premenopausal women with breast cancer: a randomized trial. JAMA 2011;306:269-76.

[72] Leonard RC, Adamson D, Anderson R, Ballinger R, Bertelli G, Coeman RE, et al. The OPTION trial of adjuvant ovarian protection by goserelin in adjuvant chemotherapy for early breast cancer [abstract 590]. J ClinOncol 2010;28 (Suppl 15):89s.

[73] Gerber B, von Minckwitz G, Stehle H, Reimer T, Felberbaum R, Maass N, et al. Effect of luteinizing hormone-releasing hormone agonist on ovarian function after modern adjuvant breast cancer chemotherapy: the GBG 37 ZORO study. J ClinOncol 2011;29:2334-41.

[74] Munster PN, Moore AP, Ismail-Khan R, Cox CE, Lacevic M, Gross-King M, et al. Randomized trial using gonadotropin-releasing hormone agonist triptorelin for the

preservation of ovarian function during (neo)adjuvant chemotherapy for breast cancer. J ClinOncol 2012;30:533-8.

[75] Partridge AH. Ovarian suppression for prevention of premature menopause and infertility: empty promise or effective therapy? J ClinOncol 2012;30:479-81.

Chapter 6

Female Salivary Testosterone: Measurement, Challenges and Applications

E.A.S. Al-Dujaili and M.A. Sharp

Additional information is available at the end of the chapter

http://dx.doi.org/10.5772/53648

1. Introduction

Testosterone (T) is one of the most important naturally circulating steroid hormones. Exerting both androgenic and anabolic activities it is secreted into the blood and in men is produced primarily by the testes. In women, by contrast, production occurs in the ovaries and particularly from peripheral conversion of the T precursors androstenedione, DHEA and DHEA-S (Burger, 2002). T is no longer regarded as a male only hormone, and similarly estradiol is no longer a female only hormone (Fausto-Sterling, 2000). While it is true that men generally have higher levels of T and lower concentrations of oestrogen and progesterone than women, all these sex steroid hormones play essential roles in both sexes (Ullis et al., 1999).

Testosterone has now been well established as having an essential function in wide-ranging areas of female health. For example, it is an important determinant of female sexuality, critical for development and maintenance of bone mineralisation, contributes to menstrual cycle regulation and to behavioural changes in premenstrual syndrome (Bachmann & Leiblum, 1991; Slemend et al., 1996). Therefore, T and other androgen replacement therapies in women with or without oestrogen have become widely recommended for a variety of women experiencing androgen deficiency syndrome (Somboonporn et al., 2006; Hickok et al., 1993).

It has been shown that sex hormones levels can be influenced by diet, exercise, age, BMI, ethnicity and others (Allen & Key, 2000; Kraemer et al., 1998). Various studies have suggested that increasing dietary fibre intake could influence total and/or bio-available T and oestradiol levels (Rock et al., 2004) or T and SHBG levels (Longcope et al., 2000). Recently, Wang et al. (2005) reported that a low-fat high-fibre diet decreased serum and urine androgens in men. The majority of these studies on T were conducted in men and the data published were conflicting. These equivocal findings resulted, at least in part, from different study designs and protocols (fibre content and type, subject compliance, lack of control affecting other dietary components) and the complex mechanisms involved in steroid metabolism. Subsequently, we have performed a pilot study to investigate the effect of increasing dietary fibre and found a moderate increase in urinary T excretion of healthy women taking a mixed high fibre diet for two weeks (unpublished observations), suggesting a potential correlation between dietary fibre intake and androgen status. This could be due to an effect on the enterohepatic cycle as hypothesised by some investigators in delaying the excretion of steroids and hence a modest increase in plasma and urinary levels (Adlercreutz et al., 1987; Groh et al., 1993). Other researchers have suggested that low-fat high-fibre diet might indirectly increase bio-available serum androgen levels by preventing the development of insulin resistance which is associated with reduced SHBG levels (Haffner et al., 1994; Pasquali et al., 1995). Conversely, some workers proposed that low-fat high-fibre diet reduced circulating steroid hormone concentrations due to higher faecal excretion of conjugated steroids (Pusateri et al., 1990) or an increase in the synthesis of SHBG (Berrino et al., 2001).

Quantitative determination of circulating T is possible from an assortment of biological material; i.e. plasma, serum, hair, saliva, and urine. However, early attempts at determining concentrations of circulating T, primarily for clinical purposes, traditionally utilised plasma or serum. As blood samples require time-consuming and often stressful venipuncture, obtaining invasive multiple samples over a period of hours can be painful and this procedure can be unattractive to participants (Dabbs, 1990). Moreover, measurement tends to be of the total rather than free, biologically active, fraction of T. Faced with these challenges there has been a growing awareness of the potential value of utilising saliva for measuring hormone concentrations (Mandel, 1993; Collins, 2000). Consequently, the use of saliva as a diagnostic tool in clinical and bio-behavioural research has grown significantly during the last two decades (Quissell, 1993). However, salivary T measurements can be markedly influenced during the process of sample collection with interference effects caused by mucopolysaccharides and leakage of blood into saliva, storage conditions and random daily fluctuations (Granger et al., 2004).

There are limited data establishing normal androgen values for women at different ages, thus hampering the ability to define those with androgen deficiency (Guay, 2002), and there is definitely a clear need for additional information on normal reference ranges of female T levels at different age groups. Moreover, little is known about detailed daily patterns in female T throughout the menstrual cycle (Davis, 1999). One of the aims of this review article is therefore to discuss the importance of estimating salivary T in women and the challenges posed by its measurement in female saliva, including a summary of our in-house ELISA technique and the optimisation needed for the estimation of salivary T. We also discuss female salivary T circadian dynamics showing our own data in this regard. Finally, we would like to highlight the importance of sampling protocol; multiple female salivary T sampling versus single saliva sampling.

2. Role of testosterone in women's health and well-being

Whilst androgens are known to play a significant role in wide-ranging aspects of male health (Nieschlag, 1998; Isidori et al., 2008), there is an increasing realisation that they are also critical for mental and sexual health as well as physical well-being in females (Christiansen, 2004; Davis & Tran, 2001). The following examples provide a non-exhaustive illustration of testosterone significance for females.

2.1. Epidemiology and clinical importance of abnormal testosterone levels in females

Female sexual dysfunction is thought to affect over 40% of women in the United States, according to a study by Laumann and colleagues (1999). As experts evaluate women with potential sexual interest disorders, there is a growing body of literature to guide them in how to understand, diagnose and treat these problems. Androgens are known to be involved in women's arousability, response, intensity and ease of orgasm, as well as in initial spontaneous desire, the active neurovascular smooth muscle response of swelling, increased lubrication and genital sexual sensitivity. T is thought to be the most important hormone for maintaining sex drive or libido in women and a deficiency can cause impaired sexual function (Snyder, 2001). In this regard, T may decrease vaginal atrophy as well as inflammation, itching and pain of the vulva (Leiblum et al., 1983). However, excessive amounts may increase the risk of endometrial cancer due to hyperinsulinemia (Ciampelli & Lanzone, 1998).

In a recent Cochrane systematic review (Somboonporn et al., 2010), it was concluded that adding T to hormone therapy has a beneficial effect on sexual function in postmenopausal women. However, the combined therapy is associated with a higher incidence of hair growth, acne and a reduction in high-density lipoprotein (HDL) cholesterol. These adverse events may vary with differing doses, routes of T administration and individual differences. Reflecting on the theoretical and conceptual challenges of relating specific hormone levels to behaviour, there is no doubt that a relationship has not been established between levels of T and symptoms of sexual dysfunction in women. In the brain, T has a role in maintaining mood and memory. Indeed, high levels of T exert a significant negative effect on mood, personal sense of well being, interpersonal relationships, self-confidence and self-worth, and depression is a major symptom associated with low levels in women (Sands & Studd, 1995). In the heart, T has relaxing (vasodilating) effect on coronary arteries (Sarrel, 1998; White et al., 1998), and thus, it can reduce symptoms of angina. Unstable hormonal fluctuations can be observed after menopause (Overlie et al., 1999). These fluctuations are usually associated with increased incidence of migraine headache, obesity, mood changes and bleeding disturbances in perimenopausal and postmenopausal women (Fettes, 1999; Vliet & Davis, 1991). It has been suggested that postmenopausal women who are not receiving some T therapy may have greater risk of developing coronary heart disease (Rako, 1998). The effects associated with administering exogenous T are not especially straightforward however. For example, when T is administered alone, it can increase the risk of atherosclerosis and decrease HDL levels (Crook & Seed, 1990). Conversely, when T is administered with oestrogens, the increased risk of heart disease diminishes (Sarrel, 1998; Davis, 2011).

In the Michigan Bone Health Study (1992–1995), the authors examined the correlates of T in pre- and perimenopausal women (i.e., age, menopausal status, body composition, and lifestyle behaviours) in aged 25–50 years (n=601). Body composition measures were found to be significantly and positively associated with total T concentrations in a dose-response manner (Sowers et al, 2001). Hysterectomy with oophorectomy was associated with significantly lower T concentrations. For bones and osteoporosis, T (and the metabolite DHT) directly stimulates receptors on the osteoblasts (bone building) cells to promote bone growth, bone mineralisation and repair of damaged bone (Gasperino, 1995; Hui et al., 2002). In light of this, T replacement may markedly decrease osteoporosis in postmenopausal women, and together with oestrogens the steroids can preserve and rebuild the cartilages between bones (Tremollieres et al., 1992). In the skin, T can improve the overall skin appearance by preserving collagen and protecting against thinning of the skin as well as sebaceous glands activity that lubricates the skin (Brincat et al., 1987). As we begin to more fully understand the above actions, the therapeutic use of exogenous T in women is becoming increasingly widespread, although not always without often unwanted side effects. Thousands of women have been treated with T, the majority experience symptom improvement, improved sexual well-being (Davis and Davison, 2012). Other possible beneficial effects of T therapy (reduced fracture risk, improved cognitive and cardiovascular function), necessitate further investigation. Reduced T levels have been found in bilateral oophorectomy, adrenal insufficiency, hypopituitarism, use of combination oral contraceptive pills or systemic glucocorticosteroids, and premature ovarian failure (Fogle et al, 2007; Labrie et al, 2011).

As women age, the dramatic drop in T level is thought to result from a decline in the adrenal production of T precursors, DHEA and DHEAS (Zumoff, et al., 1995; Davison et al., 2005). This marked fall in peripheral androgens is associated with a number of conditions including metabolic syndrome and osteoporosis (Davy & Melby, 2003). In addition, the Women's Health Initiative (2002) published their results from a prospective randomised prevention trial of more than 16000 healthy postmenopausal women which was intended to study the long term effects of HRT given as a combination of conjugated equine oestrogens and medroxyprogesterone acetate. Although decreased risks of colorectal cancers and hip fractures were reported, many women came off their hormone supplements and explored alternatives because of the reported increased risk of stroke and invasive breast cancers. Likewise, a large-scale UK study (Beral, 2003) found that current use of HRT, but not past use, was associated with an increased risk of breast cancer. Similar to many other therapeutic agents, HRT has its benefits and risks. The public is constantly in search of alternative forms of food or herbal supplements to alleviate menopausal symptoms or to prevent long-term complications of ovarian failure.

2.2. Clinical contribution of monitoring salivary T in females for pathological and physiological conditions

To date, a definite relationship has not been established between a specific level of T and symptoms of T excess or deficiency such as sexual dysfunction in women and premenstrual symptoms. There is no established level of free T below which a woman can be said to be deficient, nor any level to which a woman should be restored that determines she is replete. Thus the diagnosis of these disorders due to low testosterone remains a clinical diagnosis of exclusion. In the absence of a reliable free /total testosterone assay the limitations of available assays should be understood, and the measurement of testosterone used to exclude the use of testosterone in women in whom therapy might result in testosterone excess.

There is a paucity of research which investigates salivary female T in pathological and physiological conditions. For this reason we would like to highlight the following examples of clinical monitoring of female salivary T. Salivary T has been used to monitor treatment of children with congenital adrenal hyperplasia (CAH), Salivary T was found to be a useful additional biochemical marker with 17OHP to indicate the levels of free T (Perry et al., 2005). In a study comparing salivary and total plasma testosterone levels in healthy controls and patients with Klinefelter's syndrome (Wellen et al.,1983) provided indirect evidence that in Klinefelter patients levels of salivary T and androstenedione correlated well with the reported free plasma levels. This suggests that measurement of salivary steroids may be useful in evaluating endocrine function in both healthy and disease states. Monitoring the menstrual cycle status of female athletes by salivary steroid determination following a 21km run (De Crée et al., 1990) reported an increase of salivary T of 15.2%. These findings corroborate earlier studies, which found higher post-exercise plasma sex steroid levels.

Several studies have published data on the applicability and clinical value of salivary T measurements for the diagnosis and follow-up of therapy of idiopathic hirsutism, late-onset hypogonadism and androgen deficiency in end-stage renal disease (e.g. Shibayama et al., 2009; Luisi et al., 1982; Cardoso et al., 2011). In addition, Teoh et al. (2005) and Gayriloya and Lindau (2009) carried out physiological studies to assess population levels of salivary T in children, adult females and males. They reported high co-operation rates with the in-house salivary specimen collection.

3. Testosterone production and mechanisms of action in women

Circulating levels of plasma T in pre-menopausal women originate from multiple sites; the ovaries (20-25%), adrenal cortex (20-25%) and the remainder (50-60%) from the peripheral conversion of T precursors (androstenedione, DHEA and DHEA-Sulphate) (Burger, 2002; Longcope, 1986; Simpson, 2002). T circulates in women with around 66-74% bound strongly to sex hormone binding globulin (SHBG) and 24-30% bound weakly to albumin with only about 1-3% being free in the blood (Pardridge & Demers, 1991; Vermeulen, 1998).

Under certain conditions the bio-available T dissociates from its carrier protein (mostly albumin) and becomes free. Manni and colleagues (1985) indicated that albumin-bound T was available to tissues such as the brain in conditions where the free T level was negligible and in the absence of albumin. This hypothesis was contested by Ekins (1990) and Mendel (1989) based on the assumption that steroids can act only through their genomic mechanism. Besch et al. (1982) stated that only the non-protein-bound or 'free' fraction of a hormone, such as a steroid enters the cell of the target tissue and interacts with its specific receptor protein. As an adjunct to this latter point it should be noted that around 50% of pre-menopausal (and almost 100% of post-menopausal) T is synthesised by peripheral conversion, distinct from any endocrine function (Labrie et al., 2000). In addition, the fact that many steroids are now shown to exert some effects through the non-genomic pathway (see below) leads us to suppose that some actions, particularly in the female, are mediated by the albumin-bound fraction of T. Moreover, in a recent review Lepage (2006) demonstrated clearly the importance of measuring the bio-available T as compared to total and free T. Thus, free and non-SHBG-bound (sometimes called bio-available) T measures are likely to be the most reliable indicators of tissue exposure to T (Collins, 2000). As an adjunct, recent finding suggest that female androgens made locally in large amounts in peripheral tissues from DHEA/S act in the same cells where synthesis takes place (Labrie et al., 2003). It was therefore concluded that the measurement of androgen glucuronides instead of T perhaps better reflects the androgenic activity in women (Labrie et al., 2006).

Steroid hormones in the periphery are believed to equilibrate rapidly between tissues and blood (Goncharov et al., 2006; Miler et al., 2004; Schurmeyer & Nieschlag, 1982). Total concentrations of T in peripheral tissue and body fluids are mainly dependent upon the levels of binding proteins such as sex hormone binding globulin (SHBG) and albumin. These binding proteins can act as a reservoir for the steroid and protect it against extensive metabolism of active (free) steroids during passage of the blood through the liver (Mendel, 1989). It is now widely accepted that the free steroid form represents the biologically active fraction. However, it is believed that the albumin bound T (bio-available) can bind to the receptor (possibly the membrane bound) and exert its activity because the affinity of the steroid towards its receptor is far greater than its affinity to albumin (Author's unpublished data; Heinlein & Chang, 2002; Fix et al., 2004). In fact, T can also be regarded as a circulating prohormone that can be converted either to DHT for androgenic activity or to oestradiol which is the principal endogenous ligand for oestrogen receptors (Hiipakka & Liao,1998; McPhaul & Young, 2001).

T, like other steroids, may exert its action in living cells by either the well-known genomic pathway, involving hormones binding to a cytosolic receptor and subsequent modulation of gene expression followed by protein synthesis (genomic actions). Or through pathways that do not act on the genome (non-genomic actions) (Lösel et al., 2003). T has recently been reported to exert effects through interactions with receptors in the cell membrane (Heinlein & Chang, 2002). Rapid effects of androgens have been shown on calcium fluxes (Guo et al., 2002), intracellular phosphorylation cascades (Castoria et al., 2003), secretion of GnRH by pituitary cells (Shakil et al., 2002) and others. It seems that in these cells, androgens can exert their effect at very low concentrations that are not sufficient to stimulate gene transcription.

Androgen dynamics in women are usually controlled by 4 temporal phenomena: ovarian function, hypothalamic-pituitary-adrenal axis, age decline of adrenal androgens and depletion of ovarian follicles after menopause (Burger & Casson, 2004). T and its precursor, DHEA/S are now widely accepted as vital for normal female development (lower certain body fat, maintain muscle mass, healthy-skin, boost energy levels and mood), sexual health (substrate for oestrogen production, enhance sex drive and relieve menopausal symptoms) (Laumann, et al., 1999; Davis & Tran, 2001) and might have a role to play in alleviating the aging process of men and women (Kirkwood, 2005; Ullis et al., 1999).

4. Measurement of female salivary testosterone: Challenges and problems

Quantitative determination of circulating T can be achieved utilising a variety of different procedures such as; radioimmunoassay, luminescence immunoassay, fluorescence immunoassay, enzyme-linked immunosorbant assay, gel filtration, equilibrium dialysis and centrifugal ultrafiltration for serum free T, protein precipitation, gas-chromatography mass-spectrometry (including isotope dilution) and more recently LC/MS-Tandem spectrophotometry (Edwards, 1985; Kemeny, 1991; Sinha-Hikim et al., 1998), each with their own inherent strengths and weaknesses.

Once a medium in which to analyse T has been selected (saliva in this case) the question then becomes what type of assay should be employed? Although the bewildering array of techniques can make selecting the most appropriate test perplexing, as Edwards (1985) stated 'A systematic and objective approach will...indicate the most appropriate technique for the particular application in mind' (p.2). In both saliva and blood, RIA was until comparatively recently the method of choice for determining concentrations of circulating T. Despite a number of limitations, traditional analogue RIA is still widely used (Rosner, 2001). Several authors, however, have ardently expressed concern that this method is insensitive at the lower end of the T range; precisely where female salivary T falls (Sinha-Hikim et al., 1998). This situation arises because most T RIA's were designed for the measurement of serum levels in men and thus lack the sensitivity required for the precise measurement of the low levels prevalent in women.

Even now, simple and routine methods for determining free steroid concentrations in plasma have not been fully developed and widely validated. Consequently, most current procedures involve technically demanding and time consuming centrifugal ultrafilitration or equilibrium dialysis (Miller et al., 2004; Hammond et al., 1980; Riad-Fahmy et al., 1982); processes which in themselves yield results with varying degrees of accuracy. In an effort to circumvent the problem of not easily being able to measure free-T some authors use mathematical equations, such as the free androgen index, mass action formulation, or the Sodegaard equation (Ho et al., 2006; Vermeulen et al., 1999). All are mathematical formulae of varying complexity for working out the free component of T based on the measurement of total T and, as a minimum, SHBG. However, because these equations rely on an affinity constant (SHBG in the case of T) and because estimations of the affinity constant varies widely, there are very real problems with these approximations (Besch et al., 1982; Rinaldi et al., 2002). As Vermuelen et al. (1999) point out, total serum T concentration is subject to variations in the concentration of the binding proteins such as SHBG and CBG; it is not, therefore, a reliable index of bio-available T. Faced with these challenges, there has been a growing awareness of the potential value of utilising saliva for measuring hormone concentrations (Mandel, 1993). Consequently, the use of saliva as a diagnostic tool in bio-behavioural and clinical research has grown significantly during the previous two decades (Quissell, 1993).

In a variety of research arenas, accurate measurement of female free-T is widely regarded as problematic (Matsumoto & Bremner, 2004). In a clinical paper on screening for androgen insufficiency, Guay (2002) argued that a major problem in assessing female T is the inaccuracy of the measurements by current assays. Recent articles published by Taieb et al. (2002) and

Herold and Fitzgerald (2003) illustrate that when measured by automated processes, T concentrations may be inaccurate to the order of magnitude of 200-500%. This issue of measurement therefore acts as one potentially serious limiting factor in the confidence that we can place in the results of hormone-behaviour studies, clinical studies and for female's screening before T therapy. Although, as technology advances and measurement continues to become somewhat more straightforward there is still a need for highly sensitive, reliable, and efficient immunoassays with accessible reagents and materials for the determination of T in females (Granger et al., 1999; Guay, 2002).

Given the difficulties associated with accurately measuring female free and bio-available T, the enzyme-linked immunosorbant assay (ELISA) protocol has a number of features to recommend it over RIA. For example, reagents are cheap in comparison with RIA, the laboratory in which our research is undertaken employs staff with substantial expertise in ELISA development, validation and trouble-shooting. Moreover, there is no hazard of radiation, and because of the low concentrations of antigens in saliva HIV and hepatitis infections are much less of a danger from saliva than from blood (Major et al., 1991). Indeed, unless visibly contaminated with blood, human saliva is not considered a class 2 biohazard, affording researchers and institutions administrative and safety benefits. As a consequence of these factors the ELISA method stands out as the most appropriate routine method of choice for use in the majority of research institutes conducting bio-behavioural research and clinical work on T.

There are a number of features that are required of an effective assay. As Kemeny and Chantler (1988) note, the type of assay should be closely tailored to the particular task for which it is required; and the requirements of diagnostic laboratories are often very different than those of bio-behavioural research laboratories. For example, in bio-behavioural studies that require assessing chronobiological changes in the very low levels of free salivary T in females, issues such as ease of use and speed are less important characteristics than sensitivity and accuracy. Subsequently, one of the additional aims of this chapter is to describe the development, optimisation, and validation of an extremely sensitive in-house ELISA, designed specifically for determining salivary T in women. In particular, the ELISA is evaluated for its accuracy, specificity, and precision.

Salivary sampling regimens have several obvious and distinct advantages over blood sampling. They accommodate frequent and easy collection by non-invasive, relatively stress free-techniques, thereby facilitating short term dynamic tests, pharmacokinetic analyses, and studies of chronobiological changes (Riad-Fahmy et al., 1982). In addition, it has been reported that the majority of subjects find little difficulty in salivating directly into collection containers, providing adequate volumes (between 3mL and 5mL) for determining a steroid hormone profile in less than 5 minutes (Dabbs, 1991). Nonetheless, a number of challenges and problems associated with saliva methodology do exist (Granger et al., 2004). For example, compliance with salivary sampling protocols has been identified as a potential challenge. Compliance to collection protocols is essential for accurate determination of T levels in saliva and concerns amount collected, condition of sample and precautions taken prior to collection (i.e. rinsing of the mouth, not eating etc.). In relation to collection, compliance has been investigated by the use of an electronic monitoring device, and it was reported that only 74% of subjects were found to comply with the sampling instructions and 26% failed at least once to obtain the correct saliva sample (Kudielka et al., 2003; Broderick et al., 2003). Our own experience is that engagement with participants and the provision of detailed oral and written instructions alongside the opportunity to practice with an investigator present to answer questions and provide guidance ameliorates significantly issues of compliance.

Although diurnal and monthly patterns of salivary T generally parallel serum values, absolute ranges show variability across several studies. Few studies of normal individuals, controlling for known variables, such as pH, time of day, month and medications, have been performed using the recently developed high sensitivity enzyme immunoassays, such as those sold by Diagnostic Systems Laboratories (Webster, TX), Salimetrics (State College, PA) and American Laboratory Products Co. (ALPCO) (Windham, NH). Below are several factors which need to be taken into consideration either when using commercial kits or developing in-house assay methodology.

4.1. Blood-saliva correlation

As Albumin is a small protein, with a molecular weight of approximately 69,000, it can pass through the salivary membrane. Conversely, SHBG (to which the majority of circulating T is bound) is a large carrier protein with a molecular weight of 150-200,000. As this steroid-binding protein cannot pass easily through the salivary membrane, one of the advantages in using saliva as the biological fluid in study centres would be around the claim that it contains concentrations of analyte similar to, or even identical with, the non-protein bound (free) concentrations in blood (Baxendale, Reed, & James, 1980; Vittek et al., 1985; Longcope et al., 1987). These claims generally relate to males, however. Although there are fewer studies examining this association in females, it has been suggested that correlations between T levels in serum and saliva may be significantly lower than in males (Granger et al., 1999; Miller et al., 2004). Shirtcliff and co-workers (2002) published a study which appears to cast doubt on the veracity of this correlational relationship in females, stating that regardless of assay method, salivary T levels are modestly correlated with serum levels for males but not necessarily females. The absolute concentration, whilst reflecting accurately the unbound fraction in the plasma (and also the fraction which is not bound to SHBG) is approximately twice the concentration of free-T in plasma, in contrast to the findings in male subjects (Baxendale, Jacobs & James, 1982). One major implication of these findings is that substitution of saliva for serum T levels in at least biobehavioural studies may estimate the T-behaviour relationship differently for females than males because substitution of saliva assay results for serum values markedly underestimates known T-behaviour associations. In addition, there might be some ethnic variation in total and free T concentration in that Heald et al. (2003) found that both total and calculated free T were lower in Pakistani men than in Europeans.

4.2. Contamination of salivary samples

Clinical researchers have established that collection techniques can affect the integrity of salivary samples, which subsequently interferes with ability to accurately determine hormone levels. For example, given the difference in T concentration between blood and salivary samples, leaking of blood or serum into the mouth (i.e. due to gum disease, injury, consuming very chewy meals, caffeine intake, or vigorous cleaning) can affect the integrity of quantitative estimates of salivary concentrations (Granger et al., 2004; Lac et al., 1993). In response to a question about the incidence of haemoglobin contamination in salivary samples, at a round table discussion on assay development and collection procedures (Tenovus workshop, 1982), Schürmeyer suggested that researchers might reasonably expect a contamination incidence of around 5-10%. The majority of bio-behavioural studies investigating the role of T in women propose that single time-point or very limited sampling is sufficient. Whilst this issue is explored in more detail later in this chapter, it is worth noting here that potential contamination of salivary samples by blood further complicates the use of single samples. In addition, it is noted that where samples have been found with aberrant levels, researchers have on occasion been treated by diluting the samples (i.e. Gladue et al., 1989). Whilst this step may be appropriate for male salivary samples, dilutions of female salivary samples which may already contain levels of T at the utmost sensitivity of the assay are rendered un-determinable.

Whilst the contamination of salivary samples by blood is widely recognized as a potential problem in the scientific fields driving assay development there appears to be something of a malaise regarding the issue in a wide range of bio-behavioural studies. Indeed, with only a handful of notable exceptions a large number of authors have neglected to report how they have dealt with this serious confound. In contrast, Mazur et al. (1980, 1987) and Gladue et al. (1989) paid careful attention to the issue of contamination, adopting what, at the time, must have appeared a sound approach. In utilising measurement strips called Hemastix® they attempted to ascertain which, if any, of their salivary samples may have become contaminated with blood. Unfortunately, Kivlighan et al. (2004) cast doubt on the suitability of this approach and reported that the confounding effects of blood leakage cannot be adequately screened or controlled by visual inspection of sample discoloration or using the Hemastix® approach. Other methods have recently been developed to assess blood contamination in salivary samples. For example, Salimetrics now offer an assay to determine blood contamination in salivary samples (Schwartz & Granger, 2004), although this approach adds substantially to the cost of assaying samples. Perhaps the best approach to reducing blood contamination is avoiding its occurrence in the first place. In our own lab, and following suggestions by Adlercreutz (1990), our subjects were asked to adhere to a number of steps including refraining from brushing their teeth prior to sample collection, rinsing their mouths thoroughly several times prior to collection, not consuming large meals, and not smoking or drinking caffeine. These steps effectively reduced the amount of samples seen in the assays with abnormal levels; indeed following these steps parallel to detailed instructions enhanced collection to the extent that blood contamination in well over 10,000 samples was effectively reduced to an incidence of below 1%.

4.3. Collection methods

With the increased use of salivary measures in clinical practice, bio-behavioural and clinical research, several research teams have sought to advance our understanding of the circumstances and conditions that may influence the validity of salivary assessments (e.g. Lipson & Ellison, 1989; Shirtcliff et al., 2001). The use of a range of stimuli has been reported to stimulate salivary flow where necessary; i.e. paraffin wax, rubber bands, sugar-free gum, cotton swabs, and citric acid (Malamud & Tabak, 1993; Navazesh, 1993). Granger and co-workers (2004) found that materials commonly used in the literature to absorb saliva (cotton and polyester swabs) or stimulate saliva (powdered drink-mix crystals, citric acid and chewing gum) have the potential to change salivary T results. Typically, saliva is collected by having a participant deposit between 3-5mL into a collection container (less may be required in some circumstances); this step is usually reported as taking between 3-8 minutes. The saliva is then stored frozen prior to assay. While clinical subjects may be willing and able to provide un-stimulated samples that can be immediately frozen, this protocol is often unpractical for field collection (Lipson & Ellison, 1989). As such, collection of saliva samples under these conditions may necessitate certain changes from common clinical practices. Although collection of saliva is often referred to as un-stimulated, this is somewhat misleading. If the salivary gland is un-stimulated it does not produce saliva; what is meant essentially is saliva produced by minimal stimulation (Read, 1989). Small amounts of saliva can be collected without the need to externally stimulate production, but the amount usually collected often requires subjects to stimulate saliva production in some way. This issue is particularly pertinent when investigating changes in concentration of salivary hormones over a certain period of time or prior to competition, where time constraints exist and feelings of stress or anxiety may make saliva production more troublesome. We have optimised our own salivary samples collection method (see Table 1) that ensures the quality of saliva, reproducibility, minimises blood contamination and stress during collection.

A Precautions
DO NOT exercise 24 hours prior to or on the day of salivary sample collections. (Exercise is defined as anything more than low-moderate physical activity e.g. swimming, cycling, yoga, sex etc.)
DO NOT consume alcohol 24 hours prior to or on the day of salivary sample collections or drink coffee, milk, yoghurt or meals within 45mins of collection
Each time you collect a saliva sample the method should be identical.
Procedure:
B Step by step guide to successful saliva sample colection
Step 1 - Do not eat or brush your teeth 60 minutes prior to saliva sample collection.
Step 2 - Rinse and swill mouth out thoroughly three times with tap or bottle water.
Step 3 - Chew a quarter of a stick of sugar free gum provided, as this will aid the production of saliva.
Step 4 - Retain the sugar free gum in your mouth, and spit away the first mouthful of saliva into the waste container provided. This will remove unwanted cellular elements in the mouth and from the chewing gum.
Step 5 - Continue chewing the gum and spit into the collection container provided, until you have deposited 3-5 millilitres (ml) of saliva. Ensure the cap is replaced tightly.
Step 6 - Please mark the date and time of sample on the label of the collection container.
Step 7 - Please store saliva samples in the fridge 4°C. Samples will then be collected by the researcher and frozen until analysed.

Table 1. Optimised in-house method of salivary samples collection

4.4. Storage of saliva samples

It is now known that bacterial growth can occur if saliva samples are stored above 4˚C (i.e. at room temperature) for extended periods of time. In a recent report, it was found that bacterial growth in saliva increased by incubation at room temperature over 10 days, and this caused a significant decrease in salivary levels of both cortisol and T (Whembolua et al., 2006). Some workers have shown that salivary steroid levels (cortisol, progesterone and 17-OH-P) decreased significantly in the course of 3 weeks under different storage conditions (native or centrifuged saliva, saliva with triflouroacetate and saliva combined with 0.05% NaN_3), and that the decrease was clinically significant from the second week onwards (Groschl et al., 2001). After repeated freezing and re-thawing, only cortisol decreased significantly ($p<0.001$) presumably due to enzymatic conversion to metabolites. On the other hand, a study by Granger et al. (2004) investigating the week-to-week change in salivary T levels of samples stored at 4˚C for 4 weeks, -20˚C and -40˚C up to 24 months found that there was a linear increase in T levels across the 4 weeks for samples stored at 4˚C (R^2=0.88, $p<0.05$). By the end of 4 weeks, there was an increase of 330% in T concentration using a Salimetric assay. However, they reported a dramatic decrease in measured T levels over the 6 months and 24 months in pooled samples stored at -20 and -40˚C (R^2=0.85, $p<0.05$). Clearly, in order for researchers to have confidence in their assay results a good deal of attention has to be paid to issues of collection, storage and compliance.

5. Direct vs. In-direct technique

Solid phase and coated-technology assays can adopt either a direct or an in-direct approach to determining levels of T. Whilst several assays, including commercially available kits, employ a direct method (that is, salivary samples are not treated in any way prior to assay) there are a number of limitations with this approach, especially when examining female androgens. Whilst the benefits of utilising saliva over serum have previously been described, saliva is a far from inert substance; it contains a variety of contaminants, such as bacteria, leukocytes, mucins, and very importantly for enzyme assays, endogenous enzymes. All of which can interfere with assays based on the ELISA technique. As a consequence, salivary samples are rendered extremely susceptible to interfering agents such as pH imbalance which yields results that are, unpredictably, either too high or low (alkaline samples, for example, tend to yield low results). Schwartz et al. (1998) reported that when pH falls below 4 or rises above 9, then assay performance is likely to be compromised. At a round table discussion of sex hormones and corticosteroid assays, Adlercreutz (1990) citing a range of studies, noted that T assays do not work well in non-extracted plasma. Moreover, Jones et al. (2004) reported that some samples from female subjects gave falsely high results when measured with direct immunoassay.

Taib et al. (2003) found that 7 out of 10 immunoassay kits tested had overestimated T concentrations by up to 46%, and that the target values were missed by 200-500%. This has prompted some authors to doubt the validity of female T assays and suggest perhaps guessing levels in women to be cheaper and more accurate! (Herold & Fitzgerald, 2003). However, Dabbs and colleagues (1995) reported on the reliability of salivary T assays evaluated by nine laboratories and found acceptable overall agreement (r=0.87 for men and r=0.78 for women). We suggest that one of the reasons commercial assays invariably produce T results that appear high compared with in-house protocols is because of the cross-reactivity with DHEA/DHEA-S. The importance of the cross-reactivity findings depends not only on the % cross-reactivity, but on the relative concentration of the compound compared against T. For example, DHEA-S occurs in plasma at approximately 500 times the amount of T. Hence, a cross-reactivity of 0.72% is potentially of more importance than the 2.3 % cross-reactivity found in DHT, which occurs at levels below T in plasma. Using the extraction procedure removes the ability of DHEA-S to interfere with the 'in-house' assay optimised in our laboratory.

6. Development of ELISA based assays for the measurement of testosterone in saliva

A simple, reliable, easy to perform, sensitive and highly specific ELISA type assay for the measurement of female salivary T has been developed in our lab and utilized in several wide-ranging research projects investigating T levels in the menstrual cycle, circadian rhythm and bio-behavioural studies. This has enabled us to screen large number of samples within a short time at relatively low cost and with high sensitivity and assured specificity. The principle of the salivary T assay optimised in our laboratory is based on the in-direct, competitive binding technique (Al-Dujaili, 2006; Al-Dujaili et al., 1988; O'Sullivan et al., 1979). Essentially, the T present in salivary samples competes with a fixed and limited amount of T coated on the micro-titre plate, for binding sites on an antibody. Because the concentration of the T coated to the wells is held constant, while the concentration of T in the salivary samples vary, the amount of enzyme labelled second antibody bound to the first antibody is inversely proportional to the concentration of the unlabelled analyte present in the sample.

Extensive experimentation was conducted in our laboratory to optimise this assay. Because of the often extremely low levels of T in female saliva, one of the particular requirements for quantitative determination is that the assay be especially sensitive. However, the ELISA process sits within a complex web of inter-locked parameters, and achieving this sensitivity requires a constant balancing act between reagents and conditions to arrive at and maintain the final protocol. For example, one of the ways to minimise the impact of interfering factors is to extract the samples prior to assay. In line with guidelines taken from Al-Dujaili et al. (1988) all assay reagents and conditions have been optimised to produce the required sensitivity, precision, accuracy and reliability including the amount of testosterone-bovine serum albumin (BSA) conjugate needed to coat the plate, volume of sample, amount of antibody, incubation temperature and incubation times. Below are our optimized protocols for sample preparation, plate preparation and ELISA procedure:

6.1. Sample preparation

1. Frozen samples are thawed, centrifuged at 3500rpm for 10mins, and aliquoted.
2. Aliquots centrifuged at 6000rpm for 2mins.
3. 0.5mL of sample combined with 4mL of diethylether.
4. Vortex mix for 10mins and freeze at -80°C.
5. Decant unfrozen ether and place in 45°C water bath until evaporated under nitrogen gas.
6. Reconstitute with 0.5mL assay buffer.
7. Stand at room temp for 30mins and finally vortex mix to equilibrate.

6.2. Plate preparation

1. Coat plates with T conjugate and leave to incubate overnight at 4°C
2. Wash three times with wash buffer
3. Block for 1hr at 37°C
4. Discard blocking buffer

6.3. Optimized ELISA Procedure

1. 100μL of standard and previously extracted and reconstituted sample into wells in duplicate. Standards run at 0.00, 1, 5, 10, 50, 250, 1000pg/mL
2. Add 100μL of antibody in assay buffer
3. Shake and incubate at 37°C for 1hr
4. Discard and wash 4 times
5. Add 100μL of enzyme (horseradish peroxidase- linked second antibody)
6. Shake and incubate at 37°C for 1hr
7. Discard and wash 4 times
8. Add 100μL of substrate (tetramethylbenzidine)
9. Incubate at room temperature for 15mins
10. Add 50μL of stop solution (H_2SO_4)
11. Read at 450nm on MRX Dynex plate reader

The validity of the salivary assay for T was confirmed by Al-Dujaili (2006) using the same antibody and technique in urine and additionally by the correlation between the results obtained with the in-house ELISA and those assayed by Salimetrics ELISA kit ($Salim_{ELISA}$ =

http://dx.doi.org/10.5772/53648

1.12x In-house $_{ELISA}$ – 0.042, $R^2 = 0.95$, n= 58). Cross-reactivity data with major interfering steroids were minimal (see Table 2) except for testosterone-3-glucuronide (58.8%), dihydrotestosterone (2.3%) and androstenedione (4.6%). The average recovery of T in this assay was 104.0% (range 97.5% to 110%). The average intra-assay coefficient of variation was 5.78%. Inter-assay imprecision of 8.7% was determined from the mean of averaged duplicates for 50 separate runs for male and female aliquots. Both inter and intra assay coefficients of variation are at levels comparable with the best commercially available assay kits. Assay sensitivity was determined and an un-related *t*-test revealed the differences between the zero standard and 0.5 pg/mL concentration were significantly different: t (1, 11) = 9.098, $p<0.001$. By this method the assay sensitivity is 0.5 pg/mL(1.74 pmole). The working sensitivity of the assay, corresponding to the mass of testosterone required to give a decrease in the %B of tracer of 2.5SD of the zero point signal was 1.24 pg/mL(4.33pmole). See typical standard curve in figure 1. The applications of our salivary T ELISA can be seen in a wide-range of clinical and bio-behavioural studies (e.g. Moore at al., 2011; Conway et al., 2007; Deady et al., 2006; Sharp & Al-Dujaili, 2010). In addition, applications of the assay are discussed in sections 8 and 9 of this chapter.

Steroid hormone	% Cross- reactivity
Testosterone	100
Testosterone-3-glucuronide	58.8
Nandrolone	12
Dihydrotestosterone	2.3
Androstenedione*	4.6
DHEA	1.05
DHEA-sulphate*	0.72
Cortisol	0.001
Cortisone	0.03
Pregnenolone	0.05
Progesterone	0.02
Corticosterone	0.24
Prednisolone	0.3
Estradiol-17B	0.52
11-Deoxy-Cortisol	0.2
17-OH-Progesterone	0.02
11-deoxy-Corticosterone	0.06
Cholesterol	0.04

Table 2. Cross-reactivity between Testosterone and related steroid hormones

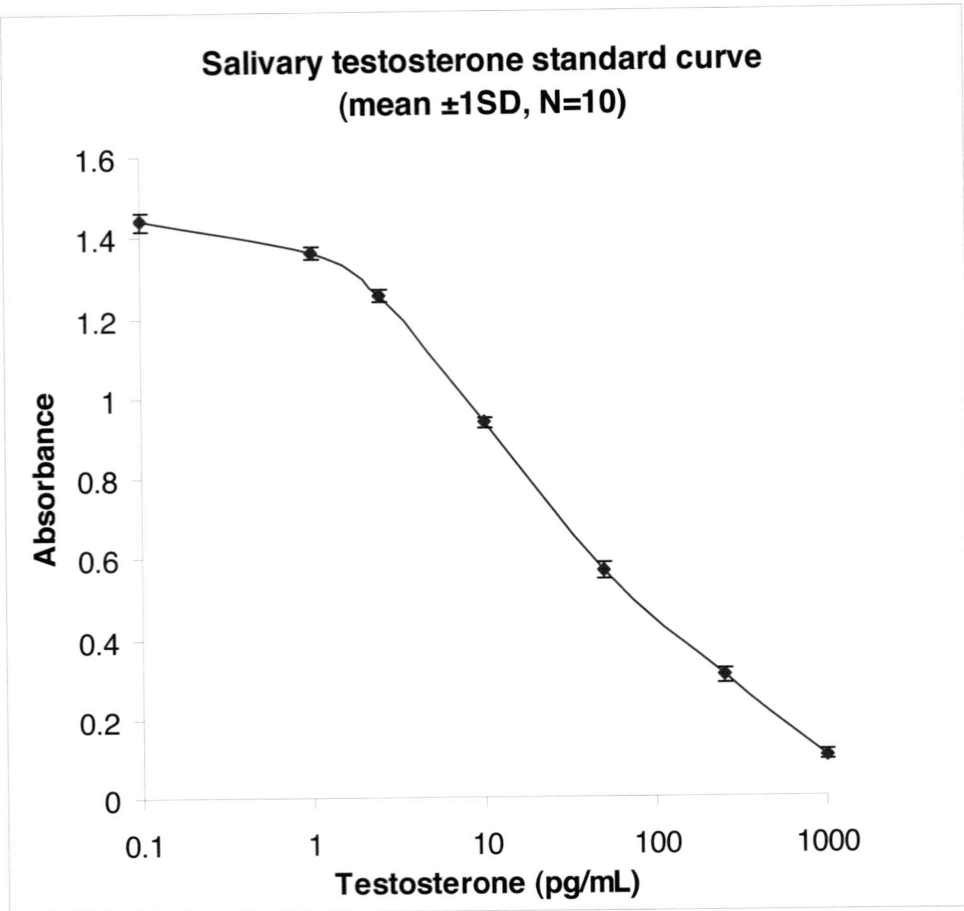

Figure 1. Typical testosterone ELISA standard curve (mean with SD, N=10)

7. Female salivary testosterone: Single vs. multiple sampling

Establishing a baseline for salivary T is not entirely straightforward. Whilst T production is partially under genetic control (Meikle et al., 1988) it is also responsive to a range of biological, environmental, and psychosocial stimuli; the relative influences of which are not yet fully understood, in either males or females. Amongst those factors identified as having a role in modifying T levels are: fasting, diet, sexual activity, alcohol, competition, behaviour intended to increase status, aggression, physical exercise, cognition, stress, immune function, and mood. In line with this, T concentrations have been shown to vary with time of day (Ahokoski et al., 1998; Walker et al., 1980), season of the year (Dabbs, 1991), sexual activity (Morris et al., 1987), and they fluctuate, in males at least, in a pulsatile fashion over minutes and hours (Veldhuis et al., 1987). Moreover, among women, T concentrations are thought to increase around the middle of the menstrual cycle (Massafra et al., 1998; Vermeulen & Verdonck, 1976; section 9 of this chapter).

Dabbs (1990) encapsulates some of the difficulties in designing suitable salivary sampling regimens when he states, '...variability introduces error into behavioral studies, where stable measures are needed to characterise individual differences and changes over time. Without more information on these changes one cannot know how many participants to run, how many measurements to take, and when to take measurements' (p.83). For a T baseline to be meaningful additionally depends, at least in part, on what purpose it is required to serve. In certain clinical practices, for example, researchers have advocated collecting single samples each day over the course of a week and pooling the samples to provide a weekly average. In order to ascertain if an individual has levels of T that might indicate a risk of a particular clinical condition this approach is appropriate. However, when attempting to examine chronobiological changes in relation to behavioural indices this sampling protocol would be unsuitable.

Comparatively little accurate research is available concerning detailed daily patterns of T in females; particularly the biologically active free and bio-available components, as measured in saliva. In the absence of reliable information, studies investigating the relationship between androgens and female behaviour have formulated methods that tend to employ either single time-point or very limited sampling protocols. However, given that females may also experience temporal fluctuation in T levels, similar to males, this salivary sampling protocol may be inappropriate. In order to address questions of salivary sampling schedules for one of our research programmes in female hormone/dominance research, we sought to provide a comprehensive picture of potential circadian activity and episodic fluctuation in female salivary T over one and then two non-consecutive days.

7.1. Methodology

Subjects were seventy-three healthy females (age range=18-29 with a mean age of 23.5). None were hirsute, had serious acne or were overweight. Particular attention was paid to factors that can affect circulating SHBG levels (i.e. history of kidney or liver disease, restriction of calorific intake) and none of the participants has administered any form of hormonal medication during the previous 9 months. Eight 4mL salivary samples were collected throughout the course of the day; one every two hours from 9am until 11pm. Following the same protocol, fifty-three healthy female participants (age range=18-28; mean=24.7) with a history of regular menstrual cycles lasting between 26-34 days also collected saliva on a second non-consecutive day. T concentrations were determined utilising our 'in-house' ELISA, described earlier in the chapter.

7.2. Findings

T concentration showed a circadian rhythm similar to that found in males. Perhaps more importantly, throughout the course of the day T concentrations were highly variable with episodic fluctuation of individual data points exceeding 83% of 9am levels. Mean T concentrations over day 1 and 2 were 140.5 and 148.2 picomoles/L respectively.

Consistent with findings from previous studies, and resulting at least in part from the spread of samples collected across menstrual cycle phase, there was considerable inter-individual variation in levels of T. Even so, table 3 illustrates that within the group mean, female participants demonstrate a clear circadian profile, with levels higher in the early morning and lower at 9pm, before starting to rise at 11pm. In the current data set percentage change from mean 9am levels reached a level of 34.4% at 9pm with individual percentage change from mean 9am levels reaching over 100%.

	9am	11am	1pm	3pm	5pm	7pm	9pm	11pm
T (pmole/L)	205.8	0.188	176.2	176.1	152.4	150.6	136.2	141.4
Mean (SEM)	(11.0)	(10.7)	(10.8)	(11.5)	(10.8)	(10.5)	(9.5)	(10.9)

Table 3. Female Circadian Salivary Testosterone (Mean ± SEM, n=71)

	9am	11am	1pm	3pm	5pm	7pm	9pm	11pm
Day1 T (pmole/L)	160.9	144.6	149.9	148.3	136.5	140.6	126.8	118.9
Mean (SEM)	(13.8)	(12.1)	(12.7)	(13.0)	(10.8)	(12.0)	(12.1)	(13.4)
Day2 T (pmole/L)	171.9	171.8	166.5	166.1	130.1	125.4	128.9	125.6
Mean (SEM)	(14.9)	(12.6)	(12.9)	(13.2)	(12.9)	(12.1)	(12.6)	(11.1)

Table 4. Testosterone Over Two Non-Consecutive Days (Mean ± SEM, n=53)

Contrary to the oft-cited claim that T is less labile in the afternoons our own results indicated that individual variability is at its most pronounced between 1pm and 7pm, which is the time it has been suggested studies take place in order to account for circadian variation and during which time 1 sample is presumed to represent basal levels. For study 2, Table 4 illustrates that across both days T followed a circadian profile appears only marginally similar.

7.3. Implications

In utilising single salivary measurements as somehow representative of basal female T levels we argue that studies attempting to correlate biological markers with behavioral indices have introduced a potentially serious confound into their methodological design. This confound is occasioned not only by normal circadian activity which, when considered in isolation we propose may be the wrong component of analysis on which to base the design of these studies, but results from the temporal fluctuation evident in individual salivary T. By adopting a more comprehensive sampling regimen than has previously been available the two studies reported here provide a more detailed representation of circadian activity in the free component of female T. Study 1 revealed evidence of a pronounced, though far from uniform, circadian profile in female T, the magnitude of which from 9am to 9pm was approximately 34%. In a study on circadian and menstrual variation Dabbs and de La Rue (1991) reported that morning T levels were 80% higher than evening samples. The magnitude of this circadian profile appears surprisingly large, however. It is, for example, much greater than the male equivalent (Bremner et al., 1983) and more than double the magnitude of our circadian findings. It is worth considering why.

Findings from early bio-behavioral studies attempting to assess the free (and/or bio-available) component T tended to suffer from limitations in the assay technology available to them. In the case of the Dabbs and de La Rue study (*ibid.*) the assay performance appeared to be a major limiting factor in placing any confidence in the findings. Not only did the extraction step recover only 85% of the original analyte, but within and between-assay coefficients of variation (CV) of 13.4% and 14.8% respectively appear excessively high. Moreover, with only two samples collected per day, the collection schedule was extremely limited. Indeed, rather than collect samples at predetermined times the participants followed their own schedules. As such, collection of the evening samples had an 85-minute standard deviation. These limitations provide a basis for recommending caution when interpreting the magnitude of their circadian findings.

The year before, Dabbs (1990) had written another paper on the circadian activity of T in both men and women and found a much smaller circadian profile. With specific reference to the female participants there were serious methodological anomalies. Data were presented from three independent studies: one group of participants collected salivary samples at 7am and 10am; a second group collected samples at 7am, 10am, and 10.30am. A final group collected samples at 10am, 4pm, and 10pm. Dabbs reported that female T levels were high in the early morning followed by a drop in the afternoon and early evening: 'Mean testosterone concentration dropped about 50% from morning to evening for both sexes, with largest drops early in the day' (p.83). However, in creating a circadian profile, the data from these separate studies were combined. In adopting this approach Dabbs fashioned a situation whereby a 7am sample for subject A must have been compared against a 10pm sample from subject B. Given the widespread acknowledgment of, often extreme, inter-individual variation in T levels, this procedure seems curious, at best. Moreover, despite earlier in the paper providing several references which pointed to the fluctuation of hormone levels with time of year, the data Dabbs collected, and subsequently combined, were collected at differing times of the year (autumn and spring). Indeed, as Dabbs notes, the results emanated from separate studies in which 'Data were collected over a 2½ year period' (p.83). Concerning the validity of findings from these studies there are additional questions concerning the assay performance and procedures. Firstly, in choosing to analyse aliquots of differing amounts of saliva (from 0.05mL to 0.4mL) Dabbs effectively altered the concentration of T being determined. He proceeded to suggest that the assay was run under analogue conditions (that is, one standard curve is provided and against which all results are determined). Secondly, the assay performance itself had an inter-assay variation in excess of 20% after recovering only 80-85% of the analyte following extraction. If these events were not problematic enough, Dabbs states 'There were changes in assay materials and in lab technicians and procedures over the course of the studies' (p.84). We argue, that these limitations essentially render the results impossible to interpret.

Interestingly, and we would argue critically, Dabbs makes the following point, 'This kind of variability should give us pause in working with single measurements from each subject, where it is not possible to recognise a score as deviant from a subject's mean' (1990, p.85). In attempting to determine the validity of utilising single salivary samples for determining baselines there are two issues that arise from this comment. Dabbs appears to be suggesting here that single time-point sampling can be problematic, if for no other reason than assay techniques can and do throw up erroneous results that can be extremely difficult to detect unless they are considered in relation to other scores from the same subject. The second issue is still whether circadian variation or episodic fluctuation confounds study design. It is not possible to make a judgement based on these two studies; firstly because of the considerable limitations in the study (design, measurement, methodology, interpretation) but also due to the lack of a comprehensive sampling regimen. It is further worth noting that Dabbs (1991) appear to contradict his earlier position, stating '…single measurements are reliable enough for use in behavioral research' (p.815).

In order to control for circadian activity several authors have indeed attempted to collect samples during the course of the afternoon, when T levels have been assumed to be less labile than in the mornings. In this regard Booth et al. (1989) state that '…it is helpful that matches are played in the afternoon' (p.558). Echoing this theme, Mazur, Booth, and Dabbs (1992) made explicit reference to their attempts to '…ensure that reported effects are not artefacts of…diurnal variation' (p.72). Recently, a study on the relationship between T and personality characteristics in which single T measures were collected, Sellers et al. (2007) stated 'To minimize the effects of diurnal fluctuations in T levels, all participants were assessed between the hours of Noon and 4pm' (p.5). Zitmann and Nieschlag (2001) put forward an alternative proposal arguing, in their review paper of T and behavioral characteristics, that T samples should be collected during the morning in order to minimise the effects of diurnal variation. Of the three published hormone-competition studies involving female participants, Mazur et al. (1997) claimed that by collecting samples between 1pm and 10pm they had effectively controlled for diurnal variation in T, which they clearly had not.

As a result of the more comprehensive circadian profile from our own data we are able to demonstrate that, far from being relatively stable, women experience considerable moment-to-moment variability in T levels. Even so, within the group mean of study 1 the significant differences generally existed between time points at the beginning of the day and late afternoon (i.e. 5pm) onwards. One interpretation of this finding would be that single measurements, especially if collected during early to mid-afternoon, would suffice in bio-behavioral research; collection at one moment in time being likely to yield much the same T level as any other. However, in the present study the lack of a statistically significant difference between T levels in the afternoon (between 1pm and 5pm) owes as much to the high standard deviations produced by the often extreme inter-individual variation as it does to a lack a difference in levels of T between time points. It is our contention, therefore, that when considered in isolation, mean circadian data may mislead researchers into believing that single sampling is appropriate in the design of bio-behavioral studies. We maintain that the episodic fluctuation (or, perhaps more correctly, random variability as the mechanism for this fluctuation is currently unknown in females) occurs at an order of magnitude that reduces confidence in the stability of a single salivary sample. It is for this reason we propose researchers utilize multiple samples in the determination of baseline T. Indeed, as Riad-Fahmy (1982) note, 'The wide episodic fluctuations in circulating steroid levels make analysis of single samples useful only in screening procedures' (p.367).

7.4. Reliability across days

Dabbs (1990) reported correlations for female T across two consecutive days as ranging from r=.55 though r=.73. Study 2 sought to examine the stability of T levels on two non-consecutive days demonstrated the relative lack of stability in levels of free T providing evidence that, contrary to earlier reports, the day-to-day stability of female T may not be especially high. In particular, the reliability between those subject who collected data on day 4 and then 14 of their cycle the reliability is, at some time points, low. There is some question as to whether levels of free T change across the menstrual cycle. Several studies have reported that T varies in a predictable manner throughout the course of a menstrual cycle (Alexander et al., 1990; Bloch et al., 1998), although the magnitude and subsequent relationship to behaviour is, at present, unclear and we address this in the following section. In a study examining plasma T changes across the menstrual cycle, Vermeulen and Verdonk (1976) stated, 'It is evident from this study that T...plasma levels do show statistically significant cyclical variations with maximal variations around ovulation' (p.493). Just over ten years later this finding was echoed in a study by Morris, et al. (1987), in which they indicated a rise in T levels around the mid- point of the cycle. Dabbs and de La Rue (1991), whilst finding a mid-cycle rise in salivary T, suggested that, as this variation was smaller than circadian variation, 'Menstrual cycle effects can be ignored in most research relating psychological and behavioural variables to individual differences in testosterone' (p.182). Our data appear to cast doubt on these recommendations.

In providing a more comprehensive profile of the temporal activity of female salivary free T the two studies reported here deal with an issue not satisfactorily addressed in the extant literature. Study 1 demonstrated that not only is there a distinct circadian rhythm but individual temporal variability can be pronounced. We contend it is this temporal variability that researchers need to account for in the design of salivary sampling protocols, and not only circadian activity. Study 2 demonstrated that this temporal profile, whilst similar over non-consecutive days 48hrs apart, reveals low reliability when samples are collected on more disparate occasions. Hence, a sample collected at 10am on day 1 may well not correspond particularly closely to a sample collected at 10am on a second day, especially if those days occur during different phases of a menstrual cycle. And yet, this is precisely the type of sampling regimen evident in the hormone-competition literature (e.g. Bateup et al., 2002). Combined, these data support the position that our understanding of the relationship between T and behavior in women is seriously hindered by the use of single-time point sampling methodology. Hence, over and above reporting evidence of circadian activity, the highly erratic nature of female salivary T levels throughout the day is an important consideration in sampling design. Indeed, these results suggest that females also exhibit episodic or random fluctuation at levels which call into question the use of single T measurement in female bio-behavioural studies.

8. Establishing female salivary testosterone circadian rhythm profiles in the menstrual cycle: Evidence of decline during ageing

In an attempt to further our understanding of circadian and menstrual dynamics the aim of the study was to establish circadian profiles and normal levels of salivary T in healthy women from the age of 19 through 69 at 3 points during the menstrual cycle, by means of a highly sensitive ELISA (described in section 7). Also, we wanted to investigate whether salivary T levels decline with age.

Five main groups of females: ages, 19-29, 30-39, 40-49 (pre and postmenopausal), 50-59 and 60-69 years were investigated. All subjects provided 8 saliva samples per day on the 4th, 14th and 21st day of their cycle according to their first day of menses, and post-menopausal women collected saliva samples on the 4th, 14th and 21st day of the calendar month. The women were not on any medication including the contraceptive pill and HRT, and did not suffer from any major illness. T levels were determined by our in-house ELISA method. The data indicated that female salivary T concentration showed a circadian rhythm similar to that found in males, although at lower levels (Fig. 2). Perhaps, more importantly, throughout the course of the day T levels were highly variable with episodic fluctuations of individual data points exceeding the 09.00 hours levels on some days (see Fig. 3). There was marked variation in T concentration between day 4, 14 and 21 of the cycle, though not statistically significant except for the age group of 30-39 year ($p<0.02$,) (see Fig. 4). When a repeated measure ANOVA with time and day as within subject factors and age group as between subject factors was applied, it was found that there was a significant difference in salivary T levels for age groups 19-29 and 40-49 years ($p = 0.01$), and between 30-39 and 40-49 years ($p = 0.02$). A Bonferroni correction was used for multiple comparisons.

Normal ranges for salivary T in females from the age of 19 through 69 year old at 3 different distinct days of the cycle (4, 14 and 21) for menstruating women, and 3 calendar days for post-menopausal women have been established. The results indicate that female salivary T concentration show a circadian rhythm similar to that found in males, although perhaps more importantly, throughout the course of the day T levels were highly variable with episodic fluctuations of individual data points exceeding the 09.00 hours levels. These findings lead us to suggest that normal ranges of T should only be determined from multiple samples as single measurements may be potentially misleading as they are subject to too much error variance. This view was reported by the authors in another study (Sharp & Al-Dujaili, 2004) and supported by Hoffman (2001) who suggested that because of diurnal and monthly variations, several steroid hormones need multiple samples to give meaningful results.

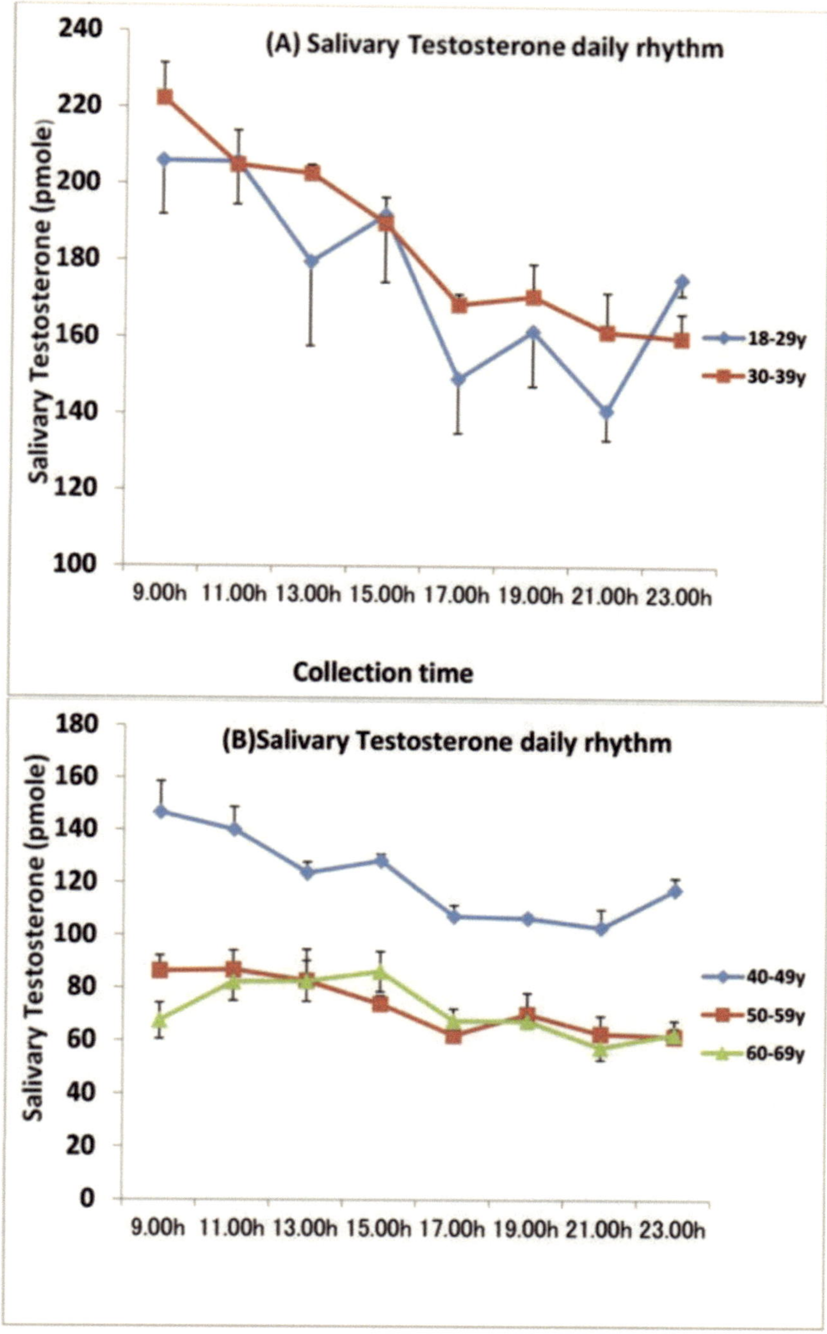

Figure 2. Female Salivary daily Testosterone rhythm throughout the menstrual cycle for A) pre-menopausal women (age group 19-29, 30-39 years) and B) postmenopausal women (age groups 44-49, 50-59 and 60-69). Some pre-menopausal women 40-44 years data were included in the graph of 40-49 years. All data represent mean ±sem of day 4, 14 and 21 of the cycle.

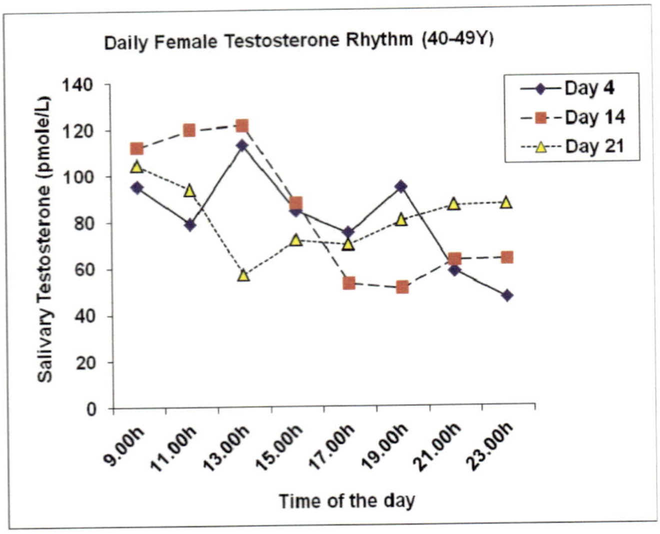

Figure 3. Female salivary testosterone levels in women at 40-49 years showing episodic fluctuations of individual data points exceeding the 09.00 hours levels on some days (Data are mean of 12 females).

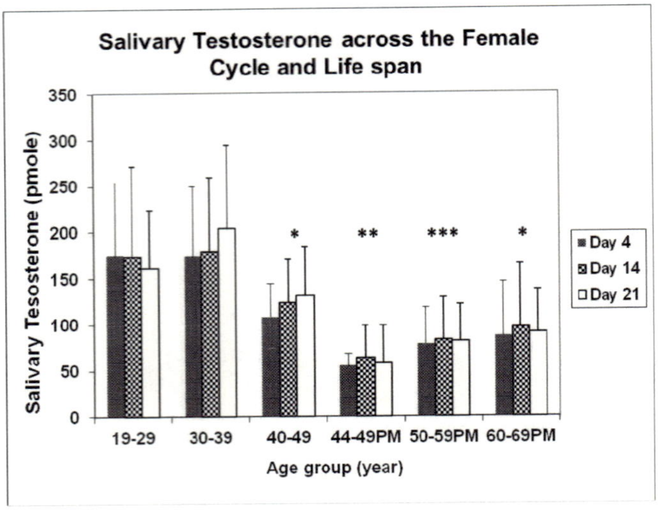

Figure 4. Summary of Salivary Testosterone results in females: Average testosterone concentration per day in pmole. (* = $P< 0.05$, ** = $p< 0.01$, *** = $p< 0.001$). Student paired t-tests were done between these groups and group 19-29years)

In terms of absolute salivary T levels obtained by our ELISA method and bearing in mind the high specificity of the T antibody employed, the values seem to be somewhat higher than those reported elsewhere, particularly for younger women. We believe that this could be due to the fact that our ELISA might be measuring some of the bio-available T concentration (i.e. the free fraction plus the albumin-bound T: Pardridge & Demers, 1991). A view supported by earlier findings by Ruutiainen et al. (1987) who found that concentrations of salivary T (without chromatographic prepurification) in hirsute women exceeded free T in plasma by 10-fold. However, Swinkels and co-workers (1991) found that salivary T levels were 3-fold higher than plasma free T due to the metabolism of androgen precursors (e.g., androstendione) during passage through the salivary gland. We believe that both of the above mechanisms may be involved.

Our results demonstrated an effect of age on salivary T similar to that found in serum in which there is a significant decline in salivary T level between younger groups of females and those after menopause and older groups. These results were also found by other researchers (e.g. Labrie et al., 1997). However, some workers (Burger, 2002) stated that serum T does not change significantly in relation to the menopausal transition but it falls slowly with age. Such difference could be explained by the fact that they were measuring serum total T rather than the biologically active hormone. Another study by Campbell and Ellison (1992) found that salivary T was higher in anovulatory cycles compared with ovulatory cycles, and that T levels tend to be higher at the midcycle phase.

The results of this study have clearly demonstrated that there was a significant decline in female salivary T across age groups and particularly after the age of 39 years. These findings are supported in a study by Labrie and colleagues (1997) in which they compared serum T levels in women of 20-30 years old with 70-80 years old, and found that there was a marked decline in C19 steroids in the older group with smaller changes after the age of 60 years. Other studies (e.g. Zumoff et al., 1995; Longcope, 1998) have also shown a decline in serum T after the age of 30 years and just before the menopause varying from 15-50%. We have also shown that there was a significant drop in female salivary T concentration in post-menopausal women compared to menstruating women within the age group of 40-49 years ($p< 0.02$ to $p<0.05$). However, Burger et al. (2000) showed no change in serum total T levels 5 years before and 7 years after the menopause. Our results, on the other hand, showed a slight increase in salivary T at the age group of 60-69 years compared to other post-menopausal women. This was mainly due to 2 subjects (ages 61 and 64) who consistently exhibited higher T values that could be due to undeclared use of HRT or non-compliance with instructions. Several studies have shown possible vital roles for androgens - and in particular T- in women (Synder, 2001; Braunstein, 2002; Burger, 2002). Specifically, to increase libido, increasing bone mineralization, effect on muscle mass and strength and sense of general well being. We also think that it is absolutely necessary to assess female T before any hormone replacement therapy, and our results demonstrate without doubt that some women had seriously low T levels that might precipitate deleterious effects on the health and life quality of these women.

In conclusion, our results suggest that females do exhibit episodic fluctuations in daily salivary T throughout the menstrual cycle, and there is marked variation in T concentration between day 4, 14 and 21 of the cycle. Moreover, single T measurements appear to be of little value representing only the level at the time they were collected. There is however, a significant decline in female salivary T after the age of 39 years. The data obtained will hopefully allow clinicians to have much greater confidence in their ability to determine the necessity of androgen replacement therapy (HRT) for post-menopausal women and those with suspected insufficiency. It is extremely important for women embarking on taking any form of HRT to consult their physician who can now assess by simple screening method the endogenous level of T in order to administer the correct dose of HRT. This might minimise any side effects.

9. Summary

We commenced our chapter with an up-to-date revision on the role of testosterone (T) in women's health, illustrating both the complexity and breadth of physiological and psychological actions. Although not exhaustive in scope it is clearly evident from these examples that T can no longer be considered as male only hormone and a greater emphasis on the role of T in female behaviours is warranted. Second, we described T production in females and discussed recent advances in our understanding of mechanisms of action such as non-genomic pathways. Here we also considered the importance of incorporating both free and bio-available fractions in the measurement of salivary T. Third we discussed the use of saliva as a diagnostic fluid and highlighted that despite its utility there are a number of problems and challenges related to the collection, storage and measurement of androgens in saliva, which researchers must be aware of if we are to have confidence in studies across several disciplines and particularly in those bio-behavioural studies which seek to draw often controversial inferences about the role of women in society based upon levels of circulating T. Fourth we dealt with the assay technology generally and more specifically the development and optimization of our own enzyme-linked immunosorbant assay (ELISA), specifically designed for use in the quantitative determination of female salivary T. Finally, we discussed the circadian dynamics of female salivary T. Very little research is available about detailed daily patterns of T in females; particularly the biologically active free component, as measured in saliva. In the absence of reliable information, hormone replacement therapy programmes and bio-behavioural studies involving female participants have tended to formulate salivary sampling strategies taken directly from research involving males. We were able to draw upon our own innovative work on the circadian dynamics of female T to illustrate the limitations of single or limited time-point sampling by demonstrating the large intra and inter subject variability of diurnal rhythms and further show that merely sampling in the afternoon as a means of reducing error is fraught with complications. Our findings allowed us to highlight the need for comprehensive multiple sampling design for effective protocols. Following this examination of circadian dynamics we also described our work on menstrual fluctuations in salivary and circadian dynamics across the lifespan, which demonstrated the significant difference in T levels across the menstrual cycle and decline across age. We hope that the ELISA protocol described here, the challenges in measurement and collection discussed and our findings on circadian dynamics in women are of some assistance to researchers in helping them reflect upon and design meaningful studies involving women and T.

Author details

E.A.S. Al-DujailI[1*] and M.A. Sharp[2]

*Address all correspondence to: ealdujaili@qmu.ac.uk

1 Dietetics, Nutrition and Biological Sciences, Queen Margaret University, Edinburgh, UK

2 School of Health and Life Sciences, Glasgow Caledonian University, Glasgow, UK

References

[1] Adlercreutz, H. (1990) Use of sex hormone and corticosteroid assays in the diagnosis of endocrine disorders in women: Introduction to a round table discussion. *Proceedings of the 4th Symposium on the Analysis of Steroids* (pp. 387-395), Pécs, Hungary.

[2] Adlercreutz, H., Höckerstedt, K., Bannwart, C., Bloigu. S., Hämäläinen, E., Fotsis, T. & Ollus, A. (1987). Effect of dietary components, including lignans and phytooestrogens on enterohepatic circulation and liver metabolism of oestrogens and on sex hormone-binding globulin (SHBG) *Journal of Steroid Biochemistry,* 27: 1135-1144.

[3] Ahokoski, O., Virtanen, A., Huupponen, R., Scheinen, H., Salminene, E., Kairisto, V., & Irjala, K. (1998). Biological day-to-day variation and daytime changes in testosterone, follitropin, lutropin and oestradiol-17β in healthy men. *Clinical Chemistry and Laboratory Medicine,* 36, 485-491.

[4] Al-Dujaili, E.A.S. (2006). Development and validation of a simple and direct ELISA method for the measurement of urinary testosterone excretion. *Clinica Chimica Acta,* 364 (1-2): 172-179.

[5] Al-Dujaili, E.A.S., Denyer, M., Milne, C., Philo, R., Pritchard, J., & Allen, A. (1988) *Serozyme: A manual non-isotopic immunoassay system.* In Immunometric assays; overview & new developments, Proceedings of NEQAS meeting (1-8), Cardiff, Wales.

[6] Alexander, G.M., Sherwin, B.B., Bancroft, J., & Davidson, D.W. (1990). Testosterone and sexual behaviour in oral contraceptive users and nonusers: A prospective study. *Hormones and Behavior.* 24, 388-402.

[7] Allen, N.E., Key, T.J. (2000). The effects of diet on circulating sex hormone levels in men. *Nutrition Res. Reviews,* 13(2): 159-184.

[8] Anderson, K.E., Rosner, W., Khan, M.S., New, M.I., et al. (1987) Diet-Hormone Interactions: protein/charbohydrate ratio alters reciprocally the plasma levels of testosterone and cortisol and their respective binding globulins in man. *Life Sciences,* 40: 1761-1768

[9] Bachmann, G.A., Leiblum, S.R. (1991). Sexuality in sexagenarian women. *Maturitas,* 13: 45-50.

[10] Bateup, H.S., Booth, A., Shirtcliff, E.A., & Granger, D.A. (2002). Testosterone, cortisol, and women's competition. *Evolution and Human Behaviour,* 23, 181-192.

[11] Baxendale, P.M., Reed, M.J., & James, V.H.T. (1980). Testosterone in saliva of normal men and its relationship with unbound and total testosterone levels in plasma. *Journal of Endocrinology,* 87, 46.

[12] Baxendale, P.M., Jacobs, H.S., &James, V.H. (1982) Salivary testosterone: relationship to unbound plasma testosterone in normal and hyperandrogenic women. Clin Endocrinol (Oxf), 16(6): 595-603.

[13] Beral, V. (2003). Breast cancer and hormone-replacement therapy in the Million Women Study. *Lancet,* 362: 419-27

[14] Berrino, F. et al. (2001) Reducing bioavailable sex hormones through a comprehensive change in diet: the diet and androgens (DIANA) randomised trial. *Cancer Epidemiology Biomarkers & Prevention* Vol. 10: 25-33.

[15] Besch, N.F., Ruetzel, C.H., Younes, M.A., Huang, N.H., Besch, P.K., & Read G.F. (1982). *Non-chromatographic determination of salivary testosterone in women*: In G.F. Read, D. Riad-Fahmy, R.F Walker, & K. Griffiths (Eds.). Ninth Tenovus Workshop: Immunoassays of Steroids in Saliva. (pp. 221-227), Cardiff, Wales: Alpha Omega, 1982.

[16] Booth, A., Shelley, G., Mazur, A., Tharp, G., & Kittok, R. (1989). Testosterone, and winning and losing in human competition. *Hormones and Behavior,* 23: 556-571.

[17] Bloch, M., Schmidt, P.J., Su, T.-P., Tobin, M.B., & Rubinow, D.R (1998). Pituitary-adrenal hormones and testosterone across the menstrual cycle in women with premenstrual syndrome and controls. *Biological Psychiatry.* 43, 897-903.

[18] Braunstein, G.D. (2002). Androgen insufficiency in women: Summary of critical issues. *Fertility and Sterility,* 77 (Suppl. 4), S94-S99.

[19] Bremner, W.J., Vitiello, M.V., & Prinz, P.N. (1983). Loss of circadian rhythmicity in blood testosterone levels with ageing in normal men. *Journal of Clinical Endocrinology and Metabolism,* 56 (6), 1278-1281.

[20] Brincat, M., Moniz, C.F., Kabalan, S., Versi, E., et al. (1987). Decline in skin collagen content and metacarpal index after the menopause and its prevention with sex hormone replacement. *Br J Obstet Gynaecol* 94: 126-129.

[21] Brown, G.L., McGarvey, E.L., Shirtcliff, E.A., Keller, A., Granger, D.A., & Flavin, K. (2008). Salivary cortisol, dehydroepiandrosterone, and testosterone interrelationships in healthy young males: a pilot study with implications for studies of aggressive behavior. *Psychiatry Res.* May 30;159(1-2):67-76.

[22] Broderick, J.E., Arnold, D., Kudielka, B.M., & Kirschbaum, C. (2003). Salivary cortisol compliance: comparison of patients and health volunteers. *Psychneuroendocrinology,* 29: 636-650.

[23] Burger, H.G. (2002). Androgen production in women. *Fertil. Steril.,* 77 (supplement 4), S3-S5.

[24] Burger, N., & Casson, P. (2004). The pathophysiology of androgens in women. In Testosterone; action, deficiency and substitution, Nieschlag, E & Behre HM (Eds), 4th edition, Cambridge, page 543-569.

[25] Burger, H.G., Dudley, E.C., Cui, J., Dennerstein, L., & Hopper, J.L. (2000). A prospective longitudinal study of serum testosterone, dehydroepiandrosterone sulphate and sex hormone-binding globulin levels through the menopause transition. *J Clin Endocrinology Metab.,* 85, 2832-8.

[26] Campbell, B.C. & Ellison, P.T. (1992). Menstrual variation in Salivary Testosterone among regularly cycling women. *Hormone Research,* 37, 132-136.

[27] Cardoso EM, Contreras LN, Tumilasci EG. et al. (2011) Salivary testosterone for the diagnosis of androgen deficiency in end-stage renal disease. Nephrol Dial Transplant 26(2): 677-683

[28] Castoria, G., Lombardi, M., Barone MV, Bilancio A, et al. (2003). Androgen-stimulated DNA synthesis and cytoskeletal changes in fibroblasts by a nontranscriptional receptor action. *J Cell Biol.* 161(3):547-556

[29] Christiansen, K. (2004). *Behavioural correlates of testosterone. In Testosterone: Actions, deficiency and substitution,* Nieschlag E and Behre HM (Eds), 3rd Edition, page 125-172, Cambridge University Press, Cambridge.

[30] Ciampelli, M., & Lanzone, A. (1998). Insulin and polycystic ovary syndrome: a new look at an old subject. *Gynecol Endocrinol.* 12(4):277-292

[31] Collins, J.J. (2000). Salivary hormone testing: Science, benefits, limitations and clinical applications. *Anti-Ageing Medical News;* Winter 2000 issue: 1-6.

[32] Conway, C.A. et al. (2007). Salience of emotional displays of danger and contagion in faces is enhanced when progesterone levels are raised. *Hormones and Behavior,* 51(2): 202-206.

[33] Crook, D., & Seed, M. (1990). Endocrine control of plasma lipoprotein metabolism: effects of gonadal steroids. *Bailieres Clin Endocrinol Metab,* 4: 851-875.

[34] Dabbs, J.M. Jr. (1990). Salivary testosterone measurements: reliability across hours, days, and weeks. *Physiology and Behavior,* 48, 83-86.

[35] Dabbs, J.M. Jr. (1991). Saliva testosterone measurements: collecting, storing, and mailing saliva samples. *Physiology and Behavior* 49 (4), 815–17.

[36] Dabbs, J.M., Campbell, B.C., Gladue, B.A., Midgley, A.R., Read, G.F., Swinkels, L.M. & Worthman, C.M. (1995) Reliability of salivary testosterone measurements: a multi-center evaluation. *Clinical Chemistry* 41: 1581-1584.

[37] Dabbs, J.M. Jr. & de la Rue, D. (1991). Salivary Testosterone measurements among women: relative magnitude of circadian and menstrual cycles. *Hormones Research*, 1 (35), 182-184.

[38] Davis SR (2011) Cardiovascular and cancer safety of testosterone in women. Curr Opin Endocrinol Diabetes Obes. Jun;18(3):198-203.

[39] Davis, S.R. (1999). Androgen replacement in women: a commentary. *Journal Clin Endocrinology Metab*, 84(6), 1886-1891.

[40] Davis SR and Davison SL. (2012) Current perspectives on testosterone therapy for women. Menopausal Medicine May 2012: S1-S4.

[41] Davis, S., & Tran, J. (2001). What are "normal" testosterone levels for women? *J Clin Endocrinol Metab*, 86: 1842

[42] Davison, S.L., Bell, R., Donath, S., Montalto, J.G., & Davis, S.R. (2005). Androgen levels in adult females: changes with age, menopause and oophorectomy. *J Clin Endocrinol Metab* 90: 3847-3853.

[43] Davy, B.M. & Melby, C.L. (2003). The effect of fibre-rich carbohydrates on features of syndrome X. *J AM Diet Assoc*, 103: 86-96.

[44] Deady, D.K., Law Smith, M.J., Sharp, M.A., & Al-Dujaili, E.A.S. (2006). Maternal personality and reproductive ambition in women is associated with salivary testosterone levels. *Biological Psychology*, vol. 71, no. 1, 29-32.

[45] De Crée C, Lewin R and Ostyn M. (1990) The monitoring of the menstrual status of female athletes by salivary steroid determination and ultrasonography. European Journal of Applied Physiology and Occupational Physiology 60, Number 6: 472-477

[46] Edwards, R. (1985). *Immunoassay: An Introduction*. London: William Heinmann.

[47] Ekins, R. (1990). Hirsutism: free and bound testosterone 9letter). *Ann Clin Biochem*, 27: 91-93.

[48] Fausto-Sterling, A. (2000). *Sexing the Body: Gender politics and the construction of sexuality*. New York: Basic Books.

[49] Fettes, I. (1999). Migraine in trhe menopause. *Neurology*, 53(Suppl 1): S29-S33.

[50] Fix, C., Jordan, C., Cano, P., Walker, W.H. (2004). "Testosterone activates mitogen-activated protein kinase and the cAMP response element binding protein transcription factor in Sertoli cells". *Proc Natl Acad Sci USA* 101 (30): 10919–10924.

[51] Fogle RH, Stanczyk FZ, Zhang X, Paulson RJ. (2007) Ovarian androgen production in postmenopausal women. J Clin Endocrinol Metab. 92(8):3 040-3043.

[52] Gasperino, J. (1995). Androgenic regulation of bone mass in women. A review. *Clin Orthop* 311: 278-286.

[53] Gavrilova N and Lindau ST (2009) Salivary Sex Hormone Measurement in a National, Population-Based Study of Older Adults. J Gerontol B Psychol Sci Soc Sci 64B (suppl 1): 94-105

[54] Gladue, B.A., Boechler, M., & McCaul, K.D. (1989). Hormonal response to competition in human males. *Aggressive Behavior*, 15, 409-422.

[55] Groh, H., Schade, K. & Horhold-Schubert, C. (1993). Steroid metabolism with intestinal micro-organisms. *Journal of Basic Microbiology*, 33, 59-72.

[56] Guay, A.T. (2002). Screening for androgen deficiency in women: Methodological and interpretative issues: The Princeton consensus statement on definition, classification, and assessment. *Fertility and Sterility*, 4 (Suppl. 4) S83-88.

[57] Guo, Z., Benten, W.P., Krucken, J., & Wunderlich, F. (2002). Non-genomic testosterone calcium signaling. Genotropic actions in androgen receptor-free macrophages. *J Biol Chem*, 277: 29600-29607.

[58] Granger, D.A., Schwartz, E.B., Booth, A., & Arentz, M. (1999). Salivary testosterone determination in studies of child health and development. *Hormones and Behavior*, 35, 18-27.

[59] Granger, D.A., Shirtcliff, E.A., Booth, A., Kivlighan, K.T., Schwartz, E.B. (2004). The trouble with salivary testosterone, *Psychoneuroendocrinology*, 29: 1229-1240.

[60] Groschl, M., Wagner, R., Rauh, M., & Dorr, H.G. (2001). Stability of salivary steroids: the influences of storage, food and dental care. *Steroids* 66: 737-741.

[61] Haffner, S.M., Valdez, R.A., Mykkanen, L. et al. (1994). Deceased testosterone and DHEA sulphate concentrations are associated with increased insulin and glucose concentrations in non-diabetic men. *Metabolism*, 43: 599-603.

[62] Hammond, G.L., Nisker, J.A., Jones, L.A., & Siiteri, P.K. (1980). Estimation of the percentage of free steroid in undiluted serum by centrifugal ultrafiltration-dialysis. *Journal of Biological Chemistry*, 255 (11), 5023-5026.

[63] Heald, A.H., Ivison, F., Anderson, S.G., Cruickshank, K., Laing. I,, & Gibson, M. (2003). Significant ethnic variation in total and free testosterone concentration. *Clin Endocrinology* 58: 262-266.

[64] Heinlein, C.A. & Chang, C. (2002). The roles of androgen receptors and androgens binding proteins in non-genomic androgen actions. *Mol Endocrinol*. 16: 2181-2187.

[65] Herold, D.A., & Fitzgerald, R.L. (2003). Immunoassays for testosterone in women; Better than a guess? *Clinical Chemistry* 49: 1250-1251

[66] Hickok, L.R., Toomey, C., Speroff. L. (1993). A comparison of estrified oestrogens with and without methyltestosterone: effects on endometrial histology and serum lipoproteins in postmenopausal women. *Obstet Gynecol.* 82: 919-924.

[67] Hiipakka, R.A., & Liao, S. (1998). "Molecular mechanism of androgen action". *Trends Endocrinol. Metab.* 9 (8): 317–324.

[68] Ho, C.K., Stoddart, M., Walton, M., Anderson, R.A., & Beckett, G.J. (2006). Calculated free testosterone in men: comparison of four equations and with free androgen index. *Ann Clin Biochem.* 43(Pt 5):389-397.

[69] Hoffman, L.F. (2001). Human saliva as a diagnostic specimen. *Journal of Nutrition,* 131, 1621S-1625S.

[70] Hui, S.L., Perkins, A.J., Zhou, L., Longcope, C., Econs, M.J., & Johnston, C.C. (2002). Bone loss at the femoral neck in perimenopausal white women: effects of weight change and sex hormone levels. *J Clin Endocrinol Metab,* 87:1539-1543.

[71] Isidori, A.M., Giannetta, E., Greco, E.A., Gianfrilli, D. et al. (2008). Effects of testosterone on body composition, bone metabolism and serum lipid profile in middle-aged men: a meta-analysis. *Clinical Endocrinology* 63(3), 280–293.

[72] Jones, J., Murphy, E., Alaghband-Zadeh, J. (2004). *Modified method for extracted assay for female testosterone measurement on the Abbott Architect analyser.* Conference Proceedings. 23rd Joint Meeting of the British Endocrine Societies with the European Federation of Endocrine Societies, Brighton, UK.

[73] Kemeny, D.M. & Chantler, S. (1991). An introduction to ELISA. In D.M. Kemeny & S.J. Challacombe. (Eds.). *ELISA and other solid phase immunoassays: Theoretical and practical aspects.* Chichester: John Wiley & Sons.

[74] Kemeny, D.M. (1991). *A Practical Guide to ELISA.* Exeter: Pergamon Press.

[75] Kirkwood, T.B. (2005). Understanding the odd science of aging. *Cell,* 120: 437-447.

[76] Kivlighan, K.T, Granger, D.A., Schwartz, E.B., Nelson, V., Curran, M., & Shirtcliff, E.A. (2004). Quantifying blood leakage into the oral mucosa and its effects on the measurement of cortisol, dehydropiandrosterone, and testosterone in saliva. *Hormones and Behavior,* 46, 39-46.

[77] Kraemer, W., Volek, J.S., Bush, J.A., et al. (1998). Hormonal responses to consecutive days of heavy resistance exercise with or without nutritional supplementation. *J Applied Physiology,* 85 (4): 1544

[78] Kudielka, B.M., Broderick, J.E., Kirschbaum, C. (2003). Compliance with saliva sampling protocols: electronic monitoring reveals invalid cortisol daytime profiles in noncompliant subjects. *Psychosomatic Med,* 65: 313-319

[79] Labrie, F., Belanger, A., Belanger, P., Berube, R., Martel, C., Cusan, L. (2006). Androgen glucuronides, instead of testosterone, as the new markers of androgenic activity in women. *J Steroid biochem Mol Biol,* 99: 182-188.

[80] Labrie, F., Belanger, A., Cusan, L., Gomez, J.L., & Candas, B. (1997). Marked decline in Serum concentrations of adrenal C19 sex steroid precursors and conjugated androgen metabolites during aging. *Journal Clin Endocrinology Metab.*, 82 (8), 2396-2402.

[81] Labrie, F., Luu-The, V., Labrie, C., Pelletier, G., & El-Alfy, M. (2000). Intracrinology and the skin. *Horm Res.* 54(5-6):218-229.

[82] Labrie, F., Luu-the V, Labrie, C., Belanger, A., Simard, J., Lin, S.X., & Peletier, G. (2003) Endocrine and intracrine sources of androgens in women: inhibition of breast cancer and other roles of androgens and their precursor DHEA. *Endocrine Rev*, 24: 152-182.

[83] Labrie F, Martel C, Balser J. (2011) Wide distribution of the serum dehydroepiandrosterone and sex steroid levels in postmenopausal women: role of the ovary? Menopause 18: 30-43.

[84] Lac, G., Lac, N., & Robert, A. (1993). Steroid assays in saliva: a method to detect plasmatic contaminations. *Arch Int Phsiol Biochim Biophys*, 101: 257-262.

[85] Laumann, E.O., Paik A, Rosen RC. (1999). Sexual dysfunction in the United States: prevalence and predictors. *Journal of the American Medical Association* 281 (6): 537-544.

[86] Leiblum, S., Bachmann, G., Kemmann, E., Colburn, D., & Swartzman, L. (1983) Vaginal atrophy in the postmenopausal woman. The importance of sexual activity and hormones. *JAMA*. 249(16):2195-2198

[87] Lepage, R. (2006). Measurement of testosterone and its sub-fractions in Canada. *Clinical Biochem*, 39: 97-108.

[88] Longcope, C. (1986). Adrenal and gonadal androgen secretion in normal females. *Clinic Endocrinol Metabolism*, 15: 213-228.

[89] Longcope, C., Feldman, H.A., McKinlay, J.B., Araujo, A.B. (2000). Diet and sex hormone-binding globulin. *J Clin Endocrinol Metab*. 85(1):293-296

[90] Longcope, C., Hui, S.L., & Johnston, C.C. (1987). Free estradiol, free testostereone, and sex hormone-binding globulin in perimenopausal women. *J Clin Endocrinol Metab*, 65: 513-518.

[91] Longcope, C. (1998). Androgen metabolism and the menopause. *Semin Reprod. Endocrinology*, 16, 111-115.

[92] Lipson, S.F., & Ellison, P.T. (1989). Development of protocols for the application of salivary steroid analyses to field conditions. *Am J Human Biol*, 249-255.

[93] Lösel, R.M., Falkenstein, E., Feuring, M., Schultz, A., Tillmann, H.C., Rossol-Haseroth, K., & Wehling, M. (2003). Nongenomic Steroid Action: Controversies, Questions, and Answers. *Physiol Rev*, 83: 965–1016.

[94] Luisi, M, Gasperi, M, Silvestri, D, Bernini, GP et al. (1982) Applicability of salivary-testosterone measurements for the follow-up of therapy of idiopathic hirsutism. Journal of Steroid Biochemistry 17: 581–583

[95] Major C. V., Read S. E., Coates R. A., Francis A., McLaughlin B. J., Millson M., Shepherd F., Fanning M., Calzavara L., MacFadden D., Johnson J. K., (1991) Comparison of saliva and blood for human immunodeficiency virus prevalence testing. *Journal of Infectious Diseases*, 163, 699-702.

[96] Malamud, D., & Tabak, L. (eds.) (1993) *Saliva as a Diagnostic Fluid*. New York: New York Academy of Sciences.

[97] Mandel, I.D. (1993). Salivary diagnosis: Promises, promises. In D. Malamud, & L.A. Tabak. (Eds.). Saliva as a diagnostic fluid. *Annals of the New York Academy of Sciences*, 694 (pp. 1-10). New York, NY: New York Academy of Sciences.

[98] Manni, A., Pardridge, W.M., Cefalu. W. et al. (1985). Bioavailability of albumin-bound testosterone. *Journal of Clinical Endocrinology and Metabolism*, 61 (4), 705-710.

[99] Massafra, C., De Felice, C., Agnusdei, D.P., Gioia, D., & Bagnoli, F. (1998). Androgens and Osteocalcin during the menstrual cycle. *Journal of Clinical Endocrinology and Metabolism*, 84 (3), 971-974.

[100] Matsumoto, A.M., Bremner, W.J. (2004). Serum testosterone assays - Accuracy matters. *J Clin Endocrinol Metab*, 89: 520-524.

[101] Mazur, A. & Lamb, T. (1980). Testosterone, status, and mood in human males. *Hormones and Behavior*, 14, 236-246.

[102] Mazur, A., Susman, A.J., & Edelbrock, S. (1997). Sex difference in testosterone response to a video game contest. *Evolution and Human Behavior*, 18, 317-326.

[103] Mazur, A., Susman, A.J., & Edelbrock, S. (1997). Sex difference in testosterone response to a video game contest. *Evolution and Human Behavior*, 18, 317-326.

[104] Mazur, A., Booth, A., & Dabbs Jr., J.M. (1992). Testosterone and chess competition. *Social Psychology Quarterly*, 55 (1), 70-77.

[105] McPhaul, M.J., Young, M. (2001). "Complexities of androgen action". *J. Am. Acad. Dermatol.* 45 (3 Suppl): S87–S94

[106] Meikle, A.W., Stringham, J.D., Bishop, D.T., & West, D.W. (1988). Quantitating genentic and non genetic factors influencing androgen production and clearance rates in men. *Journal of Clinical Endocrinology and Metabolism*, 67, 104-109.

[107] Mendel, C.M. (1989). The free hormone hypothesis: a physiologically based mathematical model. *Endocrin Rev*, 10: 232-274.

[108] Miller, K.K., Rosner, W., Lee, H., Heir, J., Sesmilo, G., Schoenfeld, D., & Kilbanski, A. (2004). Measurement of free testosterone in normal women and women with androgen deficiency: comparison of methods. *J Clin Endocrinol Metab*, 89: 525-533.

[109] Moore, F.R, Al Dujaili, E.A.S., Cornwell, R.E., Law Smith, M.J., Lawson, J.F., Sharp, M. & Perrett, D. I. (2011) Cues to sex- and stress-hormones in the human male face: functions of glucocorticoids in the immunocompetence handicap hypothesis. *Hormones and Behavior,* 60: 269-274.

[110] Morris, N.M., Udry, J. R., Khan-Dawood, F., & Dawood, M.Y. (1987). Marital sex frequency and midcycle female testosterone. *Archives of Sexual Behavior,* 16 (1), 27-37.

[111] Navazesh, M. (1993). Methods for collecting saliva. In D. Malamud, & L.A. Tabak. (Eds.). Saliva as a diagnostic fluid. *Annals of the New York Academy of Sciences,* 694 (pp 72-77). New York, NY: New York Academy of Sciences.

[112] Nieschlag, E., & Behre, H.M., (1998) eds. *Testosterone: action, deficiency, substitution.* 2nd ed. Berlin: Springer-Verlag, 1998:58-66.

[113] O'Sullivan, M.J., Bridges, J.W., & Marks, V. (1979). Enzyme immunoassay: a review. Annals of Clinical Biochemistry, 16, 221-239.

[114] Overlie, I., Moen, M.H., Morkrid, L., Skjaeraasen, J.S., & Holte, A. (1999). The endocrine transition around menopause- a five years prospective study with profiles of gonadotropines, oestrogens, androgens and SHBG among healthy women, Acta Obstet Gynecol Scand 78: 642-647.

[115] Pardridge W.M., & Demers L.M. (1991). Bioavailable testosterone in salivary glands. Clin Chemistry 37: 139-140.

[116] Pasquali R, Casimirri F, De Iasio R, Mesini P, Boschi S, Chierici B, Flamia R, Biscotti M and Vicennati V (1995) Insulin regulates testosterone and sex hormone-binding globulin concentrations in adult normal-weight and obese men *Journal of Clinical Endocrinology and Metabolism* 80, 654-658.

[117] Perry RJ, Mayo A, Deeb A, MacIntyre H, Wallace AM, et al (2005) Salivary testosterone measurement for monitoring treatment of children with congenital adrenal hyperplasia (CAH). *Endocrine Abstracts* 9: P143

[118] Pusateri, D.J., Roth, W.T., Ross, J.K. & Shultz, T.D. (1990). Dietary and hormonal evaluation of men at different risks for prostate cancer: plasma and faecal hormone-nutrient interrelationships *American Journal of Clinical Nutrition,* 51: 371-377.

[119] Quissell, D.O. (1993). Steroid hormone analysis in human saliva. *Ann N Y Acad Sci.* 694:143-145.

[120] Rako, S. (1998). Testosterone deficiency: a key factor in the increased cardiovascular risk to women following hysterectomy or with natural ageing. *J Women Health,* 7: 825-829.

[121] Read, G.F. (1989). *Hormones in saliva.* Tenovuo, J.O. (Eds.). Human Saliva: Clinical Chemistry and Microbiology. Boca Raton, FL: Press Inc.

[122] Riad-Fahmy, D., Read, G.F., Walker, R.F., & Griffiths K. (1982). Steroids in saliva for assessing endocrine function. *Endocrine Reviews,* 3 (4), 367-395.

[123] Rinaldi, S., Geay, A., Dechauld, H., Biessy, C., Zeleniuch-Jacquotte, A., Kaaks, R. (2002). Validity of free testostereone and free estradiol determinations in serum samples from postmenopausal women by theoretical calculations. *Cancer Epidemiol Biomerkers Prev*, 11: 1065-1071.

[124] Rock, C.L., Flatt, S.W., Thomson, C.A., Stefanick, M.L., Newman, V.A. et al. (2004). Effects of a High-Fiber, Low-Fat Diet Intervention on Serum Concentrations of Reproductive Steroid Hormones in Women With a History of Breast Cancer. *J Clin Oncology*, 22: 2379-2387

[125] Rosner, W. (2001). An extraordinarily inaccurate assay for free testosterone is still with us [Letter]. *Journal of Clinical Endocrinology and Metabolism*, 86 (6), 2903.

[126] Ruutiainen, K., Sannikka, E., Santti, R., Erkkola, R., & Adlercreutz, H. (1987). Salivary testosterone in hirsutism: Correlation with serum testosterone and the degree of hair growth. *J Clin Endocrinol Metab*, 64: 1015-1020.

[127] Sands, R. & Studd, J. (1995). Exogenous androgens in postmenopausal women. *Am J Med*. 98: 76-79.

[128] Sarrel, P.M. (1998). Cardiovascular aspects of androgens in women. *Semin Reprod Endocrinol*, 16: 121-128.

[129] Schurmeyer, T., & Nieschlag, E. (1982). Salivary and serum testosterone under physiological and pharmacological conditions. In: Read GF, Riad-Fahmy D, Walker RF, Griffiths K, editors.

[130] *Immunoassays of steroids in saliva*. Cardiff, Wales: Alpha Omega; 1982. pp 202–209.

[131] Schwartz, E.B., et al. (1998). Assessing salivary cortisol in studies of child development. *Child Development*. 69 (6): 1503–1513.

[132] Schwartz, E.B., & Granger, D.A. (2004). transferrin enzyme immunoassay for quatitative monitoring of blood contamination in saliva. *Clinical Chemistry*. 50: 654-656.

[133] Sellers, J.G., Mehl, M.R. & Josephs, R.A. (2007). Hormones and personality: Testosterone as a marker of individual differences. *Journal of Research in Personality*. 41 (1): 126-138.

[134] Shakil, T., Ehsanul hoque, A.N., Husain, M., & Belsham, D.D. (2002). Differential regulation of gonadotropin releasing hormone secretion and gene expression by androgens: membrane versus nuclear receptor activation. *Mol Endocrinol*, 16: 2592-2602

[135] Sharp, M.A. & Al-Dujaili, E.A.S. (2004). Application of testosterone ELISA for female salivary samples: Circadian rhythm studies. *Proceeding of American Endocrine Society's 86th Annual Meeting*, June, pp 539.

[136] Sharp, M.A. & Al-Dujaili, E.A.S. (2010). A Biological Basis for Status Competition in Human Females. Society for Behavioral Neuroendocrinology, Toronto, Canada.

[137] Shibayama Y, Higashi T, Shimada K, Odani A et al. (2009) Simultaneous determination of salivarytestosterone and dehydroepiandrosterone using LC–MS/MS: Method

development and evaluation of applicability for diagnosis and medication for late-onset hypogonadism Journal of Chromatography B 877: 2615–2623

[138] Shirtcliff, E.A., Granger, D.A., Schwartz, E., & Curran, M.J. (2001). Use of salivary biomarkers in biobehavioral research: Cotton based sample collection methods can interfere with salivary immunoassay results. *Psychoneuroendocrinology*, 26:165-173

[139] Shirtcliff, E.A., Granger, D.A., & Likos, A. (2002). Gender differences in the validity of testosterone measured in saliva by immunoassay. *Hormon Behav.*, 42: 62-69.

[140] Simpson, R.E. (2002). Aromatisation of androgens in women: Current concepts and findings. *Fertility and Sterility*, 77 (4), Suppl. 4, S6-S10.

[141] Sinha-Hikim, I., Arver, S., Beall, G., Shen, R. et al., (1998). The use of a sensitive equilibrium dialysis method for the measurement of free testosterone levels in healthy, cycling women and in the human immunodeficiency virus infected women. *Journal of Clinical Endocrinology and Metabolism*, 83 (4), 1312-1318.

[142] Slemend, C., Longcope, C., Peacock, M., et al. (1996), Sex steroids, bone mass and bone loss. Aprospective study of pre- and postmenopausal women. *J Clin Invest*, 97: 14-21.

[143] Snyder, P.J. (2001) Editorial: the role of androgens in women. *J Clin Endocrinol Metab*, 86: 1006-1007.

[144] Somboonporn W, Bell R, Davis S. (2010) Testosterone for peri- and postmenopausal women. In: The Cochrane Library, Issue 2, 2010. Chichester, UK: John Wiley & Sons, Ltd.

[145] Somboonporn, W., Davis, S., Seif, M.W., Bell, R. (2006). Testosterone for peri- and postmenopausal women. *Cochrane Database Syst Rev*:CD004509, The Cochrane Collaboration, John Wiley.

[146] Sowers MF, J. L. Beebe, D. McConnell, John Randolph, and M. Jannausch (2001) Testosterone Concentrations in Women Aged 25–50 Years: Associations with Lifestyle, Body Composition, and Ovarian Status. *Am J Epidemiol* 153: 256–264.

[147] Swinkels, L.M., van Hook, H.J., Ross, H.A., Smals, A.G., & Benraad, T.J. (1991). Concentrations of salivary testosterone and plasma total, non-sex-hormone-binding globulin-bound, and free testosterone in normal and hirsute women during administration of dexamethasone/synthetic corticotrophin. *Clin Chemistry*, 37: 180-185.

[148] Taieb, J., Benattar, C., Birr, A.S., & Lindenbaum, A. (2002). Limitations of Steroid Determination by Direct Immunoassay. *Clinical Chemistry*, 48, 583-585.

[149] Taieb, J., Mathian, B., Millot, F., et al. (2003). Testosterone measured by 10 immunoassays and by isotop-dilution gas chromatography-mass spectrometry in sera from 116 men, women and children. *Clinical Chemistry*, 49: 1381-1395.

[150] Teoh Y, Macintyre H, Ahmed F, Wallace M. (2005) Radioimmunoassay (RIA) method for Salivary Testosterone: Reference ranges in children, adult men and adult women. *Endocrine Abstracts* 9: P51

[151] Tremollieres, F., Pouilles, J.M., & Ribot, C. (1992). Postmenopausal bone loss. Role of progesterone and androgens. *Presse Med*, 21: 989-993.

[152] Ullis, K., Ptacek, G., & Shackman, J. (1999). *SuperT*, New York: Fireside Books a division of Simon and Schuster.

[153] Veldhuis, J.D., King, J.C., Urban, R.J. et al. (1987). Operating characteristics of the male hypothalamo-pituitary-axis: Pulsatile release of testosterone and follicle-stimulating hormone and their temporal coupling with leutinizing hormone. *Journal of Clinical Endocrinology and Metabolism*, 65, 929-841.

[154] Vermeulen, A., Verdonck, L., & Kaufman, J.M. (1999). A critical evaluation of simple methods for the estimation of free testosterone in serum. *Journal of Clinical Endocrinology and Metabolism*, 84 (10), 3666-3672.

[155] Vermeulen, A. & Verdonck, L. (1976). Plasma androgen levels during the menstrual cycle. *American Journal of Obstetrics and Gynaecology*, 125 (4), 491-494.

[156] Vermeulen, A. (1998). Plasma androgens in women. *Journal of Reproductive Medicine*, 43, 725-733.

[157] Vliet, E.L., & Davis, V.L. (1991). New prospectives on the relationship of hormone changes to affective disorders in the perimenopause. *Clin Issu Perinat Women's Health Nurse*, 2: 453-471.

[158] Vittek, J., L'Hommedieu, D.G., Gordon, G.G., Rappaport, S.C., & Southren, A.L. (1985). Direct radioimmunoassay of salivary testosterone: correlation with free and total serum testosterone. *Life Sci.*, 37: 711-716.

[159] Wang, C., Catlin, D.H., Starcevic, B. et al. (2005). Low-fat high-fibre diet decreased serum and urine androgens in men. *J Clin. Endocrinol Metab.*, 90 (6): 3550-3559.

[160] Wellen JJ, Smals AG, Rijken JC, Kloppenborg PW, Benraad TJ. (1983) Testosterone and delta 4-androstenedione in the saliva of patients with Klinefelter's syndrome. Clin Endocrinol (Oxf). 18(1): 51-59.

[161] Whembolua, G.S., Granger, D.A., Singer, S., Kivlighan, K.T., & Marguin, J.A. (2006). Bacteria in the oral mucosa and its effects on the measurement of cortisol, dehydroepiandrosterone and testosterone in saliva. *Hormones and Behvaior*, 49, 478-483.

[162] White, C.M., Ferraro-Borgida, M.J., Moyna, N.M., McGill, C.C., et al. (1998). The pharmacokinetics of intravenous testosterone in elderly men with coronary artery disease. *J Clin Pharmacol.* 38(9):792-797.

[163] Writing Group for the Women's Health Initiative Investigators. (2002). Risks and Benefits of Estrogen Plus Progestin in Healthy Postmenopausal Women: Principal

Results From the Women's Health Initiative Randomized Controlled Trial. *JAMA*, 288:321-333.

[164] Zitmann, M. & Nieschlag, E. (2001). Testosterone levels in healthy men and the relation to behavioural and physical characteristics: facts and constructs. *European Journal of Endocrinology*, 144, 183-197.

[165] Zumoff, B., Strain, G.W., Miller, L.K., & Rosner, W. (1995). Twenty four hour mean plasma testosterone declines with age in normal premenopausal women. *J Clin Endocrinol Metab*, 80: 1429-1430.

Chapter 7

Limits of Anabolic Steroids Application in Sport and Exercise

Marko D. Stojanovic and Sergej M. Ostojic

Additional information is available at the end of the chapter

http://dx.doi.org/10.5772/53015

1. Introduction

Androgens are the group of hormones that promotes the development and maintanance of male sex characteristics and are largely responsible for the developmental changes that occur during puberty and adolescence. The most important androgen secreted is testosterone. It is both an active hormone and a prohormone for the formation of a more active androgen, the 5a-reduced steroid dihydrotestosterone (DHT), which acts in the cell nucleus of target tissues, such as skin, male accessory glands, and the prostate, exerting predominantly androgenic, but also anabolic, effects. [75]. Testosterone is 19-carbon steroid formed from cholesterol via a series of enzimatic reactions in the Leydig cells of the testes and adrenal cortex in men, while in woman the primary site is the adrenal cortex [33]. Testosterone secretion is under the control of luteinizing hormone (LH) which is produced by the pituitary gland. Synthesis and release of LH is under control of the hypothalamus through gonadotropin-releasing hormone (GnRH) and inhibited by testosterone via a negative feedback mechanism [43]. Testosterone basic structure is composed of 3 cyclohexane rings and 1 cyclopentane ring with a methyl group at positions 10 and 13 [67]. Healthy men produce approximately 4.0–9.0 mg of testosterone per day with blood concentrations ranging from 300 to 1,000 ng/dL-1 (10.4–34.7 nmol/L-1), while blood concentrations for females range from 15 to 65 ng/dL -1 (0.5–2.3 nmol/L-1) [43]. Testosterone is carried to target cells through the bloodstream either free (only about 1–3% of circulating testosterone) or bound to a carrier protein. Most of the circulating testosterone (~50–60%) is bound with high affinity to sex hormone-binding globulin (SHBG), while a smaller fraction (40–50%) is bound loosely to albumin [49]. After reaching target cell, testosterone passes the membrane by simple diffusion becouse of its small molecular weight and liphophilic nature, [8]. Once entering the cell, the effects of testosterone in males and females occur by the way of two main mechanisms: genomic action by activation of the androgen receptor (directly or as DHT - 5 alpha dihydrotestosterone), and nongenomic action by conversion to estradiol and activation of certain estrogen receptors [19]. In u nutshell, the binding of the testosterone to its receptor produces conformational changes that result in the formation of a "transformed" or activated receptor with high affinity for specific DNA-binding site. This consequently recruits co-activators or co- repressors of gene expression [4]. Several non-genomic mechanisms appear to be involved regarding testosterone, including mediation by the membrane-bound sex hormone-binding globulin receptor and also a putative G-protein-coupled receptor that androgens directly bind with, as well as through stimulation of nonreceptor tyrosine kinase c-SRC. In adittion, testosterone administration has been shown to rapidly increase intramuscular calcium and extracellular signal–regulated kinase 1/2 (ERK 1/2) phosphorylation, involved in muscle hypertrophy [26]. Testosterone is metabolically inactivated in the liver and excreted in urine thru conjugation reactions, act to couple the anabolic steroid or its metabolite with glucuronic acid or sulfate [65].

Testosterone effects on body tissue are far more complicated than its production and secretion, directly or indirectly through its metabolites influencing the development and function of practicaly every organ in the body [51, 52]. Its complex biological actions regulates the development of the male phenotype, secondary sexual characteristics that transforms boys into men during embryonic life and at puberty respectively and regulates many physiological processes in the adult male including protein metabolism, sexual and cognitive functions, erythropoesis, plasma lipids and bone metabolism [11, 74]. In general, testosterone has masculinizing (growth of the male reproductive tract and development of secondary sexual characteristics) and anabolic effects (nitrogen fixation and increased protein synthesis with consequent increase in sceletal muscle mass and strength). Anabolism is defined as any state in which nitrogen is differentially retained in lean body mass through the stimulation of protein synthesis and/or a reduction in protein breakdown [54].

Medical interest in testosterone started in the mid-1930s after the chemical structure was published, and was largely based on its anabolical effect. Shortly after its synthesis, oral and injectable testosterone preparations become available to the medical community [77], with early studies mainly exploring its effects for treating hypogonadism and impotency [43]. However, it has been shown early that testosterone itself is relatively ineffective when taken orally or injected in an aqueous solution because it is susceptible to relatively rapid breakdown by the liver before it can act on the target organ. About 90% of the hormone is already metabolized before it reaches the bloodstream. Testosterone has a short free-circulating half-life due to its rapid metabolism by the cytochrome P450 family of hepatic isoenzymes [3]. In adittion, it has a therapeutic index of 1 meaning there is similarity in the proportion between the anabolic and androgenic effects. Consequently, the chemical structure of testosterone has been modified to cirkumvent this problem. It should be noted, however, that no synthetic steroid has completely eliminated the androgenic effect, which is partly due to the fact that the androgenic and anabolic effects differ only in location and not in the mechanism of the steroid hormone action. Since its discovery, numerous derivatives of testosterone have been synthesized, in order to delay the degradation of steroids, to maintain blood levels of

http://dx.doi.org/10.5772/53015

the drug for prolonged time periods, to intensify the overall effects of the compound while limiting androgenic effects and overpower the catabolic pathways by supplying the drug in mass quantity. Slight biochemical modifications has been proved to alter biological activity by modifying presystemic metabolism, half-life, AR binding affinity, AR stabilization, coactivator recruitment, nuclear translocation, DNA binding affinity, and tissue selectivity. One of the first changes made to the testosterone molecule was the addition of a methyl or ethyl group to the 17-alpha- carbon position (called alkylation), which inhibits the presystemic metabolism of the molecule, substantialy extending its half-life and making it active when administered orally [43]. Beyond alkylation, one more major modifications can be destuinguished, esterification of testosterone and nortestosterone at the 17-beta- position makes the molecule more soluble in lipid vehicles used for injection and slows the release of the injected steroid into the circulation [6]. Those synthetic compounds, which are similar in chemical structure to testosterone, are collectively called anabolic steroids.

The effect of testosterone and its derivatives on muscle mass gains has not been lost on the medical community. The therapeutic importance of anabolic steroids in treatment of catabolic conditions was recognized as early as in the 1950s, after which an enormous number of steroids were synthesized and tested for potency. For example, metandienone and stanozolol, two of the most frequently used anabolic steroids, were synthesized in 1955 and 1959, respectively [65]. Today, there are more than 100 varieties of anabolic steroids that have been developed, but only a limited number have been approved for human use. The common anabolic steroids are shown in Table 1.

Oral Agents **17- alpha-alkyl derivatives**	**Injectable Agents** **17 beta-ester derivatives**
Methandrostenolone (dianabol)	Testosterone esters: blend, cypionate, enanthate, heptylate, propionate
Methyltestosterone (android)	Nandrolone esters: decanoate (deca-durabolin) , phenpropionate
Oxandrolone (anavar)	Boldenone
Oxymetholone (anadrol)	Methenolone
Stanozolol (winstrol)	Trenbolone
Fluoxymesterone (halotestin)	Stanozolol
Danazol	Dromostanolone
Ethylestrenol (maxibolin, oraboline)	

Table 1. Anabolic Steroids in Common Use

As can be seen in Table 1., there are two major classes of AS used, based on the route of administration: Oral and parenteral AS preparations. Oral preparations are synthesized in order to offer protection to the molecule when it becomes exposed to the strong acid solutions found in the stomach, and when it contacts the enzymic mechanisms of the liver. Protection is conferred by the substitution of a methyl (CH3) or ethyl (C2H5) group for the H attached to the carbon atom (C) on the cyclopentane ring structure, in position 17. The 17α-alkylated steroids prevent deactivation by the first-pass metabolism by sterically hindering oxidation of the 17β-hydroxyl group. The effectiveness of 17- alkylated AS is due to a slower hepatic inactivation that occurs with unmodified hormone. Oral activity can also be obtained thru attachment of a methyl group at C-1, but these anabolic steroids are considered to be relatively weak in pharmacological activity. Oral preparations are proved to have a short half-life so, in order to maintain the appropriate blood concentration the drug must be taken several times a day. Parenteral preparations do not require a 17a- alkyl group, but the 17p-hydroxyl group is esterified with an acid moiety to prevent rapid absorption from the oily vehicle. Once an AS-ester hits the bloodstream, enzymes called esterases rapidly split off the fatty acid. A long fatty acid makes the AS more lipid-soluble and it will disperse from the injected oil depot more slowly (days to weeks). The duration of action of the parenteral steroids depends upon the chain length of the acid moiety and the formulation, with general tendency that the longer the chain length, the more slowly the preparation is released into circulation. Generaly, parenteral AS dosing require intramuscular dosing once every 2 to 12 weeks, depending on the carboxylic acid groups added [9].

Pharmaceutical companies initially developed these synthetic analogues of testosterone in order to treat catabolic medical conditions. A number of clinical studies have shown that the potent anabolic effects of anabolic steroids could be used to: restore hormone levels in hypogonadal men, thereby increasing fat-free mass, muscle size and strength, and bone density; improve mood and alleviate depression; increase body weight, muscle mass, and strength in eugonadal patients with secondary wasting syndromes, such as infection with HIV when maintaining lean body mass may be beneficial for long-term survival; and augment muscle mass in older men and prevent age-related sarcopenia that contributes to frailty and falls [28]. The anabolic activity of testosterone derivatives is primarily manifested in its myotrophic action, which results in greater muscle mass and increased strength. This, in adittion to the stimulatory effects of androgens on the brain, which frequently result in a feeling of euphoria, increased aggressive behavior, and diminished fatigue, has led to the widespread use of anabolic steroids by both profesionnal and recreational athletes. Athletes use them to enhance performance, driven by the potential financial and other rewards that may come with sporting success. In adittion, recreational users of anabolic steroids are the most rapidly growing group, and their aim is to combat ageing and obesity as well as to improve physical appearance in order to receive the admiration that modern society give to a 'perfectly toned' body. However, anabolic steroids have been associated with a range of transient side effects, which can be divided into several categories, including cardiovascular, hepatic, endocrine/reproductive, behavioral, dermatologic, and injection related. Data from larger observational studies suggest that the majority (88%-96%) of anabolic steroid users experience at least 1 minor subjective side effect [14]. Studies on the benefits and risks of testosterone are ongoing, but seem to consistently produce mixed results. As therapeutical use becomes more common, its controversy in the sports world has lead to considerable public outcry against its use. In this chapter we will considers available data on anabolic steroid application in sport & exercise with special attention on three distinct aspects of AS usage by professional and recreational atheletes: effects on sport performance, adverse effects and legislative considering its usage.

2. Anabolic steroids and sport performance

Soon after the development of synthetic steroids, these drugs were discovered by athletes for their muscle building and performance enhancing properties. According to anecdotal reports, it has been rumored, but never documented, that some German athletes were given testosterone in preparation for the 1936 Berlin Olympics. West Coast bodybuilders began experimenting with testosterone preparations in the late 1940s and early 1950s. It appears that the use of testosterone and its synthetic derivatives began to infiltrate sports during the 1950s, with even government instituted-top secret program implementation that provided for the administration of androgens and other doping products to male and female athletes during later period [43]. In the early 1950s, the first suspicion that anabolic steroids were actualy administered in order to improve sporting performance came with allegation that soviet weightlifters were adminestering AS to gain strength [71] News of the efficacy of these drugs apparently spread during the early 1960s to other strength-intensive sports, from the throwing events of track and field to football. Throughout the 1960s, the use of anabolic steroids increased so dramatically that In 1969 John Hendershott, the editor of Track & Field News, called these drugs the "breakfast of champions" [40]. Although the International Olympic Committee banned use of anabolic agents in 1964, the practice spread and probably reached its pinnacle in the athletic programs in Germany during the 1970s [78]. Their use nowdays is most common among weight lifters and heavy throwers, nevertheless almost all types of athletes whose event requires explosive strength, in- cluding football players, swimmers and track and field athletes, have been known to use steroids. The level of steroid use appears to have increased significantly over the past three decades [46], and is no longer limited to elite athletes or to men. Although competitive athletes report higher rates of steroid use, a significant number of recreational athletes and non-athletes appear to be using these drugs, probably to "improve" their appearance.

The effects of testosterone and its derivatives on human performance have been extensively studied. As early as 1889, Brown- Sequard, reported increases in muscular strength, mental abilities, and appetite as a qonsequence of self-injections of testicular extracts from guinea pigs and dogs [22]. Largely based on this work, two of the Austrian physiologist Oskar Zoth and Fritz Pregl began to investigates the effects of injections of testicular extracts on muscle strength and athletic performance [42]. Zoth and Pregl injected themselves with extracts from bull testicles and reported increased strength of their middle fingers. Although it is likely that these results were placebo effects, Zoth may be the first person to suggest injecting steroids in an attempt to increase performance [41].

Since the 1960s many researchers have investigated performance-enhancing effects of anabolic steroid administration in professional and recreational athletes. The strength gains and other purported performance-enhancing benefits commonly attributed to anabolic steroid use in professional and recreational athletes were challenged and often discounted by early medical studies. Upon further examination of initial studies it become apparent that most of them had major flaws in design, such as lack of control groups and a double-blind procedure, the presence of confounding factors (e.g., differences in level of exercise and in motivation), and inappropriate statistical techniques [12, 34]. In adittion, most of them have used steroid doses 5–20 times lower than those used by many athletes. As it has been proved that anabolic steroid administration increases lean body mass, muscle mass, and maximal voluntary strength in a concentration-dependent manner [13], it is no surprise that early investigations were usually unable to determine any substantiall effect of AS administration on human performance..

Considerable amount of researh investigating ergogenic effects of anabolic steroid administration were conducted before and during 1980s, with conflicting findings presented. Several studies did not report ergogenic effects of anabolic steroids on muscle strength or performance. Fowler and coworkers [31] examined the intake of 20 mg/day for 16 weeks of methyl androstenolone acetate to 47 men (10 rugby players and 37 untrained students) who either did not exercise or exercised 30 min/day, 5 days a week and reported no significant difference between groups in muscle size, body weight, or isometric strength. Weiss and Muller [72] examined the intake of 10 mg of Metandienone for 17 days in 32 high school students and did not report any enhancment of strength measured during arm extension. Casner and coworkers [18] examined the intake of 6 mg/days of Stanozolol in 27 young man conducting the weight training 3 d/wk and reported no ergogenic effects of anabolic steroid on leg, arm and trunk isometric strength. Golding and coworkers [35] administered 1o mg/day of Metandienone in three consecutive 4-week cycles interpersed with 1 week of no adminitration in 40 experienced weightlifters and reported no significant improvements in strength parameters. Stromme and coworkers [67] examined the intake 75 mg/day of mesterolone for 4 weeks and 150 mg/day for the subsequent 4-week period in 21 students engaged in weight training sessions and reported that anabolic steroids did not enhanced strength parameters measured during different flexion and extension exercises. Crist and coworkers [21] administered 100 mg/week of testosterone cipionate or placebo (3 weeks each) and reported no significant difference was observed in several isokinetic flexion/extension exercises between anabolic steroid and placebo conditions. Loughton and Ruhling [55] examined the intake of 10 mg/day of Metandienone for 3 weeks and 5 mg/day for 3 more weeks concomitant with weight training and running program and reported greater weight gains in the androgen group but nonsignificant interactions in strength performance.

Considerable amount of research during this period did report significant ergogenic effects of anabolic steroid administartion in professional or recreational athletes. Johnson and O'Shea [45] examined administration of 10 mg/day of Matandienone during the last 3 weeks of 6 week training programme to half of the 24 subjects. They reported reported significantly greater gains in isometric strength and 1 repetition maximum (1RM) squat in the steroid group. Next year, O'Shea and Winkler [60] reported enhanced muscle strength after 6 weeks of strength training with concomitant use of 10mg/day of Oxandrolone in well-trained weightlifters. Finaly, O'Shea [61] administered 10 mg/day of Dianabol for 4 weeks to half of the sample consisted of 18 weightlifters and reported significantlly higher increase in squat and bench press strength in the steroid group. Several other authors reported similar results obtained on the sample of professional or recreational athletes administering Metandienone in the same quantity as O'Shea in previously mentioned study with a similar duration of studies [15, 44, 12]. Moreover, although most research has focused on absolute strength determined by one repetition maximum or isokinetic strength, one study tested the effects of anabolic steroid use on sport performance. Rademacher and coworkers.[64] reported that in male canoeists, 6 weeks of Oral-Turinabol administration improved strength and performance measured by canoe ergometry with 6% and 9%, respectively.

Although study designs improved during 1970s and 1980s and in some cases were more realistic than previously, it could be speculated that the first rigorous study of the performance-enhancing effects of anabolic steroids was not carried out until 1996. In this seminal study by Bhasin and coworkers [11] supraphysiological dosages of anabolic steroid (testosterone enenthate- 600mg/week) were administered to forthy eugonadal men between 19 and 40 years old (within 15% of their ideal body weight) who were or were not engaged in strength training programme. Subjects sample was randomly assigned to one of four groups: placebo but no exercise; testosterone but no exercise; placebo plus exercise; testosterone plus exer- cise. The subjects who were administered both anabolic steroid and strength training were found to gained significantly greater muscle mass (+6 kg), fat free mass (6,1 kg), quadriceps and biceps area (+1174 mm2 and +501mm2, respectively) as well as 1-RM bench and press squats (+22kg and +38 kg, respectively) when compared to other groups. Moreover, injectable steroid has been shown to improve strength even without a concomitant resistance-training programme! The investigation suggests that supraphysiological doses of anabolic steroids stimulate significant alterations in muscle size and muscle strength, especially when taken in conjunction with a progresive resistance training programm. Several other studies during and after this period further examined anabolic steroid use in professional or recreational athletes, with continuous reports that anabolic steroid users had greater mass than nonusers and that longitudinally anabolic steroids increased lean body mass, muscle strength and performance. Subsequent work showed that increases in fat-free mass, muscle size, and strength are highly dose-dependent and correlated with serum testosterone concentrations [12, 76] It has been shown that improvements in body physique were greatest at higher doses, for example, at least 125 mg/week1 [43]. It appears that the most common benefit of anabolic steroid use is an increase in muscle mass and/or strength. It also appears that this effect may demonstrate a dose-response relationship, i.e. the more anabolic steroid used, the greater the effect on muscle mass and strength [13]. However, higher dosages are correlated with higher incidence of adverse effects of anabolic steroid use in humans, which we will discuss further in the next section.

Information on doses and modes of administration of AS used by athletes to increase their performance is relatively sparse. It is known that steroid regimens favored by professional and recreational athletes differ markedly from those used clinically. Athletes use suprapharmacological doses that range from 10–100-fold above normal levels [75]. Steroids are usually used in the off-season, when athletes are strength trained and when use is least likely to be detected. Typically, they take androgens in cycles of 4-12 weeks, with a period of abstinence, knowns as a "drug-free holiday" period of varying duration. The purpose for the holiday is to minimize side effects, promote recuperation of various hormonal systems, and avoid detection during competition. Although the length of each cycle is quite variable (ranges from 1 to 728 weeks), the median cycle length is reported to be 11 weeks [43]. After this period, athletes often reported a plateau in subjective benefits, which might be explained by steroid receptor saturation and downregulation. In adittion, most athletes use "stacking" regimens that involve taking multiple agents simultaneously, and/or a pyramid their doses in cycles of 6 to 12 weeks. At the beginning of a cycle, one starts with low doses of the drugs being stacked and then slowly increases the doses. In the second half of the cycle, the doses are slowly decreased to zero. Athletes tend to use both oral and parenteral (injectable) compounds, with typical regimen of 3 agents being reported [43].

3. Adverse effects of anabolic steroids

For clinical purposes, the administration of anabolic steroids can be of therapeutic benefit and reasonably safe. By contrast, for the purposes of enhancing performance in sport or for cosmetic purposes, usually because it is a clandestine activity, the athletes and bodybuilders are making subjective decisions regarding the effect these steroids are having on their health. The incidence of complications associated with the nonmedical use of anabolic steroids as performance-enhancing drugs is unclear because the denominator of drug use in athletes is not well defined. Data from larger observational studies [27] suggest that the majority (88%-96%) of anabolic steroid users experience at least 1 subjective side effect. Since anabolic steroids have effects on several organ systems, a myard of side effects can be found. Consequently, the undesirable effects arising from anabolic steroid administration have been extensively studied and reviewed [37, 66, 50]. Hovewer, it should be recognized that giving super high doses of anabolic steroids to induce side effects for ethical reasons cannot be studied in laboratory settings, with data defining cumulative effects caused by stacking remains speculative and derived from case reports and medical literature from lower level doses. Nevertheless, summarising the literature, it can be concluded that the potential adverse effects of anabolic steroid use can be divided into several categories, including cardiovascular, hepatic, endocrine/reproductive, psychological, musculoskeletal and dermatologic related.

In both the medical and lay literature one of the principal adverse effects generally associated with anabolic steroid use is the increased risk for myocardial infarction. Several case reports document myocardial infarction and stroke in 20- to 30-year-old weightlifters that used anabolic steroids, which can be attributed to the increased platelet count and platelet aggregation that occurs in people who abuse anabolic steroids [30]. Steroids also cause hypertrophy of the myocardium, which also increases the likelihood of arrhythmias, sudden death, systolic and diastolic hypertension [44]. Anabolic steroid abuse cause harmfull changes in lipoprotein profile with increased LDL levels (by 40-50%) and decreased HDL level (40-70%). The decline in HDL are most evident with the use of oral administration anabolic steroids with drugs such as stanazolol, oxymetholone and metandienone and can often be seen in a few days after the initiation of anabolic steroid use [70]. High doses of AS may increase the risk of atherosclerosis and thrombosis through their effects on clotting factors and platelets and induce vasospasm or myocardial injury because of effects on myocardial cells [56]. Finaly, high dose AS use is found to induce systemic hypertension, with magnitude and incidence of hypertension likely related to dosage and to the type of AS used [17]

Cardiovascular	Myocardial infarction; Myocardium hypertrophy; Increased LDL and decreased HDL levels; Thrombosis; Elevated blood pressure
Hepatic	Increased risk of liver tumors and liver damage
Endocrine/reproductive	**Male**: Testicular atrophy; Oligospermia; Gynecomastia; Prostatic hypertrophy **Female**: Alterations of pubic hair growth, Clitoral hypertrophy, Menstrual irregularities; Breast atrophy
Psychological	Mood swings; Aggressive behavior; Depression; Psychosis
Musculoskeletal	Increased risk of musculotendious injuries
Dermatological	Acne; Alopecia

Table 2. Adverse effects of anabolic steroid use.

Liver function disturbances and diseases in AS-abusing athletes have been of great concern since animal studies have clearly shown the deleterious effects of AS on the liver. In adittion, liver cancer occurrence in non-athletic populations being treated with testosterone for aplastic anemia has been reported [58]. Elevations in levels of liver enzymes (aspartate aminotransferase, alanine aminotransferase, and lactate dehydrogenase) are regularly reported in athletes who use steroids. Several case reports have associated the occurrence of liver disorders such as subcellular changes of hepatocytes, impaired excretion function, cholestasis, peliosis hepatis and hepatocellular hyperplasia, and carcinomas in with the abuse of AS in young, healthy athletes. Hepatic dysfunction is most commonly associated with the 17-alpha alkylated steroids, with no cysts or tumors have been reported in athletes using 17β-alkylated steroids. Thus, evidence appears to indicate that the risk for hepatic disease from anabolic steroid use may not be as high as the medical community had originally thought although a risk does exist especially with oral anabolic steroid use or abuse.

Use of steroids in men decreases levels of luteinizing hormone and follicle-stimulating hormones, which leads to decreased endogenous testosterone production, decreased spermatogenesis, and testicular atrophy. The testicular atrophy and the oligospermia usually resolve after discontinuation of the drugs, but the count and morphology of the sperm may be abnormal for up to 6 months [23]. Prostatic hypertrophy, priapism, and, rarely, carcinoma of the prostate can be associated with steroid use [72]. When AS levels are elevated, they undergo aromatization, being converted to estrogens and qonsequently can produce (i)reversible gynecomastia. Use of anabolic steroids in women, is not only associated with menstrual abnormalities but with masculinizing effects as well. Female athletes reported the development of acne vulgaris, changes in libido and alterations of the voice as the most pronounced acute effects, with long-term AS administration proved to induce loss of hair, alterations of pubic hair growth, clitoral hypertrophy, menstrual irregularities and a reduction of the breasts [43].

Hystoricaly, low doses of AS have been used to treat depression and melancholia either as monotherapy or as adjunct to standard treatment, but misuse of these agents has added a new term to the drug lexicon "roids rage" Anecdotal reports of ''roid rage,'' have attracted a great deal of attention in scientific community. Pope and Katz [63] noted that anabolic steroids produce clear psychiatric effects, particularly in individuals using excessive doses (more than 1,000 mg/wk) of these compounds and stacking the drugs. Some individuals may experience mental status and behavioral changes with anabolic steroid use iincluding irritability, aggressivity, euphoria, grandiose beliefs, hyperactivity, and reckless or dangerous behavior [20]. Other presentations have included the development of acute psychoses, exacerbation of tics, and the development of acute confusional states [38]. Kouri and coworkers [53] reported that administration of supraphysiological doses (600 mg weekly) of testosterone enanthate to healthy young men was associated with a significant increase in aggressive responses than placebo administration. A high proportion of women athletes using high doses of androgens report symptoms of hypomania and depression, rigid dietary practices, and dissatisfaction and preoccupation with their physique [36].

Some scientists believe that there is an increased risk of musculotendious injuries with steroid use in humans. It has been speculated that tendons may not increase in strength as muscles do and, when subject to increased intensity and frequency of training, may be at higher risk for rupture [7, 66]. However, although the studies in mices and rats have suggested that anabolic steroids may lead to degeneration of collagen and/or decrease in collagen synthesis [48, 57], the response in humans has been less clear. Ultrastructural analysis on ruptured tendons from anabolic steroid users have shown that anabolic steroids did not induce any ultrastructural collagen changes that would increase the risk of tendon ruptures [29].

Acne is one of the more common side effects associated with anabolic steroid administration, and it is a result of the androgenic stimulation of the sebaceous glands. One study reported that 43% of users experienced acne as a consequence from androgen use [62]. They appear to disappear upon cessation of anabolic steroids administration. Finaly, temporal hair recession and alopecia can be seen in men and women using anabolic steroids for extended periods of time.

Summarising the literature, it can be concluded that anabolic steroid users and potential users should be aware that many of the adverse effects of anabolic steroids are present and may exert profound effects on their health. More so, studies have been able to link anabolic steroids to many of the serious adverse effects listed. It would seems logical that the axiom, particularly among professional and recreational athletes who can use excessively large amounts of steroids, that the 'more you take, the more you grow' should be accompanied with 'the more you may damage your health'.

4. Anabolic steroids and doping regulations

The use of substances to enhance performance in sports is a long standing phenomenon. In 1928, the International Amateur Athletics Federation (IAAF), became the first International Sport Federation to ban the use of stimulating substances. Many other federations followed suit, but restrictions remained ineffective because no tests were made. Meanwhile the problem was made worse by synthetic substances developed in the 1930s and in growing use for doping purposes by the 1950s. The death of a Danish cyclist at the 1960 Olympic Games in Rome put pressure on sports authorities to work more aggressively to deter doping following the confirmation of amphetamine in biologic fluids collected at autopsy on this athlete [32]. The death of cyclist Tom Simpson, during the Tour de France, following the use of amphethamines, further catalysed the situation and in 1966, the first doping tests were introduced for international cycling and football. With the increasing use of performance-enhancing drugs and several high-profile deaths of athletes from various sports, the International Olympic Committee (IOC) established a medical commission in 1967 with its primary goal to create a list of prohibited substances and methods [32]. The initial goal of putting in place an antidoping structure was rapidly widened to encompass the following three fundamental principles: (1) protection of the health of athletes, (2) respect for both medical and sports ethics, and (3) equality for all competing athletes. In the same year, the International Olympic Committee drew up its first list of prohibited substances, and drug tests were first introduced at the 1968 Olympic Games in Mexico. At that time, many sports governing bodies such as UCI (cycling) and FIFA (football) based in Europe established rules regarding the use of drugs in sports.

At the 1988 Olympic games in Seoul, Canadian sprinter and then current world's fastest man Ben Johnson tested positive for stanozonol [16]. This positive test sent shock waves through the sporting community, resulting in the U.S. government passing the Anti-Drug Abuse Act, which made it illegal to distribute or possess androgens. Additionally, the IOC expanded the banned substance list to include diuretics, such as probenecid, and other products typically used to mask androgens use. In 1990, the U.S. government went a step farther when it passed the first Anabolic Steroid Control Act and inserted 27 steroids, along with their muscle building salts, esters, and isomers as class III drugs and simple possession could result in prison time [43]. Today, under the US Federal Controlled Substances Act, anabolic steroids are classified as Schedule III substances, which places them in the same category as amphetamines, methamphetamines, opium and morphine. Possession of any Schedule I substance is a felony offense with punishment up to five years in prison. If one sells steroids, or possesses enough to evidence an intent to sell, he/she faces up to five years in prison and a $250,000 fine.

During a raid at 1988 Tour de France, police found a large number of prohibited medical substances. This highly publicized scandal highlighted the need for an independent international agency that would establish unified standards for antidoping work and coordinate the efforts of sports organizations and public au thorities. The IOC took the initiative and convened the World Conference on Doping in Sport held in Lausanne, Switzerland in February 1999. Following the proposal of the Conference, the World Anti-Doping Agency (WA-DA) was established on November 10, 1999.

According to surveys and media reports, the illegal use of AS to increase muscle size and strength is widespread [28]. Current estimates indicate that there are as many as three million AS users in the United States alone and that 2.7–2.9% of young American adults have taken AS at least once in their lives [59]. Interviews of high-school students in several European countries reveal that 1–5% have used AAS [69], with similar figures found for high-school-aged students from Canada, Australia and South Africa [5]. Anabolic steroids are used for performance enhancement across the spectrum of athletes, from the elite to rising young men and women in youth programs and high school. Increasing numbers of athletes are nowdays relying on anabolic steroids to enhance their strength, endurance, and performance, despite the knowledge of the potentially serious adverse consequences these agents can have. According to the WADA statistics, AS are the most frequent adverse analytical findings for Olympic sport athletes, in-and out-of- competition. In 2003, the World-wide Out-of-Competition Testing Program conducted by the World Anti-Doping Agency detected 23 positive cases among a total of 5004 samples obtained (4229 urine, and 775 blood samples), with three refusals to provide a sample. The prevalence values for AS use among other groups of exercisers and athletes range between 6.2 and 38.4%. However, the reported response rates were at best 66%, rendering these findings highly unreliable [69]. In 2006, the 33 WADA accredited laboratories in 29 countries reported 1 966 (45.4%) of the 4 332 adverse analytical findings were anabolic steroids. It is likely that the AS use among athletes from high school to Olympics caliber is on the rise and gaining momentum, according to individuals closest to the issue [10].

Nowdays, many countries are on the way to strengthening the laws against possession and use of AS and now consider these drugs as equivalent to narcotics. An important concern is the ease with which banned substances can be obtained by athletes and the public. The results of studies by Eriksson [24,25] show the effect of AS on muscle fibres lasts much longer than believed, which suggests that athletes using anabolic agents should be disqualified for longer than 2 years. His histological observations is highly in accordance to an old observation in East Germany that "androgenic initiation" has long-lasting effects. Anabolic steroids are controlled substances and are illegal to possess or sell without a prescription for a legitimate medical condition by the prescribing physician. Androstenedione, norandrostenedione and other similar prohormones, at one time available over the counter as dietary supplements, are now defined as controlled anabolic steroids. Due to serious health risks, non-medical use of anabolic steroids is nowdays banned by most major sports organizations. International Olympic Comitee banned the use of anabolic steroids in 1976. In addition, anabolic steroids are on the WADA (World Anti-Doping Agency) prohibited list, the annual publication of all illegal performance-enhancing substances.

Acknowledgments

The chapter is dedicated to Z. Djindjic (1952-2003).

http://dx.doi.org/10.5772/53015

Author details

Marko D. Stojanovic[1,2] and Sergej M. Ostojic[1,2]

1 Center for Health, Exercise and Sport Sciences, Belgrade, Serbia

2 Faculty of Sport and Physical Education, University of Novi Sad, Serbia

References

[1] Ariel G. Residual effect of an anabolic steroid upon isotonic muscular force. Journal of Sports Medicine and Physical Fitness 1974; 14 103-11.

[2] Ariel G. The effect of anabolic steroid upon skeletal muscle contractile force. Journal of Sports Medicine and Physical Fitness 1973; 13 187-90.

[3] Bagatell CJ, Bremner WJ. Androgens in men: uses and abuses. N EngI J Med 1996; 334 707-714.

[4] Bagchi MK, Tsai MJ, O'Malley BW, Tsai SY. Analysis of the mechanism of steroid hormone receptor-dependent gene activation in cell-free systems. Endocrine Reviews 1992;13 525–35.

[5] Bahrke MS, Yesalis CE, Abuse of anabolic androgenic steroids and related substances in sport and exercise. Current Opinion in Pharmacology 2004; 4 614-620.

[6] Bartsch W. Anabolic steroids: action on cellular level. In: Kopera H, editor. Anabolic-androgenic steroids towards the year 2000. Vienna: Blackwell-MZV, 1993: 29-39.

[7] Battista V, Combs J, Warne WJ. Asynchronous bilateral Achilles tendon ruptures and androstenediol use. American Journal of Sports Medicine 2003: 31 1007–1009.

[8] Beato M, Klug J. Steroid hormone receptors: an update. Hum Reproduction Update. 2000; 6(3) 225-36.

[9] Behre HM, Nieschlag E. Testosterone buciclate (20 Aet-1) in hypogonadal men: pharmacokinetics and pharmacodynamics of the new longlasting androgen ester. J Clin Endocrinol Metab 1992;75 1204-1210.

[10] Berning, J.M., K.J. Adams, and B.A. Stamford. Anabolic steroid usage in athletics: facts, fiction, and public relations. J. Strength Cond. Res. 2004; 18(4) 908–17.

[11] Bhasin S, Storer TW, Berman N, et al. The effects of supraphysiological doses of testosterone on muscle size and strength in normal men. New England Journal of Medicine 1996;335 1-6.

[12] Bhasin S, Woodhouse L, Storer TW.. Proof of the effect of testosterone on skeletal muscle. J Endocrinol 2001;170 27–38.

[13] Bhasin S, Woodhouse L, Casaburi R, Singh AB, Bhasin D, Berrman N, Chen X, Yarasheski KE, Magliano L, Dzekov C, Dzekov J, Bross R, Phillips J, Sinha-Hikim I, Shen R, Storer TW. Testosterone dose-response relationships in healthy young men. American Jornal of Physiology- Endocrinology and Metabolism 2001; 281 E1172 – E1181,

[14] Bolding G, Sherr L, Elford J. Use of anabolic steroids and associated health risks among gay men attending London gyms. Addiction 2002; 97 195-201.

[15] Bowers RW, Reardon JP. Effects of methandrostenolone (Dianabol) on strength development and aerobic capacity [abstract]. Medicine and Science in sport& exercise 1972; 4: 54

[16] Carpenter PC. Performance-enhancing drugs in sport. Endocrinology and Metabolism Clinics of North America 2007; 36 481–495.

[17] Casavant MJ, Blake K, Griffith J, Yates A, Copley LM, Consequences of use of anabolic androgenic steroids. Pediatr Clin North Am 2007; 54 677–690.

[18] Casner SW, Early RG, Carlson BR. Anabolic steroid effects on body composition in normal young men. Journal of Sports Medicine and Physical Fitness 1971; 11 98–103.

[19] Christiansen K. Hormones and sport. Journal of Endocrinology 2001; 170, 39-48.

[20] Clark AS, Henderson LP. Behavioral and physiological responses to anabolic-androgenic steroids. Neuroscience& Biobehavioral Reviews 2003;27 413-436.

[21] Crist DM, Stackpole PJ, Peake GT. Effects of androgenic-nabolic steroids on neuromuscular power and body composiion. Journal of Applied Physiology 1983; 54 366-70.

[22] Dotson, JL and Brown, RT. The history of the development of anabolic-androgenic steroids. Pediatric Clinics of North America 2007; 54 761–769.

[23] Eklof AC, Thurelius AM, Garle M, Rane A, Sjoqvist F. The anti-doping hot-line, a means to capture the abuse of doping agents in the Swedish society and a new service function in clinical pharmacology. European Journal of Clinical Pharmacology. 2003; 59 571–577.

[24] Eriksson A, Kadi F, Malm C, Thornell LE. Skeletal muscle morphology in powerlifters with and without anabolic steroids. Histochemical and Cell Biology 2005; 124 167–75.

[25] Eriksson A. Strength training and anabolic steroids: a comparative study of the vastus lateralis, a thigh muscle and the trapezius, a shoulder muscle, of strength-trained athletes. PhD thesis, Umeå University, 2006.

[26] Estrada M, Espinosa A, Muller M, Jaimovich E. Testosterone stimulates intracellular calcium release and mitogen-activated protein kinases via a G protein-coupled receptor in skeletal muscle cells. Endocrinology 2003; 144 3586–3597.

[27] Evans NA. Gym & tonic: a profile of 100 male steroid users. British Journal of sports Medicine 1997;3154-58.

[28] Evans, NA. Current Concepts in Anabolic-Androgenic Steroids. The American Journal of Sports Medicine. 2004; 32 (2) 534-542.

[29] Evans NA, Bowrey DJ. Newman GR. Ultrastructural analysis of ruptured tendon from anabolic steroid users. Injury 1998; 29 769-773.

[30] Ferenchick G, Schwartz D, Ball M, Schwartz K. Androgenic-anabolic steroid abuse and platelet aggregation: a pilot study in weight lifters. The American Journal of Medical Sciences 1992;30378-82.

[31] Fowler WM, Gardner GW, Egstrom GH. Effect of an anabolic steroid on physical performance of young men. Journal of Applied Physiology 1965; 20 1038–1040.

[32] Fraser, AD. Doping control from a global and national perspective. Therapeutic Drug Monitoring 2004; 26 171–174.

[33] Friedl KE. Effects of Testosterone and Related Androgens on Athletic Performance in Men. In: The endrocrine System in Sports and Exercise. W.J. Kreamer and A.D Rogol, eds Malden, MA: Blackwell Publishing,2005. Pp 525-539.

[34] George AJ.. Androgenic anabolic steroids. In: Mottram DR, editor. Drugs in sport. 3rd Edition. London: Routledge 2003 p. 138–88.

[35] Golding LA, Freydinger JE, Fishel SS. Weight, size and strength: unchanged with steroids. Phys Sportsmed 1974; 2 39-43.

[36] Gruber AJ, Pope HG. Psychiatric and medical effects of anabolic-androgenic steroid use in women. Psychotherapy Psychosomatics 2000; 69 19–26.

[37] Hall RC, Hall RC. Abuse of supraphysiologic doses of anabolic steroids. Southern Medical Journal. 2005; 98(5) 550-5.

[38] Hartgens F, Kuipers H Effects of androgenic-anabolic steroids in athletes. Sports Medicine 2004;34 513-54.

[39] Haupt HA. Rovere GD. Anabolic sleroids: a review of the literature. American Journal of Sports Medicine 1984; 12 469-84.

[40] Hendershott J. Steroids: Breakfast of champions. Track and Field News 22: 3, 1969.

[41] Hoberman, J. Testosterone Dreams: Rejuvenation, Aphrodisia, Doping. Berkeley: University of California Press, 2005.

[42] Hoberman JM, Yesalis CE. The history of synthetic testosterone. Scientific American 1995 272 76–81.

[43] Hoffman, JR, Kraemer, WJ, Bhasin, S, Storer, T, Ratamess, NA, Haff, GG, Willoughby, DS, and Rogol, AD. Position stand on Androgen and human growth hormone use. J Strength Cond Res 2009; 23(5) S1–S59.

[44] Johnson LC, Fisher G, Silvester LJ, et al. Anabolic steroid: effects on strength, body weight, oxygen uptake and spermato- genesis upon mature males. Medicine and Science in Sports&exercise 1972; 4 43-5.

[45] Johnson LC, O'Shea JP. Anabolic steroid: Effects on strength development. Science 1969; 164 957–959.

[46] Johnston, L., Bachman, P., O'Malley, J., & Schulenberg, J.. Monitoring the Future: National Results on Adolescent Drug Use: Overview of Key Findings 2003. National Institute on Drug Abuse, U.S. Department of Health and Human Services. NIH Publication No. 04-5506, 2004.

[47] Karila TA, Karjalainen JE, Mantysaari MJ, et al. Anabolic androgenic steroids produce dose-dependent increase in left ventricular mass in power athletes, and this effect is potentiated by concomitant use of growth hormone. International Journal of Sports Medicine 2003;24337-343.

[48] Karpakka JA, Pesola MK, Takala TE. The effects of anabolic steroids on collagen synthesis in rat skeletal muscle and tendon. A preliminary report. American Journal of Sports Medicine 1992; 20 262-266.

[49] Kaufman JM, Vermeulen A (2005) The decline of androgen levels in elderly men and its clinical and therapeutic implications. Endocrinology Review 2005 26:833-876.

[50] Kicman AT, Gower DB. Anabolic steroids in sport: biochem- ical, clinical and analytical perspectives. Annals of Clinical Biochemistry 2003; 40 321–356.

[51] Kochakian CD. History, chemistry and pharmacodynamics of anabolic-androgenic steroids. Wien Med Wochenschr 1993;143 359-63.

[52] Kochakian CD. . Mechanisms of androgen action. Laboratory investigation 1959; 8 538-556.

[53] Kouri E, Lukas S, Pope H, Oliva P. 1995. Increased aggressive responding in male volunteers following the administration of gradually increasing doses of testosterone cypionate. Drug and Alcohol Dependance 1995; 40 73–79.

[54] Kuhn CM. Anabolic Steroids. Recent Progress in Hormone Research 2002;57 411- 434.

[55] Loughton SJ, Ruhling RO. Human strength and endurance responses to anabolic steroid and training. Journal of Sports Medicine& Physical Fitness 1977; 17 285-96.

[56] Melchert RB, Welder AA. Cardiovascular effects of androgenic-anabolic steroids. Medicine and Science in Sports& Exerc 1995; 27 1252–1262.

[57] Michna H. Organisation of collagen fibrils in tendon: changes induced by an anabolic steroid. I. Functional and ultrastructural studies. Virchows Archive B (Cell Pathology Including Molecular Pathology) 1986; 52, 75-86

[58] Nakao, A., Sakagami, K., Nakata, Y., Komazawa, K., Amimoto, T., Nakashima, K., Isozaki, H., Takakura, N. and Tanaka, N. Multiple hepatic adenomas caused by long-

term administration of androgenic steroids for aplastic anemia in association with familial adenomatous polyposis. Journal of Gastroenterology 2000; 35 557- 562.

[59] National Insitute on Drug Abuse (NIDA). About anabolic steroid abuse. NIDA Notes 15:15, 2000.

[60] O'Shea JP, Winkler W. Biochemical and physical effects of an anabolic steroid in competitive swimmers and weightlifters. Nutritional Reports International 1970; 2 351–362.

[61] O'Shea JP. The effects of an anabolic steroid on dynamic strength levels of weightlifters. Nutritional Reports International 1971; 4 363-70.

[62] O'Sullivan AJ, Kennedy MC, Casey JH, Day RO, Corrigan B, Wodak AD. Anabolic-androgenic steroids: Medical assessment of present, past and potential users. The Medical Journal of Australia 2000; 173 323-327..

[63] Pope HG, Katz DL. Psychiatric effects of anabolic steroids. Psychiatric Annals 1992;2224-29.

[64] Rademacher G, Gedrat J, Hacker R.. Die Beeinflussung des Adaptationsverhalten ausgewahlter Funktionssysteme von Ausdauersportlern wahrend einer kraftbetohnten Training-sphase durch die zusatzliche Gabe von Oral-Turinabol. In: Hacker R, Marees HD, editors. Hormonelle Regulation und psychophysische Belastung im Leistungssport. Koln: DeutscherArzte-Verlag,1991:77-84.

[65] Schänzer W. Metabolism of anabolic androgenic steroids. Clinical Chemistry 1996 ; 42(7) 1001-20.

[66] Shahidi NT . A review of the chemistry, biological action, and clinical applications of anabolic–androgenic steroids. Clinical Therapy 2001; 23 1355–1390.

[67] Srinivas-Shankar U, and Wu, FCW. Drug insight: Testosterone preparations. Nature Clinical Practice Urology 2006; 3 653–665.

[68] Stromme SB, Meen HD, Aakvaag A. Effects of an androgenic-anabolic steroid on strength development and plasma testosterone levels in normal males. Medine and Science in Sport& Exercise 1974; 6 203–208.

[69] Thiblin I, Petersson A. Pharmacoepidemiology of anabolic androgenic steroids: a review. Fundam Clin Pharmacol 2005; 19: 27–44.

[70] Thompson PD, Cullinane EM Sady SP Chenevert CSaritelli AL Sady MA Herbert PN . Contrasting effects of testosterone and stanozolol on serum lipoprotein levels. JAMA. 1989; 261(8) 1165-8.

[71] Todd T. Anabolic steroids: The gremlins of sport. Journal of Sport Hystory 1987; 14 87–107.

[72] Weiss, U and Muller, H. On the problem of influencing strength training with anabolic hormones. Schweiz Z Sportsmed 1968;16 79–89.

[73] Wemyss-Holden SA, Hamdy FC, Hastie KJ. Steroid abuse in athletes, prostatic enlargement and bladder outflow obstruction—is there a relationship? British Journal of Urology 1994; 74 476–478.

[74] Wilson JD. Androgens. In: Hardman JG, Limbird LE, Molinoff PB, Ruddon RW, eds. Goodman and Gilman's Experimental Basis of Therapeutics. New York, NY: McGraw-Hill; 1996:1441-1457.

[75] Wilson JD. Leihy MW, Shaw G. et al. Androgen physiology: unsolved problems at the millennium. Molecular and Cellular Endocrinology 2002; 198 1-3.

[76] Woodhouse LJ, Reisz-Porszasz S, Javanbakht M, Storer TW, Lee M, Zerounian H et al. Development of models to predict anabolic response to testosterone administration in healthy young men. American Journal of Physiology- Endocrinology and Metabolism 2003; 284 E1009–E1017.

[77] Yesalis CE, Courson SP, Wright JE. History of anabolic steroid use in sport and exercise. In: Yesalis CE, ed. Anabolic Steroids in Sport and Exercise. Champaign, IL: Human Kinetics 2000;51–71.

Chapter 8

Steroidogenic Enzyme 17,20-Lyase Activity in Cortisolsecreting and Non-Functioning Adrenocortical Adenomas

Hajime Ueshiba

Additional information is available at the end of the chapter

http://dx.doi.org/10.5772/53212

1. Introduction

The frequency of adrenal incidentalomas has been reported to range between 0.7% and 4% in abdominal computed tomography [1-5], or from 1.4% to 8.7% in autopsy series [6-8]. The widespread application of high resolution imaging techniques, such as computed tomography, magnetic resonance imaging and ultrasonography, has led to an increasing frequency of discovering adrenal incidentalomas. The majority of these lesions are of cortical origin, include non-functioning adenomas, adenomas associated with pre-clinical Cushing's syndrome, pheochromocytomas, adrenocortical carcinomas, myelolipomas, ganglioneuromas, metastatic tumors and cysts [9-13]. Adrenal incidentalomas are usually asymptomatic, however many of these lesions may secrete weak precursor hormones or active hormones in insufficient amounts to cause clinically apparent disease. There are reports of several cases of adrenal incidentaloma who had no clinical evidence of Cushing's syndrome and normal basal steroid hormone secretion, but non-suppressible serum cortisol after dexamethasone administration. These cases were regarded as "pre-clinical Cushing's syndrome" [14-16] and many of them treated by adrenalectomy, which restored a normal cortisol suppression to dexamethasone.

To study the differences between non-functioning adenomas and those associated with pre-clinical Cushing's syndrome, we performed a comprehensive analysis of serum steroid hormone profiles in patients with such adrenocortical tumors using a combination method of high-performance liquid chromatography(HPLC) and radioimmunoassay(RIA) [17].

2. Materials and Methods

2.1. Subjects

We studied 22 patients with incidentally discovered adrenal masses. These lesions were seen on abdominal imaging and were diagnosed clinically and/or pathologically. From our adrenal incidentaloma cases, we selected for inclusion only patients with adrenocortical adenomas. Fifteen non-functioning adenoma cases (7 males and 8 females, mean age 59.3±13.7 yr) and seven pre-clinical Cushing's syndrome cases (2 males and 5 females, mean age 54.7±12.4 yr) were studied (Table 1). As the control group, sixteen healthy adults(8 males and 8 females, mean age 51.0±7.4 yr) were used.

Non-functioning	No	Age(yr)	Sex	Side	Size(mm)	BP(mmHg)	Operation
	1	71	M	right	25x15	150-80	(+)
	2	83	M	right	30x20	160-84	
	3	74	M	right	30x20	146-86	(+)
	4	61	M	left	8x8	130-70	
	5	49	M	right	22x13	134-78	
	6	42	M	left	18x12	138-80	
	7	53	M	left	19x17	142-82	
	8	87	F	right	32x15	100-80	
	9	57	F	left	12x12	140-80	
	10	53	F	right	22x18	104-60	(+)
	11	55	F	right	12x9	120-76	
	12	49	F	right	26x19	124-80	(+)
	13	42	F	left	21x18	144-84	
	14	56	F	left	32x21	128-72	(+)
	15	57	F	left	25x29	146-84	
Pre-clinical	1	41	M	left	15x10	146-88	
Cushing	2	54	M	left	16x11	148-84	
	3	61	F	right	18x18	130-84	(+)
	4	60	F	right	17x13	160-70	(+)
	5	59	F	right	17x15	130-82	
	6	72	F	right	18x12	156-86	(+)
	7	36	F	left	22x18	124-80	(+)

Table 1. Clinical features in cases of non-functioning adenoma and pre-clinical Cushing's syndrome

http://dx.doi.org/10.5772/53212

2.2. Hormonal measurements

Blood samples were obtained from patients with adrenal masses and normal subjects between 8 and 9 a.m. after an overnight fast. Serum levels of 10 steroid hormones [pregnenolone (Preg), progesterone (P), deoxycorticosterone (DOC), corticosterone (B), 17-hydroxypregnenolone (17-OH-Preg), 17-hydroxyprogesterone (17-OHP), 11-deoxycortisol (S), cortisol (F), dehydroepiandrosterone (DHEA), △4androstenedione (△4A)] were determined by an HPLC/RIA method as previously described [17].

2.3. Statistical analyses

We analyzed product/precursor ratios as indices of the relative activities of adrenal steroidogenic enzymes. Data are shown as mean ± SD. Variables were compared by the Mann-Whitney U test with Bonferroni correction. P values less than 0.05 were considered statistically significant.

2.4. Results

Eleven cases of non-functioning adenomas (Group I) had normal levels in DHEA and △4A compared to normal controls by simultaneous analysis (Fig.1).In 4 cases of non-functioning adenomas (Group II), however, serum levels of DHEA and △4A were significantly decreased compared to normal controls by simultaneous analysis (Fig.2). Other steroid hormone levels were normal in all cases of non-functioning adenomas. Therefore, we divided these patients into two groups based on the relative activities of adrenal steroidogenic enzymes by calculating product/precursor ratios. In pre-clinical Cushing's syndrome, serum levels of DHEA and △4A were significantly decreased compared to normal control values (Fig.3) and these results were similar to values in Group II patients.

17,20-Lyase activities assessed by DHEA/17-OH-Preg and △4A/17-OHP ratios were significantly decreased in Group II of non-functioning adenoma and pre-clinical Cushing's syndrome compared to Group I patients and normal controls (Fig.4). 17-Hydroxylase activities assessed by 17-OH-Preg/Preg and 17-OHP/P ratios (Fig.5), 3β-hydroxysteroid dehydrogenase activities assessed by P/Preg, 17-OHP/17-OH-Preg and △4A/DHEA ratios (Fig.6), 21-hydroxylase activities assessed by DOC/P and S/17-OHP ratios (Fig.7) and 11β-hydroxylase activities assessed by B/DOC and F/S ratios (Fig.8) had the same levels in all cases of non-functioning adenomas and pre-clinical Cushing's syndrome compared to normal control values.

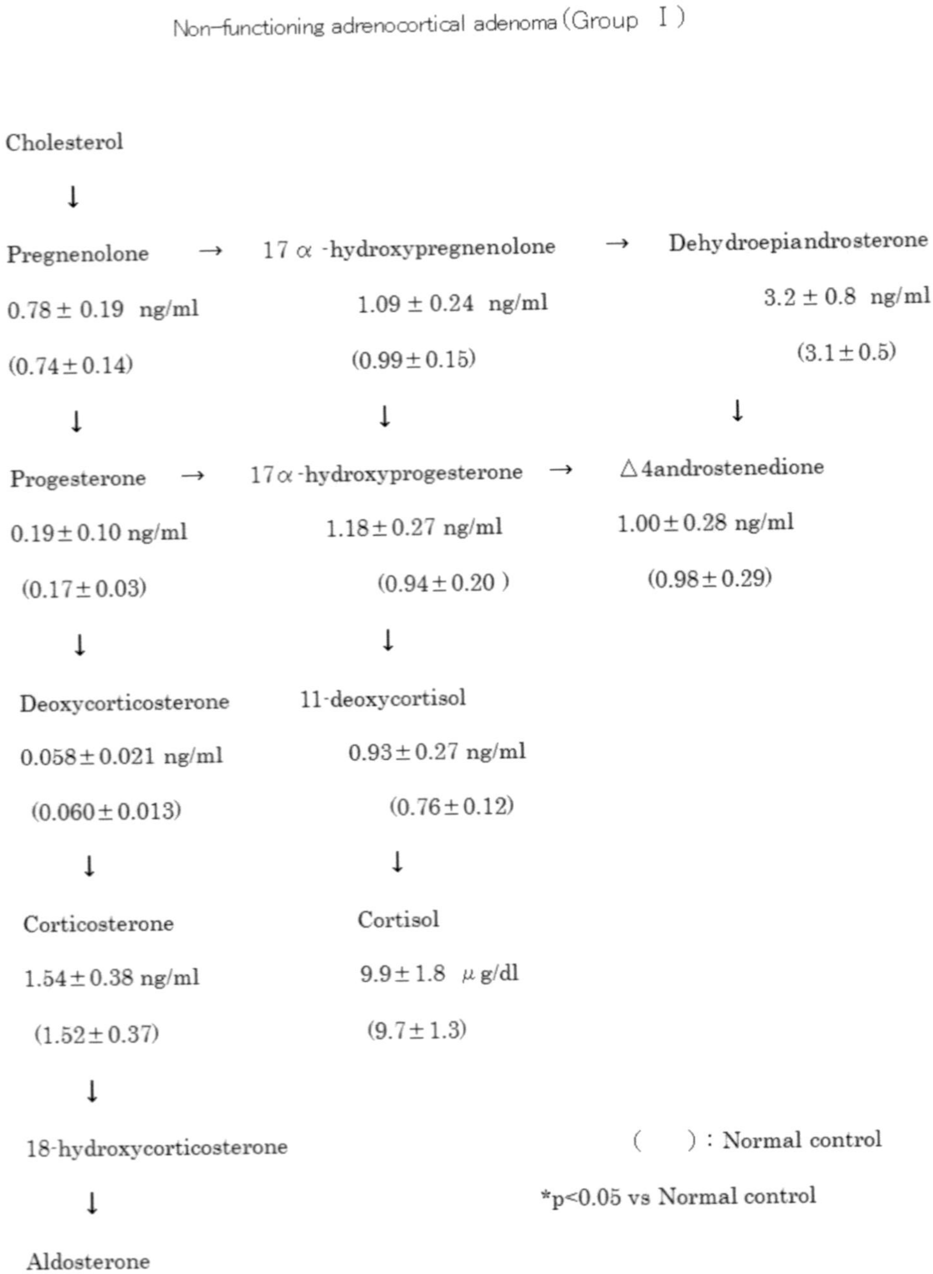

Figure 1. Serum steroid hormone profiles in non-functioning adrenocortical adenoma Group I

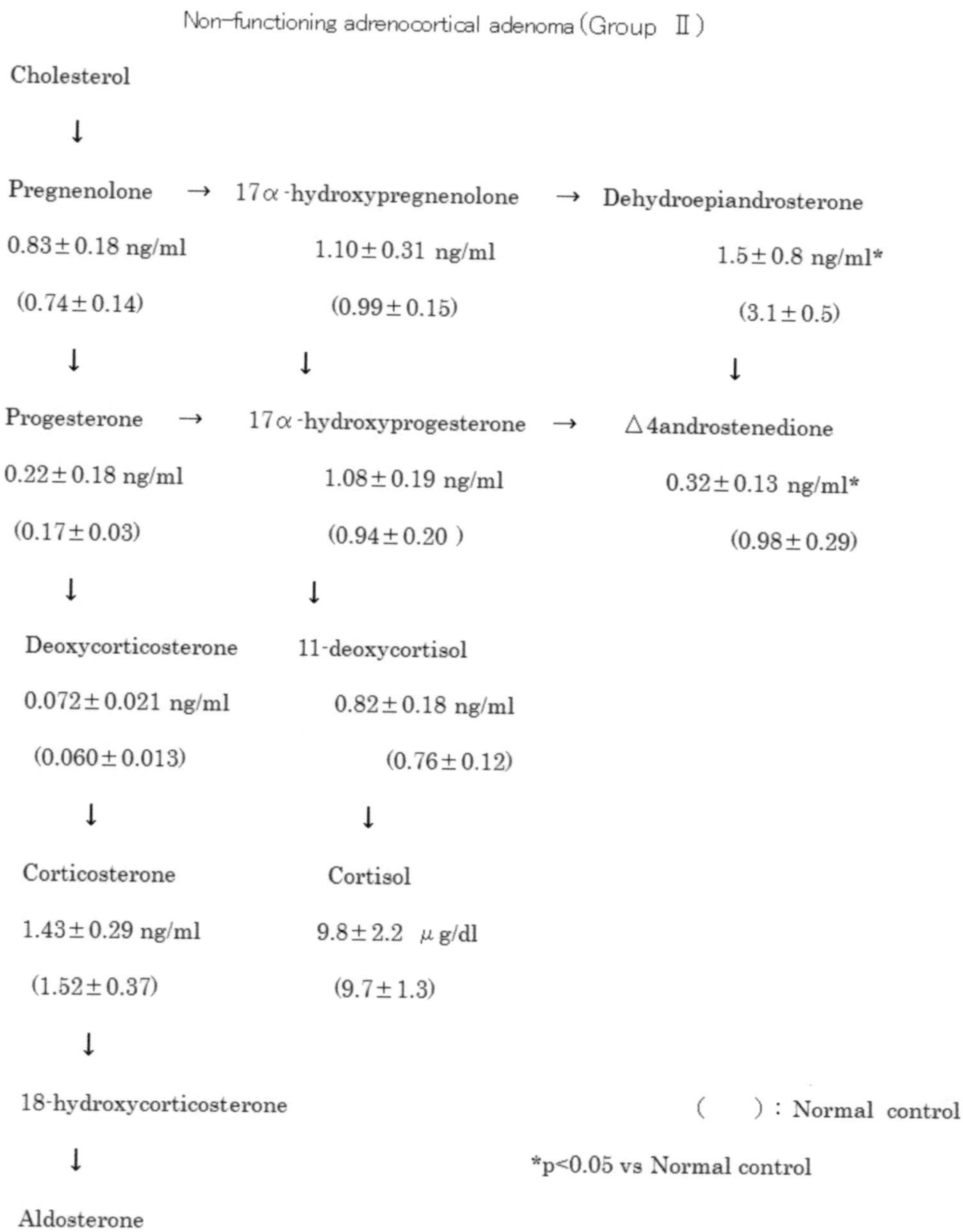

Figure 2. Serum steroid hormone profiles in non-functioning adrenocortical adenoma Group II

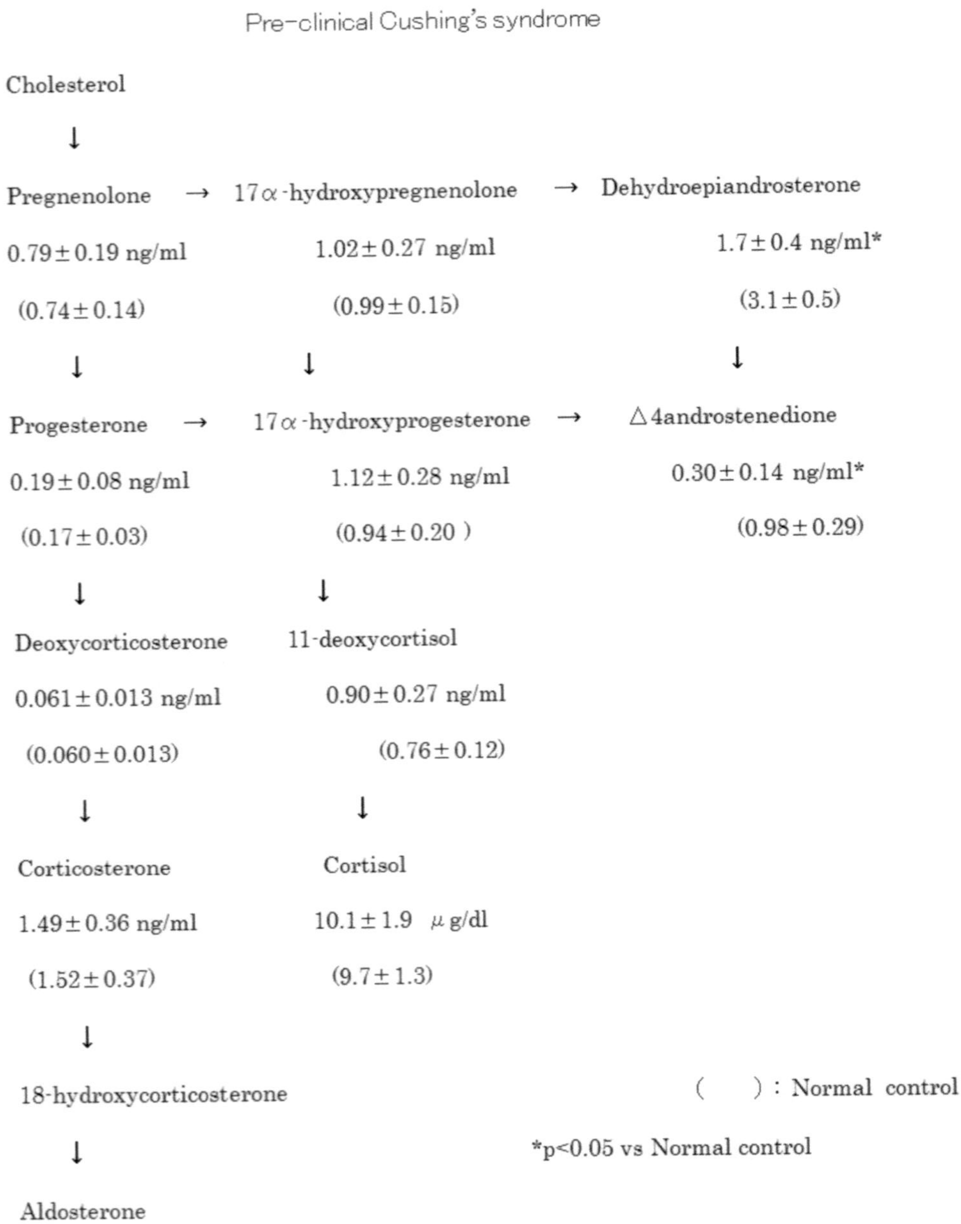

Figure 3. Serum steroid hormone profiles in pre-clinical Cushing's syndrome

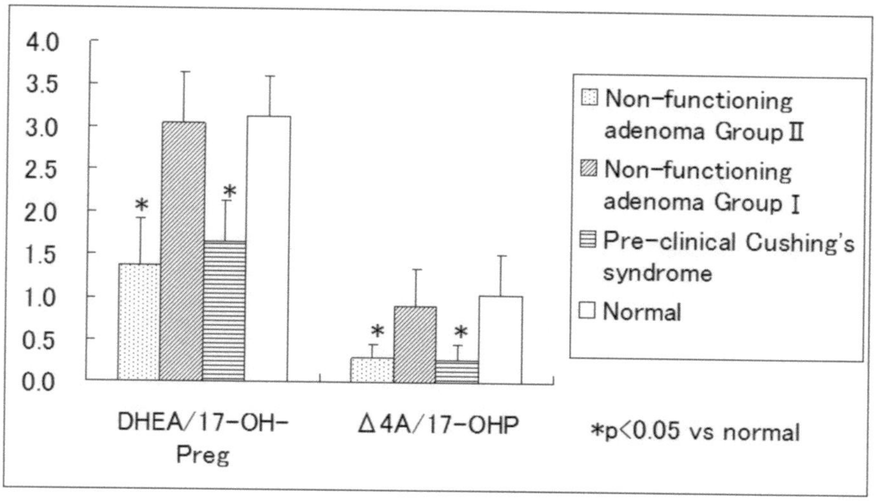

Figure 4. 17,20-Lyase activities

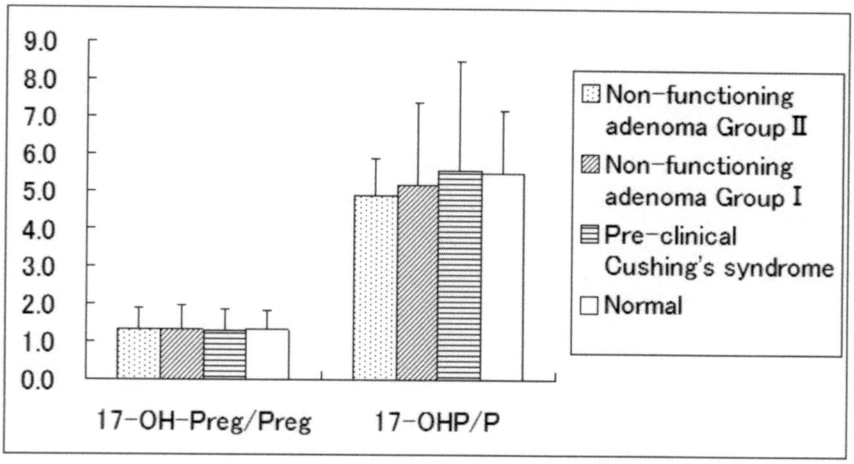

Figure 5. 17-Hydroxylase activities

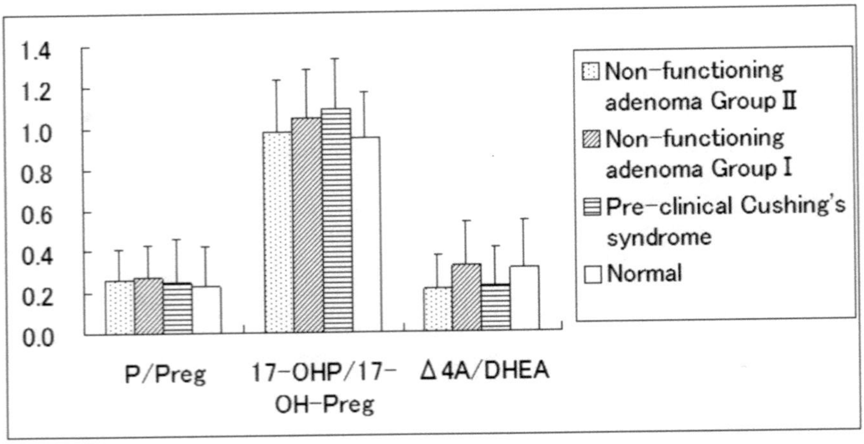

Figure 6. 3β - Hydroxysteroid dehydrogenase activities

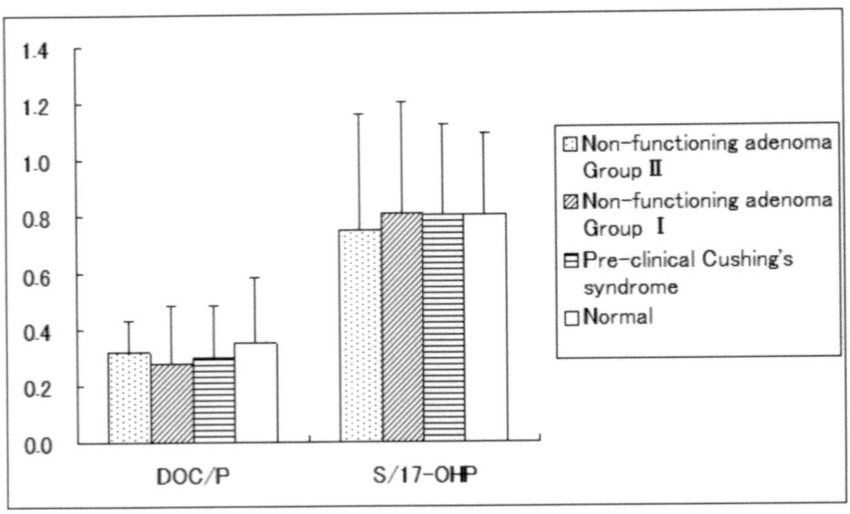

Figure 7. 21- Hydroxylase activities

http://dx.doi.org/10.5772/53212

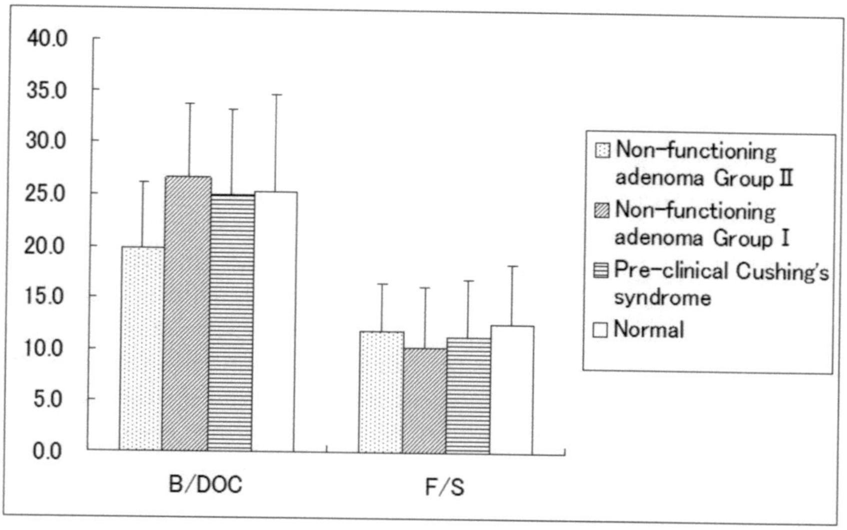

Figure 8. 11β -Hydroxylase activities

3. Discussion

We examined serum steroid hormone profiles of patients with non-functioning adrenocortical adenomas and pre-clinical Cushing's syndrome. We also assessed the steroidogenic enzymatic activities of these patients by analysis of the product/precursor ratios of C21 and C19 steroid hormones in the steroidogenic pathway. Patients with pre-clinical Cushing's syndrome and a subgroup of patients with non-functioning adrenocortical adenomas had distinctly decreased adrenal androgen secretion compared with a suppressed 17,20-lyase activity. The remaining patients with non-functioning adrenocortical adenomas had completely normal adrenal androgen values and 17,20-lyase activity.

Previous reports have shown an exaggerated response of 17-hydroxyprogesterone after ACTH stimulation in some patients with incidentally detected adrenal incidentalomas [18,19]. This response has been explained by existing 21-hydroxylase deficiency which may be a pathogenetic factor in the development of adrenal tumors. Macronodular adrenal hyperplasia is a frequent finding in patients with classic congenital adrenal hyperplasia, however,also about half of the heterozygous carriers in families with congenital adrenal hyperplasia were reported to have uni- or bilateral adrenal nodules on abdominal computed tomography in consecutive 4-mm scans [19].These investigators concluded that mild 21-hydroxylase deficiency is associated with the formation of adrenal incidentaloma. Other investigators have reported that the ACTH-stimulated 17-hydroxyprogesterone levels were abnormally increased in more than 50% of patients with non-hyperfunctioning adrenal adenomas [20]. After unilateral adrenalectomy, this hormonal abnormality disappeared in most patients with adrenal tumors. The ACTH-stimulated 17-hydroxyprogesterone levels significantly correlated with the size of the tumors. These results indicate that tumors themselves may be responsible for the increased ACTH-stimulated 17-hydroxyprogesterone levels in patients with non-hyperfunctioning adrenal adenomas.

In this study, we demonstrated that serum DHEA and △4A levels were significantly decreased in some patients with non-functioning adrenocortical adenomas(Group II) and all those with pre-clinical Cushing's syndrome. 17,20-Lyase activities were significantly decreased in Group II of non-functioning adenoma and pre-clinical Cushing's syndrome compared to Group I patients and normal controls. We found no clinical or pathological differences between Group I patients and Group II patients who had normal adrenal androgen concentrations. We have no explanation as to why there was difference between these groups. Since serum steroid hormone profiles had a similar pattern between some non-functioning adrenocortical adenomas and adenomas of patients with pre-clinical Cushing's syndrome, we suggest that the former may in time progress into pre-clinical and clinical Cushing's syndrome. There are limitations in this study such as small sample size and no tissue investigation. In the future the activity of steroidogenesis enzyme should be measured in the specimens from adrenaltissues.

Author details

Hajime Ueshiba*

Address all correspondence to: ueshiba@med.toho-u.ac.jp

Department of Internal Medicine, Toho University School of Medicine, Japan

References

[1] Belldegrun, A., Hussain, S., Seltzer, S. E., Loughlin, K. R., Gittes, R. F., & Richie, J. P. (1986). Incidentally discovered mass of the adrenal gland. *Surg Gynecol Obstet*, 163, 203-208.

[2] Glazer, H. S., Weyman, P. J., Sagel, S. S., Levitt, R. G., & Mc Clennan, B. L. (1982). Nonfunctioning adrenalmasses: incidental discovery on computed tomography. *Am J Roentgenol*, 139, 81-85.

[3] Abecassis, M., Mc Loughlin, M. J., Langer, B., & Kudlow, J. E. (1985). Serendipitous adrenal masses:prevalence, significance, and management. *Am J Surg*, 149, 783-788.

[4] Herrera, M. F., Grant, C. S., van Heerden, J. A., Sheedy, P. F., & Ilstrup, D. M. (1991). Incidentally discovered adrenal tumors: an institutional perspective. *Surgery*, 110, 1014-1021.

[5] Peppercorn, P. D., Grossman, A. B., & Rezneck, R. H. (1988). Imaging of incidentally discovered adrenal masses. *Clin Endocrinol, 48*, 379-388.

[6] Copeland, P. (1983). The incidentally discovered adrenal mass. *Ann Intern Med, 98*, 940-945.

[7] Hedeland, H., Ostberg, G., & Hokfelt, B. (1968). On the prevalence of adrenocortical adenomas in an autopsy material in relation to hypertension and diabetes. *Acta Med Scand, 184*, 211-214.

[8] Granger, P., & Genest, J. (1970). Autopsy study of adrenal s in unselected normotensive and hypertensive patients. *Can Med Assoc J, 103*, 34-36.

[9] Kloos, R. T., Gross, M. D., Francis, I. R., Korobkin, M., & Shapiro, B. (1995). Incidentally discovered adrenal masses. *Endo Rev, 16*, 460-484.

[10] Bencsik, Z., Szabolcs, I., Kovacs, Z., Ferencz, A., Voros, A., Kaszas, I., Bor, K., Gonczi, J., Goth, M., Kovacs, L., Dohan, O., & Szilagyi, G. (1996). Low dehydroepiandrosterone sulfate(DHEA-S) level is not a good predictor of hormonal activity in nonselected patients with incidentally detected adrenal tumors. *J Clin Endocrinol Metab, 81*, 1726-1729.

[11] Kasperlik-Zatuska, AA, Rostonowska, E., Stowinska-Srzednicka, J., Migdalska, B., Jeske, W., Makowska, A., & Snochowska, H. (1997). Incidentally discovered adrenal mass(incidentaloma): investigation and management of 208 patients. *Clin Endocrinol, 46*, 29-37.

[12] Barzon, L., Scaroni, C., Sonino, N., Fallo, F., Paoletta, A., & Boscaro, M. (1999). Risk factors and long-term follow-up of adrenal incidentalomas. *J Clin Endocrinol Metab, 84*, 520-526.

[13] Mantero, F., Terzolo, M., Arnaldi, G., Osella, G., Masini, A. M., Ali, A., Giovagnetti, M., Opocher, G., & Angeli, A. (2000). A survey on adrenal incidentaloma in Italy. *J Clin Endocrinol Metab, 85*, 637-644.

[14] Bogner, U., Eggens, U., Hensen, J., & Oelkers, W. (1986). Incidentally discovered ACTH-dependent adrenal adenoma presenting as "pre-Cushing's syndrome.". *Acta Endocrinol, 111*, 89-92.

[15] Rosen, H. N., & Swartz, S. L. (1992). Subtle glucocorticoid excess in patients with adrenal incidentaloma. *Am J Med, 92*, 213-216.

[16] Renicke, M., Nieke, J., Krestin, G. P., Saeger, W., Allolio, B., & Winkelmann, W. (1992). Preclinical Cushing's syndrome in adrenal "incidentaloma:" comparison with adrenal Cushing's syndrome. *J Clin Endocrinol Metab, 75*, 826-832.

[17] Ueshiba, H., Segawa, M., Hayashi, T., Miyachi, Y., & Irie, M. (1991). Serum profiles of steroid hormones in patients with Cushing's syndrome determined by a new HPLC/RIA method. *Clin Chem, 37*, 1329-1333.

[18] Seppel, T., & Schlaghecke, R. (1994). Augmented 17-alpha-hydroxyprogesterone response to ACTH stimulation as evidence of decreased 21-hydroxylase activity in patients with incidentally discovered adrenal'incidentalomas.'. *Clin Endo*, 41, 445-451.

[19] Jaresch, S., Kornely, E., Kley, H. K., & Schlaghecke, R. (1992). Adrenal incidentaloma and patients with homozygous or heterozygous congenital adrenal hyperplasia. *J Clin Endocrinol Metab*, 74, 685-689.

[20] Toth, M., Racz, K., Adleff, V., Futo, L., Jakab, C., Karlinger, K., Kiss, R., & Glaz, E. (2000). Comparative analysis of plasma 17-hydroxyprogesterone and cortisol responses to ACTH in patients with various adrenal tumors before and after unilateral adrenalectomy. *J Endocrinol Invest*, 23, 287-294.

Chapter 9

Salivary or Serum Cortisol: Possible Implications for Alcohol Research

Anna Kokavec

Additional information is available at the end of the chapter

http://dx.doi.org/10.5772/51436

1. Introduction

Alcohol consumption can induce the development of nutritional disorders as alcohol ingestion often replaces food intake [1]. The long-term intake of alcohol decreases the amount of food consumed when food is freely available [2], and the degree of malnutrition may be related to the irregularity of feeding habits and intensity of alcohol intake [3]. The repercussions of alcohol abuse (over time) can involve damage to most of the major organs and systems in the body [4]. However, despite the overwhelming evidence linking alcohol to ill health the role (if any) alcohol plays in the development of disease remains uncertain.

The hypothalamic-pituitary-adrenal (HPA) axis is responsible for the synthesis and release of steroid hormones, the most abundant being dehydroepiandrosterone (DHEA), DHEA sulfate (DHEAS), cortisol, and aldosterone [e.g. 5]. The release of either corticotropin-releasing factor or arguinine vasopressin by the hypothalamus stimulates the anterior pituitary to release adrenocorticotropin (ACTH), which promotes the synthesis and release of steroid hormones that have glucocorticoid (i.e. cortisol), mineralocorticoid (i.e. aldosterone), and androgenic (i.e. DHEA, DHEAS) functions [6].

Steroid hormones have a diverse and highly important role in the body and any dysregulation in steroid activity can lead to the development of disease. The adrenocortical system is markedly altered by food availability and an elevation in cortisol is commonly observed under fasting conditions [7-9]. Cortisol plays a major role in the regulation of carbohydrate, protein, and lipid metabolism [10,11] and during prolonged fasting by stimulating gluconeogenesis acts to protect the body from cellular damage until food once again becomes available [7,8,10-14].

It is well accepted that alcohol consumption can significantly reduce DHEAS [9, 15] and aldosterone [16, 17]. However, the literature is highly contradictory with respect to the effect of oral alcohol intake on cortisol. Investigations have shown that blood alcohol concentrations exceeding 1 g/L can elevate plasma cortisol [18]. Moreover, it has also been reported that low to moderate alcohol intake has little [19], if any effect on [20-24] or may even significantly reduce [9], cortisol concentration. Furthermore, early work showed that while alcohol consumption may promote a significant decrease in cortisol (initially) this is later followed by a significant elevation in plasma cortisol concentration [25].

In the past it has been proposed that the discrepancy in cortisol, noted in the alcohol literature, could be due to differences in stress levels associated with the testing procedure [26]. Cortisol is rapidly released in response to stress and the stress associated with blood sampling (alone) can falsely increase cortisol values during the study. Furthermore, as each individual responds differently to the blood taking procedure, the difference in stress levels between individuals may be responsible for the discrepancy in findings observed between studies employing similar blood sampling methodology [27].

Plasma free cortisol measurement is the most reliable measure of adrenal glucocorticoid activity as plasma total cortisol values may be affected by the alteration of its carrier protein, CBG [28]. However, it is not unusual in psychoneuroendocrinology for the assessment of cortisol to be made in saliva [29], as the amount of cortisol in saliva is highly correlated with the level of plasma free cortisol [8,30-32], and the level of cortisol in cerebrospinal fluid (CSF). Moreover, steroid hormone concentration in saliva is not dependent on saliva flow rate and no dilution effect has been observed [33]. Therefore, as cortisol is released in response to stress [34], salivary assessments of cortisol, due to the non-invasive nature of the sampling procedure, may provide a more reliable measure of steroid activity.

The aim of this study was to clarify the effect (if any) of consuming a small-moderate amount of white wine on cortisol by comparing the effect (if any) of consuming a small-moderate amount of white wine on salivary cortisol and serum cortisol, and salivary cortisol alone.

2. Method

2.1. Subjects

A total of 16 subjects aged 19-22 years were recruited to participate in one of two alcohol trials. Eight subjects were recruited on two separate occasions. Due to early suggestions that under conditions of stress cortisol release may be influenced by gender factors [35] only males were recruited.

Subjects were excluded if they reported to have had: a previous history of psychiatric disorder; any neurological disease; any major physical complaint, including Type 1 or Type 2 diabetes; a history of drug use; taken any prescribed medication within the last 7 days; routinely engaged in shift work; or satisfied the DSM-IV-TR diagnostic criteria for alcohol abuse and/or dependence (American Psychiatric Association, 2000).

Individuals were all white Caucasians of Australian or British origin. The height of subjects in both trials was 175-182cm. No subject was obese as the weight of all subjects when assessed was within the medically recommended range for age and height.

The majority of subjects lived at home with family (n = 11) while the remainder lived in shared accommodation (n = 5). None of the subjects reported to have a family history of alcoholism and the group of 16 males contained only one non-drinker. The age subjects first consumed alcohol was reportedly between 14.4 years and 17 years. A little less than 40% regularly consumed a mixture of alcoholic beverages (n = 6), while others preferred to drink beer (n = 7) or spirits (n = 2), only.

Subject participation was obtained by informed consent. Approval for the study was granted by La Trobe University Human Ethics Committee who determined that the procedures were consistent with ethical guidelines for human research set by the National Health and Medical Research Council of Australia.

2.2. Equipment and assays

Assessment of cortisol in saliva was made using COBAS ELECSYS 2010 immunoassay (Roche Diagnostics, Indianopolis, IN, USA). The intra-assay coefficient of variation (CV) was 6.1% at 4.68 nmol/L, 2.7% at 11.5 nmol/L, 1.5% at 15.9 nmol/L, and 2.8% at 19.8 nmol/L. Quality controls for the assessment of cortisol in saliva was performed using Bio Rad Unassayed Liquicheck Chemistry Control (Bio Rad, USA, Lot # 16340 Expiry date: 12/2007). Staff at Analytical Reference Laboratories (St. Kilda Road, Melbourne, Australia), who were blind to the experimental manipulations, performed the cortisol analyses.

Serum samples were assayed locally to determine free cortisol levels using IBL Cortisol ELISA kits (RE52061, IBL Gesellschaft Für Immunchemie Und Immunbiologie MBH, Flughafenstrasse 52a, D-22335 Hamburg, Germany). The intra-assay CV of this coated-well competitive binding radioimmunoassay was 8.1% at 43.5 ng/ml, 3.2% at 226.5 ng/ml, and 5.6 % at 403.6 ng/ml. The inter-assay CV was 6.6% at 55 ng/ml, 7.7% at 209 ng/ml, and 6.5% at 361 ng/ml.

Semi-quantitative urinalysis was performed using Labstix™ (Bayer Australia Limited), in order to measure ketones (sensitivity was 0.5-1.0 mmol/l acetoacetic acid), glucose (sensitivity was 4-7 mmol/l glucose), blood (sensitivity was 150-620 μg/l haemoglobin), protein (sensitivity was 0.15-0.30 g/l albumin), and pH. Blood alcohol level (BAL) was assessed using a Lion alcolmeter™ (Lion laboratories Limited, Cardiff. UK).

2.3. Procedure

Given the high rate of weekend binge drinking in young adults testing was scheduled midweek. Subjects were told to maintain their usual daytime and evening routines prior to participating in the study. In the 24 hours prior to testing subjects were asked to: abstain from engaging in strenuous physical activity; avoid any sudden disruption to their usual sleep/wake routine; avoid skipping meals and eating high calorie food outside of their usual meal times; and limit caffeine intake to no more than two cups per day. Alcohol was not permitted to be consumed for at least 48 hours prior to the day of testing. Lastly, prescription and over the counter (e.g. pain and cough preparations) was not permitted to be used for at least 7 days prior to the study.

Participation in both alcohol trials was preceded by a six hour fast, which commenced at 1100 h Eastern Standard Summer Time (ESST), and testing began at approximately 1700h EST. Ketone bodies were assessed using urinalysis upon arrival in order to confirm that all individuals had complied with the fasting conditions. Alcohol was not permitted to be consumed for at least 48 hours prior to testing and all subjects were breathalyzed upon arrival to ensure that all recorded a BAL of zero.

Test Beverage: The test beverage consumed in both alcohol trials was Hardy's Regional Reserve Chardonnay 2005 white wine (McLaren Vale Vineyards, South Australia), containing 13% alcohol (315 Kj per unit).

Alcohol Dosage: The National Health and Medical Research Council of Australia define low risk alcohol consumption for males as no more than four standard drinks (40g alcohol) per occasion (NHMRC, 2001). In order to secure ethics approval to conduct the study the dosage of alcohol needed to adhere to these strict safety guidelines. Those who drank alcohol reported on average to consume 9.1 standard units (SD = 8.7 U) containing 10g alcohol on an average of 6.9 occasions per month (SD = 4.4 occasions). Therefore, it was deemed appropriate to set the dosage of alcohol for this study at the maximum amount of 40g alcohol.

Trial 1 (Serum + Salivary cortisol): Upon arrival subjects (n = 8), were asked to provide a 50ml urine sample for urinalysis prior to having 10ml of blood drawn from the left forearm for assessment of serum cortisol. Simultaneous saliva sampling for assessment of salivary cortisol was conducted while blood was withdrawn to ensure any stress effects resulting from the blood taking procedure were similar when taking the salivary and serum cortisol measures. Following the blood taking procedure participants were asked to slowly ingest a total of four standard units of alcohol (40g alcohol) over a 135-min period. Simultaneous blood and saliva sampling for the assessment of cortisol and measurement of BAL was performed a further three times at regular intervals while alcohol was being consumed. The rate of alcohol consumption was monitored to ensure subjects consumed alcohol at a similar rate during the study. As cortisol is released in response to physical or mental stress subjects were required to be seated at all times during the testing procedure. Physical activity or anything of a mentally stressful nature (e.g. movies, hand held video games) was not permitted at any time. During the study subjects engaged in quiet conversation with each other or played card games. At the completion of Stage 1 all participants reported moderate intoxication. No subject experienced gastrointestinal or other distress during the course of the study.

Trial 2 (Salivary cortisol): Upon arrival participants (n = 8) were required to provide a 5-ml saliva sample for measurement of cortisol and a 50-ml urine sample for urinalysis before consuming 40 g alcohol over a 135-min period. Saliva samples for the assessment of cortisol were taken; urinalysis was performed; and blood alcohol level (BAL) was assessed at regular intervals across a 135-min period. The rate of alcohol consumption was monitored to ensure subjects consumed alcohol at a similar rate during the study. Subjects were required to be seated during the testing procedure. Physical activity or anything of a mentally stressful nature (e.g. movies, hand held video games) was again not permitted at any time during the study. Subjects engaged in quiet conversation with each other or played card games. All individuals reported moderate feelings of intoxication at the completion of the alcohol trial and no participant experienced gastrointestinal or other distress at any stage.

2.4. Statistical Analyses

Both the saliva (only) and serum+saliva trials employed a repeated measures design. The dependent variable was the level of cortisol (serum cortisol, salivary cortisol) and in both trials this was assessed across four time points (i.e. 0-min, 45-min, 90-min and 135-min). In order to achieve a moderate effect size d = 1.0, α =.05, and Power =.75 using the sample size calculations listed in [36] a total of 21 participants would need to be recruited. However, with a repeated measures design the data from each participant is used at each measurement point so in effect eight participants in a repeated measures design with four measurement points is equivalent to data for 32 participants (i.e. 8 x 4 = 32), which is in excess of the 21 participants required. Thus, it was deemed statistically sufficient to recruit 8 participants for each trial.

Pearson's product-moment correlation analysis was used to assess whether a relationship exists between serum cortisol and salivary cortisol in the serum+saliva trial. A within subjects analysis of variance (ANOVA) was used to assess change in the level of the dependent variable (serum cortisol, salivary cortisol) when white wine is consumed across the four time points in the saliva (only) and serum+saliva trials. Any minor violation of sphericity was corrected using the Huynh-Feldt Epsilon correction. Results were classed as significant if the calculated probability was less than 05. All significant ANOVA findings were assessed post-hoc using paired samples t-tests.

3. Results

The average BAL recorded during the saliva + serum trial and the saliva (only) trials reached a mean peak of 0.08 mg/100 ml (SEM =.003 mg/100 ml) and 0.07 mg/100 ml (SEM = ±.005 mg/100 ml), respectively, after four standard units of white wine (40g alcohol) had been consumed at 135-min.

The mean level of serum and salivary cortisol in the serum + saliva trial is graphically presented in Figure 1. No significant relationship was observed between the level of serum cortisol and salivary cortisol at any time point ($P > .05$). The ANOVA analysis also failed to reveal any significant differences in salivary cortisol across the 135-min alcohol consumption period ($F(3, 21) = 1.62$, $P = .22$). Inspection of the raw data showed a high degree of variability between subjects, which likely contributed to the non-significant finding. In contrast, a significant difference in serum cortisol concentration was observed across time points, ($F(3, 21) = 9.29$, $P < .01$). Post-hoc assessment confirmed that the average level of serum cortisol is significantly higher at 45-min when compared to 90-min and 135-min and at 90-min when compared to 135-min ($P < .05$).

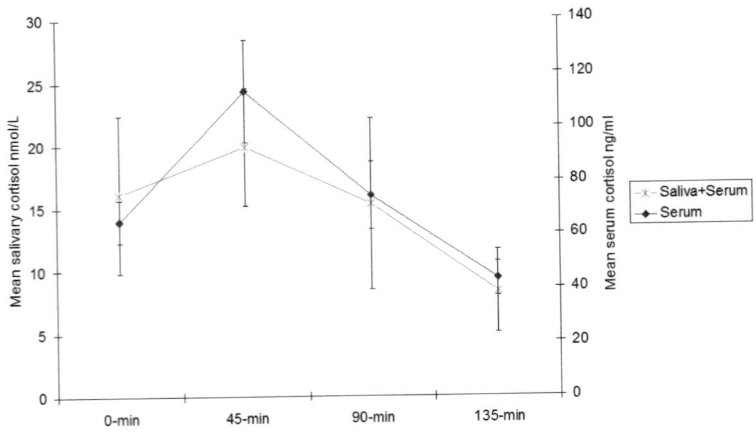

Figure 1. Mean salivary cortisol and serum cortisol obtained during the serum+saliva trial before (0-min) and after ingestion of white wine containing 40g alcohol (45-135 min). Data are shown as the mean ± SEM (n = 8).

The level of salivary cortisol in the saliva (only) trial during white wine consumption was noted to be significantly different across time points (F (3, 21) = 5.46, P =.05). Post-hoc assessment confirmed that the average level of salivary cortisol in the saliva (only) trial is significantly lower at 135-min when compared to 0-min, 45-min and 90-min and significantly lower at 45-min when compared to 90-min (P <.05). The mean salivary cortisol level measured during the saliva (only) trial is graphically compared with the serum cortisol data from the serum + saliva trial in Figure 2.

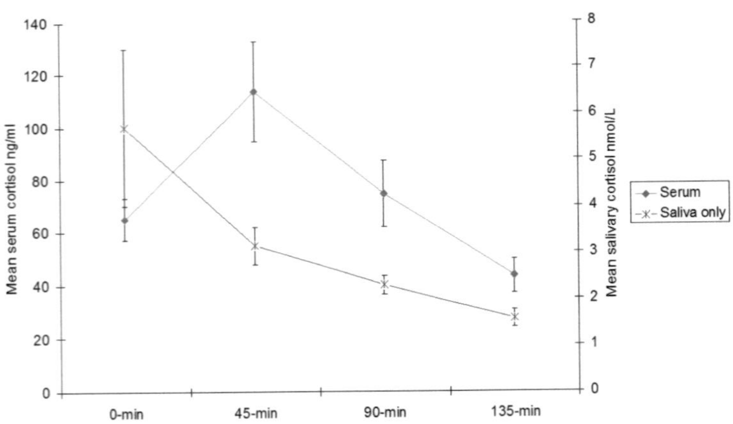

Figure 2. Mean salivary cortisol obtained during the saliva (only) trial (n = 8) and serum cortisol from the serum+saliva trial (n = 8) before (0-min) and after ingestion of white wine containing 40g alcohol (45-135 min). Data are shown as the mean ± SEM.

4. Discussion

The results of this study have shown that when alcohol is consumed under fasting conditions: the level of serum cortisol is significantly elevated almost immediately; the level of salivary cortisol when assessed during a blood taking procedure is not significantly altered over time; and the level of salivary cortisol when assessed in the absence of blood taking is significantly reduced over time.

Research has shown that blood alcohol concentrations exceeding 1 g/L can elevate plasma cortisol concentration [18]. However, other investigations using rodents and humans have indicated either no-change, or a significant decrease in plasma glucocorticoid levels following alcohol consumption [e.g. 2, 20-25). Results of this study, which was conducted under fasting conditions are consistent with the suggestion that alcohol can promote an elevation in cortisol [18] and low to moderate alcohol intake has little [19], if any effect [20-24], on cortisol.

The collection of serum cortisol and salivary cortisol was conducted simultaneously and it could be argued that while the stress of the blood sampling procedure may have raised blood levels those in saliva may not have had time to equilibrate. However, it should be noted that the entry of cortisol from blood to CSF is a fairly rapid process [37].

In the present study there appeared to be little evidence for the suggestion that an initial alcohol-induced decrease in cortisol is later followed by a significant elevation in cortisol [25] either during or following alcohol consumption in serum or salivary cortisol measures. Our early work identified some food-induced recovery in the HPA axis following alcohol consumption [9], suggesting that the addition of nutritional factors can promote an elevation in cortisol. Moreover, we have also assessed the effect of beer, an alcoholic beverage that contains some carbohydrate, on steroid activity and we noted an elevation in salivary cortisol after 40 g alcohol [38]. Thus, differences in nutritional content of the alcoholic beverage consumed may be responsible for this discrepancy in cortisol findings highlighting the importance of nutritional factors when assessing the effects of alcohol on cortisol rhythmicity.

Researchers have previously claimed that differences in stress levels associated with the blood taking procedure [26] can falsely increase cortisol values. During the serum+saliva trial the level of serum cortisol was significantly elevated at 45-min while the level of salivary cortisol remained statistically unaltered. In contrast, the level of salivary cortisol in the saliva only trial is significantly reduced, which is consistent with previously published data obtained under similar experimental conditions [9, 38].

It has been suggested that as each individual may respond differently to the blood taking procedure the high degree of variability in stress response may be an important factor that could contribute to non-significant findings [27]. A large degree of inter-subject variability was noted in the salivary cortisol data during the serum+saliva trial, which most likely explains the non-significant result. The sample size in the present study, while statistically large enough, is relatively small given the high degree of variability observed. Therefore, the salivary cortisol data in the serum+saliva trial may need to be interpreted with caution.

An increase in the level of cortisol in CSF, in the absence of any elevation in plasma cortisol, has been reported previously [33]. In the serum+saliva trial there did not appear to be any significant relationship between serum cortisol and salivary cortisol, which suggests that the mechanisms underlying the release of cortisol in saliva and serum may not be the same. It has been suggested that the brain has the ability to synthesize steroid hormones such as dehydroepiandrosterone sulfate de novo [39]. However, whether this is also true for cortisol requires further investigation.

Cell membranes are highly permeable to alcohol and there is evidence that alcohol can increase membrane fluidity by expanding the volume and disordering the lipid components of the neuronal membrane [40]. The entry of alcohol into cells increases the concentration of solute and a hypernatremic dehydration condition may develop as cells gradually become saturated with alcohol. Both alcohol and cortisol can promote the release of K^+ from intracellular stores. However, the K^+ loss induced by alcohol is much larger [41] that is compensated by a Na^+ gain that more than doubles the glucose consumption by cells at higher alcohol concentrations [42, 43]. It has been suggested that the alcohol-induced increase in K^+ efflux is most likely due to extracellular K^+ directly antagonising the intoxicating effect of alcohol in the CNS [44]. The alcohol-induced increase in K^+ efflux increases glial depolarization [45] and glucose demand by neurons and astrocytes as additional glucose is required by astrocytes to take up the excess K^+ and store it [46]. An increase in K^+ efflux can stimulate GABA release [47], in order to protect against brain impairment caused by an increase in neuronal depolarization [48]. Alcohol's potentiation of GABA is specifically linked to the $GABA_A$ receptor gated chloride channel [49] and this may be due to Cl^- being needed by astrocytes in order to maintain electrical neutrality [46].

An increase in K^+ efflux could eventually develop into an extracellular acidosis [50], which in turn could promote a significant alteration in the activity of the HPA axis as a result of chronic osmotic stimulation [51]. A decrease in HPA axis activity under these conditions would be beneficial to the survival of the organism because cortisol decreases GABA activity at higher concentrations [52, 53], which could potentially increase the risk of brain injury due to an increase in neuronal depolarization [48]. Additionally, cortisol (similar to alcohol) can promote the loss of body potassium due to the release of K^+ from intracellular stores [41] and reduce glucose utilization and transport in neurons and astrocytes [54-56], which could increase the risk of hypoglycemia and hypoxia [57]. Thus, the significant decrease in salivary cortisol noted in the saliva (only) trial may have occurred due to an alcohol-induced alteration in HPA axis activity as outlined in the Salt and Water hypothesis [for review see 58].

5. Conclusions

The data here supports the suggestion that stress is an extraneous factor that can influence the cortisol data [26]. It was argued that consuming white wine under fasting conditions most likely promotes an alcohol-induced reduction in HPA activity [58]. The data in the present study has confirmed there is a need for strict methodological controls to be included

http://dx.doi.org/10.5772/51436

in any study assessing the effects of alcohol on the HPA axis. Cortisol is the body's major stress hormone. However, the role of cortisol in the human body is varied with cortisol also having a significant effect on energy regulation [10, 11]. Therefore, care should be taken when designing studies aimed at assessing the effect of alcohol on steroid hormones as any alteration in participant stress and/or nutritional status has the potential to increase inter-subject variability and potentially obscure the true effects of alcohol on the HPA axis [27].

Acknowledgements

I am grateful to Amy Lindner for assistance with subject recritment, Bronwyn Stevens for her assistance before and during the experimental trials and Maureen Todkill and Janelle Perkins for their assistance with the blood sampling procedure.

Author details

Anna Kokavec*

Address all correspondence to: a.kokavec@latrobe.edu.au

1 School of Psychological Science, La Trobe University, Bendigo, Australia

References

[1] Orozco, S., & De Castro, J. M. (1991). Effects of alcohol abstinence on spontaneous feeding patterns in moderate alcohol consuming humans. *Pharmacol Biochem Behav*, 40, 867-873.

[2] Strbak, V., Benicky, J., Macho, L., Jezova, D., & Nikodemova, M. (1998). Four-week ethanol intake decreases food intake and body weight but does not affect plasma leptin, corticosterone, and insulin levels in pubertal rats. *Metabolism*, 47, 1269-73.

[3] Santolaria, F., Perez-Manzano, J. L., Milena, A., Gonzalez-Reimers, E., Gomez-Rodriguez, M. A., Marinez-Riera, A., Aleman-Valls, M. R., & De la Vega-Prieto, M.J. (2000). Nutritional assessment in alcoholic patients. Its relationship with alcoholic intake, feeding habits, organic complications and social problems. *Drug Alcohol Dep.*, 59, 295-304.

[4] Victor, M., Adams, R. D., & Collins, G. H. (1989). *The Wernicke-Korsakoff Syndrome and other Related Neurologic Disorders Due to Alcoholism and Malnutrition.*, FA Davis, Philadelphia.

[5] Endoh, A., Kristiansen, S. B., Casson, P. R., Buster, J. E., & Hornsby, P. J. (1996). The zona reticularis is the site of biosynthesis of dehydroepiandrosterone and dehydroe-

piandrosterone sulfate in the adult human adrenal cortex resulting form its low expression of 3hydroxysteroid dehydrogenase. *J Clin Endocrinol Metab.*, 81, 3558-65.

[6] Jacobson, L., & Sapolsky, R. (1991). The role of the hippocampus in the feedback regulation of the hypothalamic-pituitary-adrenocortical axis. *Endocrinol Rev.* , 12, 118-34.

[7] Vance, M. L., & Thorner, M. O. (1989). Fasting alters pulsatile and rhythmic cortisol release in normal man. *J Clin Endocrinol Metab.*, 68, 1013-8.

[8] Akanji, A. O., Ezenwaka, C., Adejuwon, C. A., & Osotimehin, B. O. (1990). Plasma and salivary concentrations of glucose and cortisol during insulin-induced hypoglycaemic stress in healthy Nigerians. *Afr J Med*, 19, 265-9.

[9] Kokavec, A., & Crowe, S. F. (2001). The effect of a moderate level of white wine consumption on the hypothalamic-pituitary-adrenal axis before and after a meal. *Pharmacol Biochem Behav.*, 70, 243-50.

[10] Dallman, M. F., Akana, S. F., Strack, A. M., Hanson, E. S., & Sebastian, R. J. (1995). The neural network that regulates energy balance is responsive to glucocorticoids and insulin and also regulates HPA axis responsivity at a site proximal to CRF neurons. *Ann NY Acad Sci.*, 771, 730-42.

[11] Dallman, M. F., Strack, A. M., Akana, S. F., Bradbury, M. J., Hanson, E. S., Scribner, K. A., & Smith, M. (1993). Feast and famine: Critical role of glucocorticoids with insulin in daily energy flow. *Frontiers Neuroendocrinology*, 14, 303-47.

[12] Choi, S., Horsley, C. S., & Dallman, M. F. (1996). The hypothalamic ventromedial nuclei couple activity in the hypothalamo-pituitary-adrenal axis to the morning fed and fasted state. *J Neurosci.*, 16, 8170-8180.

[13] Lane, M. A., Ingram, D. K., Bal, S. S., & Roth, G. S. (1997). Dehydroepiandrosterone sulfate: A biomarker of primate aging slowed by calorie restriction. *J Clin Endocrinol Metab.*, 82, 2093-6.

[14] Tegelman, R., Lindeskog, P., Carlstrom, K., Pousette, A., & Blomstrand, R. (1986). Peripheral hormone levels in healthy participants during controlled fasting. *Acta Endocrinol.*, 113, 457-62.

[15] Andersson, S. H., Cronholm, T., & Sjovall, J. (1986). Effects of ethanol on the levels of unconjugated and conjugated androgens and estrogens in plasma of men. *J Steroid Biochem.*, 24, 1193-8.

[16] Guillaume, P., Jankowski, M., Gianoulakis, C., & Gutkowska, J. (1996). Effect of chronic ethanol consumption on the atrial natriuretic system of spontaneously hypertensive rats. *Alcohol Clin Exp Res*, 20, 1653-61.

[17] Wigle, D. A., Pang, S. C., Radakovic, N. N., Sarda, I. R., Watson, J. D., Roy, R. N., & Flynn, T. G. (1993). Chronic ethanol ingestion modifies the renin-aldosterone axis independent of alterations in the regulation of atrial natriuretic peptide. *Alcohol Clin Exp Res.*, 17, 841-6.

[18] Guillaume, P., Gutkowska, J., & Gianoulakis, C. (1994). Increased plasma atrial natriuretic peptide after acute injection of alcohol in rats. *J Pharmacol Exp Ther.*, 271, 1656-65.

[19] Jenkins, J. S., & Connolly, J. (1968). Adrenocortical response to ethanol in man. *BMJ.*, 2, 804-5.

[20] Davis, J. R., & Jeffcoate, W. J. (1983). Lack of effect of ethanol on plasma cortisol in man. *Clin Endocrinol.*, 19, 461-6.

[21] Gianoulakis, C., Guillaume, P., Thavundayil, J., & Gutkowska, J. (1997). Increased plasma atrial natriuretic peptide after ingestion of low doses of ethanol in humans. *Alcohol Clin Exp Res.*, 21, 162-70.

[22] Ida, Y., Tsujimaru, S., Nakamaura, K., Shirao, I., Mukasa, H., Egami, H., & Nakazawa, Y. (1992). Effects of acute and repeated alcohol ingestion on hypothalamic-pituitary-gonadal and hypothalamic-pituitary-adrenal functioning in normal males. *Drug Alcohol Dep.*, 31, 57-64.

[23] Joffe, B. I., Kalk, W. J., Shires, R., Lamprey, J. M., Baker, S., & Seftel, H. C. (1984). The 8-hour metabolic profile after drinking ethanol. *J Endocrinol Invest.*, 7, 239-41.

[24] Waltman, C., Blevins, L. S., Boyd, G., & Wand, G. S. (1993). The effects of mild ethanol intoxication on the hypothalamic-pituitary-adrenal axis in nonalcoholic men. *J Clin Endocrinol Metab.*, 7, 518-22.

[25] Linkola, J., Fyhrquist, F., & Ylikahri, R. (1979). Renin, aldosterone and cortisol during ethanol intoxication and hangover. *Acta Physiol Scan.*, 106, 75-82.

[26] Cicero, T.J. (1981). Neuroendocrinological effects of alcohol. *Ann Rev Med*, 32, 123-42.

[27] Guaza, C., Torrelas, A., & Borrell, J. (1983). Adrenocortical response to acute and chronic ethanol administration in rats. *Psychopharmacology*, 79, 173-6.

[28] Laudat, M. H., Cerdas, S., Fournier, C., Guibanc, D., Guilhaume, B., & Luton, J. P. (1988). Salivary cortisol measurement: a practical approach to assess pituitary-adrenal function. *J Clin Endocrinol Metab.*, 66, 343-8.

[29] Kirschbaum, C., & Hellhammer, D. H. (1994). Salivary cortisol in psychoneuroendocrine research: recent developments and applications. *Psychoneuroendocrinology*, 19, 313-33.

[30] Read, G. F., Riad, Fahmy. D., Walke, R. F., & Griffiths, K. (1982). Immunoassay of steroids in saliva. *Cardiff:*.

[31] Umenda, T., Hiramatsu, R., Iwaoka, T., Shimadda, T., Miura, F., & Sato, T. (1981). Use of saliva for monitoring unbound free cortisol levels in serum. *Clin Chim Acta.*, 110, 245-51.

[32] Vining, R. F., Mc Ginley, R. A., Maksujtis, J. J., & Yho, K. (1983). Salivary cortisol: a better measure of adrenal cortical function than serum cortisol. *Ann Clin Biochem.*, 20, 329-35.

[33] Guazzo, E. P., Kirkpatrick, P. J., Goodyer, I. M., Shiers, H. M., & Herbert, J. (1996). Cortisol, dehydroepiandrosterone (DHEA), and DHEA sulfate in the cerebrospinal fluid of man: Relation to blood levels and the effects of age. *J Clin Endocrinol Metab.*, 81, 3951-60.

[34] Virgin, C. E., Ha, T. P. T., Packan, D. R., Tombaugh, G. C., Yang, S. H., Horner, H. C., & Sapolsky, R. M. (1991). Glucocorticoids inhibit glucose transport and glutamate uptake in hippocampal astrocytes: Implications for glucocorticoid neurotoxicity. *J Neurochem.*, 57, 1422-8.

[35] Kirschbaum, C., Wüst, S., & Hellhammer, D. H. (1992). Consistent sex differences in cortisol responses to psychological stress. *Psychosomatic Med.*, 54, 648-57.

[36] Hinkle, D. E., Wiersma, W., & Jurs, S. G. (2002). *Applied Statistics for the Behavioral Sciences.*, Wadsworth Publishing.

[37] Martensz, N. D., Herbert, J., & Stacey, P. M. (1983). Factors regulating levels of cortisol in cerebrospinal fluid of monkeys during acute or chronic hypercortisolaemia. *Neuroendocrinology*, 36, 39-48.

[38] Kokavec, A., Lindner, A. J., Ryan, J. E., & Crowe, S. F. (2009). Ingesting alcohol prior to food can alter the activity of the hypothalamic-pituitary-adrenal axis. *Pharmacol Biochem Behav.*, 93, 170-176.

[39] Majewska, M.D. (1992). Neurosteroids: endogenous bimodal modulators of the GABAA receptor. *Mechanism of action and physiological significance. Prog Neurobiol.*, 38, 379-95.

[40] Tarter, R. E., Arria, A. M., & Van Thiel, D. H. (1989). Neurobehavioral disorders associated with chronic alcohol abuse. In Goedde HW, Agarwal DP (Eds), Alcoholism: Biomedical and Genetic Aspects. *Pergamon Press Inc.*

[41] Streeton, D. H. P., & Solomon, A. K. (1954). The effect of ACTH and adrenal steroids on K transport in human erythrocytes. *J Gen Physiol.*, 643-661.

[42] Nelson, N. (1944). Photometric adaptation of Somogyi method for determination of glucose. *J Biol Chem.*, 153, 375-382.

[43] Ponder, E. (1946). Prolytic ion exchanges produced in human red cells by methanol, ethanol, guaiacol, and resorcinol. *J Gen Physiol.*, 30, 479-459.

[44] Israel, Y., Kalant, H., & Laufer, I. (1965). Effects of ethanol on Na, K, Mg-stimulated microsomal ATPase activity. *Biochem Pharmacol.*, 14, 1803-1814.

[45] Hosli, L., Hosli, E., Andres, P. F., & Landolt, H. (1981). Evidence that the depolarization of glial cells by inhibitory amino acids is caused by an efflux of K+ from neurones. *Exp Brain Res.*, 42, 43-48.

[46] Kandel, E. R., Schwartz, J. H., & Jessell, T. M. (1991). *Principles of Neural Science. New Jersey.*

[47] Szerb, J. C., Ross, T. E., & Gurevich, L. (1981). Compartments of labeled and endogenous gamma-aminobutyric acid giving rise to release evoked by potassium or veratridine in rat cortical slices. *J Neurochem.*, 37, 1186-1192.

[48] Hamberger, A., Nystrom, B., Sellstrom, A., & Woiler, C. T. (1976). Amino acid transport in isolated neurons and glia. *Adv ExpMed Biol.*, 69, 221-236.

[49] Mehta, A. K., & Ticku, M. K. (1988). Ethanol potentiation of GABAergic transmission in cultured spinal cord neurons involves -aminobutyric acidA-gated chloride channels. *J Pharmacol Exp Ther.*, 246, 558-564.

[50] Velisek, L. (1998). Extracellular acidosis and high levels of carbon dioxide suppress synaptic transmission and prevent the induction of long-term potentiation in the CA1 region of rat hippocampal slices. *Hippocampus.*, 8, 24-32.

[51] Jessop, D. S., Chowdrey, H. S., & Lightman, S. L. (1990). Inhibition of rat corticotropin-releasing factor and adrenocorticotropin secretion by an osmotic stimulus. *Brain Res.*, 523, 1-4.

[52] Majewska, M. D., Bisserbe, J. C., & Eskay, R. (1985). Glucocorticoids are modulators of GABAA receptors in brain. *Brain Res.*, 339, 178-182.

[53] Randall, R. D., Lee, S. Y., Meyer, J. H., Wittenberg, G. F., & Gruol, D. L. (1995). Acute alcohol blocks neurosteroid modulation of synaptic transmission and long-term potentiation in the rat hippocampal slice. *Brain Res.*, 701, 238-248.

[54] Kadekaro, M., Ito, M., & Gross, P. (1988). Local cerebral glucose utilization is increased in acutely adrenalectomized rats. *Neuroendocrinology*, 47, 329-336.

[55] Horner, H., Packan, D., & Sapolsky, R. (1990). Glucocorticoids inhibit glucose transport in cultured hippocampal neurons and glia. *Neuroendocrinology*, 52, 57-64.

[56] Virgin, C. E., Ha, T. P. T., Packan, D. R., Tombaugh, G. C., Yang, S. H., Horner, H. C., & Sapolsky, R. M. (1991). Glucocorticoids inhibit glucose transport and glutamate uptake in hippocampal astrocytes: Implications for glucocorticoid neurotoxicity. *J Neurochem.*, 57, 1422-1428.

[57] Tombaugh, G. C., Yang, S. H., Swanson, R. A., & Sapolsky, R. M. (1992). Glucocorticoids exacerbate hypoxic and hypoglycemic hippocampal injury in vitro: Biochemical correlates and a role for astrocytes. *J Neurochem.*, 59, 137-146.

[58] Kokavec, A., & Crowe, S. F. (2001). Consequences of imbibing alcohol in the absence of adequate nutrition: the salt and water hypothesis. *Med Hyp.*, 57, 667-672.